# THE NUTRITION FACTOR

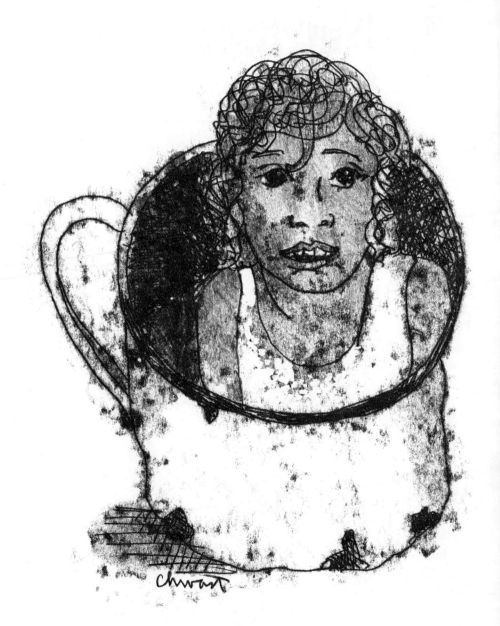

# Alan Berg

PORTIONS WITH ROBERT J. MUSCAT

# The Nutrition Factor

ITS ROLE IN NATIONAL DEVELOPMENT

A STUDY SPONSORED JOINTLY
BY THE FOUNDATION FOR CHILD DEVELOPMENT
AND THE BROOKINGS INSTITUTION

THE BROOKINGS INSTITUTION

*Frontispiece drawing by Seymour Chwast*
*Endsheet photographs (clothbound edition) by the author*

*Copyright © 1973 by*
THE BROOKINGS INSTITUTION
*1775 Massachusetts Avenue, N.W., Washington, D.C. 20036*

*Library of Congress Cataloging in Publication Data appear on the last page of this book.*

THE BROOKINGS INSTITUTION is an independent organization devoted to nonpartisan research, education, and publication in economics, government, foreign policy, and the social sciences generally. Its principal purposes are to aid in the development of sound public policies and to promote public understanding of issues of national importance.

The Institution was founded on December 8, 1927, to merge the activities of the Institute for Government Research, founded in 1916, the Institute of Economics, founded in 1922, and the Robert Brookings Graduate School of Economics and Government, founded in 1924.

The Board of Trustees is responsible for the general administration of the Institution, while the immediate direction of the policies, program, and staff is vested in the President, assisted by an advisory committee of the officers and staff. The by-laws of the Institution state, "It is the function of the Trustees to make possible the conduct of scientific research, and publication, under the most favorable conditions, and to safeguard the independence of the research staff in the pursuit of their studies and in the publication of the results of such studies. It is not a part of their function to determine, control, or influence the conduct of particular investigations or the conclusions reached."

The President bears final responsibility for the decision to publish a manuscript as a Brookings book or staff paper. In reaching his judgment on the competence, accuracy, and objectivity of each study, the President is advised by the director of the appropriate research program and weighs the views of a panel of expert outside readers who report to him in confidence on the quality of the work. Publication of a work signifies that it is deemed to be a competent treatment worthy of public consideration; such publication does not imply endorsement of conclusions or recommendations contained in the study.

The Institution maintains its position of neutrality on issues of public policy in order to safeguard the intellectual freedom of the staff. Hence interpretations or conclusions in Brookings publications should be understood to be solely those of the author or authors and should not be attributed to the Institution, to its trustees, officers, or other staff members, or to the organizations that support its research.

# Foreword

In recent years, experts and policy makers concerned with the problems of the developing countries have been changing their view of the malnutrition problem; what was once seen only as a welfare problem is beginning to be regarded also as a major obstacle to development. With broadening understanding of the effects of malnutrition on human growth and performance, and ultimately on national economic growth, foreign assistance agencies and governments in many low income countries are turning to nutrition in their search for ways to overcome chronic poverty.

This study contributes to that search by examining malnutrition as an impediment to national development, assessing the means currently available for dealing with malnutrition, and suggesting a future course of action. It focuses on policy and planning, moving consideration of nutrition beyond its usual clinical and laboratory confines and reflecting the author's experience and contributions to nutritional thinking over the past decade. The author has sought to develop a practical, systematic approach to program development and further research in an area heretofore largely unexplored.

Alan Berg undertook this study during his tenure as a senior fellow in the Brookings Foreign Policy Studies program and as a Belding Scholar of the Foundation for Child Development. His research was sponsored jointly by Brookings and the Foundation, whose primary goal is to improve the provision of health and social services to young children. An exploration of malnutrition's effect on child development has an important bearing on that objective. Mr. Berg wishes to thank the Foundation and Robert J. Slater, its president, for their encouragement and support of his work.

Several of the ideas developed in this book were presented earlier in articles and papers by the author. For permission to use parts of that material, Mr. Berg is grateful to *Foreign Affairs, Harvard Business*

*Review, International Development Review, American Journal of Clinical Nutrition,* and *Interplay,* and to the Swedish Nutrition Foundation, the American Medical Association, the MIT Press, and the United Nations.

For their comments on various drafts of the study and for helpful advice, he wishes to thank Thomas Arndt, Sol Chafkin, Dana Dalrymple, Martin Forman, Paul Isenman, Jerome Kahan, F. James Levinson, Richard Manoff, David Mathiasen, John Mellor, V. Ramalingaswami, Irwin Rosenberg, Vernon Ruttan, Walter Rybeck, Nevin Scrimshaw, and Carl Taylor.

Mr. Berg wishes to acknowledge special debts to Henry Owen, director of the Brookings Foreign Policy Studies program, for his guidance throughout the study; to Robert J. Muscat, who collaborated in the writing of Chapters 2, 4, and 5 and Appendix D, and who was his most incisive critic in other portions of the study; to Ann M. Watkins for her intelligent, imaginative, and industrious research assistance; and to Derrick Jelliffe, whose influence was instrumental in the development of Chapter 7. Judith Foster typed the manuscript and Daphne Carter helped with the documentation. The manuscript was edited by Alice M. Carroll and the index prepared by Joan C. Culver.

The views expressed are those of the author and should not be attributed to the staff members, officers, or trustees of the Brookings Institution or to the Foundation for Child Development.

KERMIT GORDON
*President*

*January 1973*
*Washington, D.C.*

# Contents

## Text Tables

## Appendix Tables

## Figures

# THE NUTRITION FACTOR

## CHAPTER ONE

# The Malnutrition Problem

"I think it could be plausibly argued," wrote George Orwell in *The Road to Wigan Pier*, "that changes of diet are more important than changes of dynasty or even of religion."[1] As with other things Orwellian, people are starting to take heed. In policy-making quarters in several parts of the world, nutrition has begun to strike a sensitive chord. Disturbing research findings about the effects of malnutrition on childhood death rates, on the frequency and severity of illness, on physical growth, on productivity, and on mental development have stirred concern. For years it has been assumed that, given educational opportunities and other environmental advantages, a child had every reason to be as bright, imaginative, and productive as other children of his age. Now it is being suggested that the child behind the empty-eyed face commonly seen in poor countries may be backward.

The greater interest of policy makers in nutrition also reflects their growing disenchantment with accepted economic development dogma. To masses of people in low-income countries, the so-called Development Decade of the 1960s did not fulfill its promise. Rising expectations are giving way to rising frustrations. New solutions are being sought.

At the same time, nutrition is becoming a more relevant policy issue—and remedial action more feasible—as countries are relieved of the pressure of an inadequate food supply. Several countries whose food shortages in the mid-1960s prompted U.S. congressional hearings on the apparent inevitability of famine in the 1970s have achieved or are approaching self-sufficiency in cereal grain production. For many of them, growing enough food is no longer the most immediate concern. In fact, there is or soon will be broadened choice of land use. Should a country use the land to plant crops for export, to increase production of domestically needed industrial raw materials, or to raise more nutritious foods to improve the local diets?

Nutrition, as a result of all this, is being discussed outside its traditional confines of scientific forums. Senior planning officials of fifty-five countries, for instance, gathered with nutrition experts in late 1971 at the Massachusetts Institute of Technology for the first International Conference on Nutrition, National Development, and Planning. Added stimulus comes from a special UN commission on malnutrition convened by Secretary-General U Thant and from World Bank President McNamara's policy pronouncements favoring greater emphasis on the problem.[2]

The new interest in nutrition, however, is mixed with curiosity, and the attention devoted to it is often mixed with skepticism. Interest rarely has been translated at the operating level into action; few countries have nutrition programs, and fewer still have nutrition plans or policies. Partly this reflects the traditional view of malnutrition as a welfare rather than as a development problem.[3] Welfare is not ignored by development planners; but, except in emergencies, it falls outside their primary focus of attention.

Also, for those unfamiliar with the field, malnutrition is not dramatically visible. Unlike famine, which attracts national and international attention—and usually prompts substantial response—most malnutrition is unobtrusive. The day-in, day-out erosion of health it causes may reach epidemic proportions—malnutrition has been identified as the world's number-one health problem[4] and is associated with more deaths and disease than the occasional famines*—but it lacks drama. (Once certain forms of malnutrition become severe, they become less unobtrusive. The despair one feels when seeing a blind child prompts voluntary donations to special schools for the blind; but a drive to provide the vitamin A—at less than 2 cents a child per year—that would have prevented the blindness does not arouse like concern.)

The most telling reason for the neglect of the problem of malnutrition may be the isolation of the power structure from its effects. Malnutrition does not raise the pervasive concern of the politically and socially vocal classes that an ailment like malaria, which knows no class bounds, arouses. Nor has it the urgency of a contagious disease—like smallpox.

Communication of the problem from the nutrition to the development communities also has been an impediment. Most advocates of better nu-

---

* This is not to deny the nutritional significance of famines and other disasters, a subject treated in Appendix A.

trition are scientists—pediatricians, biochemists, pathologists, plant geneticists, physiologists, microbiologists, and food technologists—who seldom think and talk in the same language as those who are responsible for
development policies. Nutritionists often are ill-equipped to deal with the
kinds of questions posed by the development planner, whom they see as
hard-fisted and insensitive to human need; the planner, in turn, is uncomfortable in dealing with the nutritionist, who often appears to him to be
professionally parochial and unable to see the problem in broad perspective.

Unfortunately, nutrition has no group of programmers or operational
entrepreneurs—common in other fields—to push through its findings. Nor
have leadership entities emerged to pave the way for action of consequence. (For more than two decades UN technical agencies have tried to
fill this need. They have successfully attracted attention to the problem,
but they have not been able to mobilize a serious attack on malnutrition.)
The difficulties are in part organizational. Because nutrition cuts across
conventional functional responsibilities and national organization charts,
it is difficult to discuss within a standard operational framework. Its
blurred and sometimes pejorative public connotation does nothing to compensate for that ambiguousness; to many, the word *nutrition* conjures up
images of vitamin pills and canned peaches, and the nutritionist is seen as
a medical clinician or a dietician–home economist. Clearly there is a label
problem.

## The Malnourished

Given the limited resources at the disposal of developing countries and
the plethora of needs competing for them, why should a government finance major programs to combat malnutrition? To most planners in developing countries the answer is not at all clear. The magnitude of the
malnutrition problem can best be appreciated by considering the amount
of child mortality, the relationship of malnutrition to that mortality, and
the extent of malnutrition among the survivors.

Available child mortality data are probably understated; in many instances children who are born today and die tomorrow are not recorded.
One Latin American clergyman reportedly did not register children until
they were two years old "because so many die before that it isn't worth
it."[5] In parts of Ghana the naming of a child is postponed eight days; if it

does not survive that long, it is not counted as a birth. Generally, the more poverty stricken the area, the higher the death rate, and the higher the death rate, the poorer the available records.

Nonetheless, figures still show that child mortality in developing countries is of staggering proportions.* Children under five years of age in Brazil constitute less than one-fifth of the population but account for four-fifths of all deaths; in India, for 65 percent of the deaths; in Egypt, for 68 percent. (In the United States, children at this age account for 8.8 percent of the population and 4.8 percent of deaths.) In Pakistan the percentage of one-to-four-year-olds who die is 40 times higher than in Japan and 80 times higher than in Sweden. In rural Punjab, one of India's strongest and healthiest areas, the death rate at that age is 72 times higher than in Sweden; in Egypt, 107 times higher; and in The Gambia, 111 times higher.†

If India's child death rate were the same as Taiwan's, 5.6 million fewer Indian children would die every year. A Guinean at birth can expect a life span of 26 years, one-third the life expectancy of a Japanese.

There is little dispute that "malnutrition is the biggest single contributor to child mortality in the developing countries."‡[6] In parts of Latin America, where the making and selling of minicaskets are common sights, malnutrition has been identified as the primary or an associated cause in 57 percent of all deaths of one-to-four-year-olds; it is an important factor in more than half of infant deaths and a contributor to the immaturity responsible for half to three-quarters of deaths in the first month of life.[7]

Malnutrition causes otherwise minor childhood diseases to become killers. For example, respiratory and gastrointestinal infections in Nicaragua are responsible for 15.3 percent of all deaths compared to 0.4 percent in North America. In Guatemala, 500 times as many preschool-aged children die of diarrheal diseases as in the United States. The death rate from measles, an especially virulent killer when accompanied by malnutrition, was more than a thousand times greater in Guatemala than in the United States in 1965.

Deaths are measurable. The toll among the survivors is less dramatic and less visible. Yet, more than two-thirds of the 800 million children now

* See Appendix B, Tables B-1 and B-2.
† Child mortality statistics generally group all children from one up to four or five years old. Breakdowns within the age group are seldom available. In nutrition parlance the group commonly is referred to as "preschool" children, something of a misnomer since many of the nutritionally most needy will not later attend school.
‡ See Appendix B, Tables B-3 and B-4.

growing up in developing countries are expected to "encounter sickness or disabling diseases either brought on or aggravated by protein-calorie malnutrition."[8] In Latin America, South Africa, and India, studies have shown that 20–30 percent of the time the young child is experiencing acute infection.[9] The UN World Health Organization (WHO) states that, on the average, 3 percent of children under five in low-income countries suffer from severe protein-calorie malnutrition (third degree malnutrition, or below 60 percent of standard body weight per age).[10] Thus at any given time there are approximately 10 million severely malnourished preschool-aged children. Commonly 25 percent, or an additional 80 million preschoolers, are estimated to be suffering from moderate malnutrition (second degree, or 60–75 percent of norm), and an additional 40–45 percent, or 130–160 million children, it is generally agreed, have mild malnutrition (first degree, or 75–90 percent of norm).

Whatever the technique for measuring the extent of malnutrition—food-balance sheets, food consumption surveys, consumer expenditure surveys, medical nutrition surveys—the different methods present a consistent and reasonably reliable picture of a problem of major magnitude: when adults are included, something on the order of a billion and a half persons.[11]

## Solutions to the Problem

This study focuses on the effect of malnutrition on nations—and ways in which the problem can be addressed. It begins with the assumptions that man is the key to development, that the quality of human existence is the ultimate measure of development, and that among the factors affecting the human condition, food–nutritional adequacy is perhaps the major determinant.

It is important, however, that the concentration on nutrition in these pages be viewed in the intended context. Although the well-being of man, and ultimately of nations, may be enhanced by better nutrition, it also depends heavily on economic, educational, environmental, and other opportunities not elaborated on here. This study should be regarded, therefore, as a discussion of one aspect of the process of development. Nutrition is not the centerpiece of development, but it is an important part and is deserving of more attention than it has received.

The relationship of malnutrition to development—by weighing the effect of malnutrition on the individual projected to national dimensions (including the relationship of the nutrition problem to population growth) —is examined in the following two chapters.

Some may take issue with the "development" approach; it is commonly argued that the existence of widespread malnutrition is grounds enough for large nutrition programs and that children should not have to justify their claim to sustenance on societal economic grounds. Obviously, malnutrition is intolerable; and that so many of the malnourished are small children only adds poignancy to the problem. Over the years, however, this case as a "moral imperative" has gained for nutrition programs no more than a token portion of development resources.

Although the magnitude and implications of malnutrition are clear, the best approach to its solution is much less clear. Development planners who have given attention to the subject commonly suggest that better nutrition is an automatic outgrowth of economic development and that total energies should be devoted to increasing income. Or they point to the emphasis already being given to increasing agricultural production and suggest that expanding food supplies is the best route to satisfying nutritional need.

Income and agriculture, discussed in Chapters 4 and 5, obviously are powerful influences on nutritional status. The poor worldwide tend to spend a high proportion of their income, and a higher than average proportion of any increase in income, on food. So any income gain generally has direct nutritional consequences. Similarly, major increases in food production generally can be a significant force for improving the nutrition of the poor.

Although the positive effects of income and agriculture on nutrition are touched on in the following chapters, they are not dealt with in depth because of the abundant literature already devoted to them. A number of less familiar but nonetheless important factors shape and sometimes offset the positive effect of income and agricultural growth on nutritional status. And since these qualifications are generally neglected, the discussions in the income and agriculture chapters cover them in greater detail. In short, although much of the conventional wisdom on income and agriculture's effect on nutrition is accepted here, these positive relationships are not given "equal time." The need at this stage is to deepen our understanding of some of the limitations of these forces—with a view to examining the range of complementary measures that need to be woven into nutrition strategies.

The subsequent five chapters examine such complementary measures. Since much malnutrition is attributable to inadequate understanding of food needs, nutrition education—its practice, its limitations, and its potential—as a means of changing food practices to improve nutrition is discussed in Chapter 6.

Of all the food practices that require changing, perhaps the most critical are those related to breast feeding and the provision of nutritious food solids to children and expectant and nursing mothers at appropriate times. Breast feeding is the most important influence on an infant's nutritional status, yet its recent dramatic decline has received surprisingly limited attention. Chapter 7 analyzes this disturbing trend and its costs to society and suggests possible remedies.*

Opportunities to provide nutritious solid foods at an early age, and beyond, have been enhanced by the recent development of new technologies. Many nutritious foods can now be produced at extraordinarily modest costs and in some instances in ways that require no change of eating habits or income levels. Chapter 8 looks at both the new fortified and formulated foods and the new ingredients now available that make these foods possible.

The means of getting the new foods to those in need poses in many ways more difficult problems than the technology to develop the foods. Chapter 9 examines the role of the marketplace as a distribution mechanism and Chapter 10 direct government feeding programs. Both mechanisms present significant problems—and opportunities.

Although each option is discussed in a separate chapter, it should be understood that most nutrition programs must combine several "best solutions." Because each nutritional deficiency affects different people in different ways, it is most unlikely that all can be countered with a single stroke. A case study in Chapter 11 suggests one country's experience in pulling together the various strands into a national nutrition program. The final chapter draws general conclusions about nutrition programs and policies and looks at future needs.

Basic to every approach described in this study is the consideration of malnutrition as a problem whose causes and solutions are embedded in the broader socioeconomic system. A framework for national planning for better nutritional status is offered in Appendix D. The appendix sets forth a method rather than a master plan for instituting a nutrition pro-

* Also see Appendix C.

gram, suggesting the variety of factors that each nation might assess as it tries to define the elements of a realistic program.

In a systematically planned search for remedies to nutrition problems, many nonstandard nutritional measures will be considered. Protected water supplies, waste disposal and other forms of environmental sanitation, immunization against certain diseases, for instance, all relate to the incidence of malnourishment, its relative severity, and the reduction of mortality. Although such measures (which have been widely analyzed for other purposes in other studies[12] and thus are not elaborated on here) are not normally thought of as nutrition measures, they may be significant determinants of nutritional status or, more likely, essential in combination with the food-related measures that this study focuses on.

Throughout this study the emphasis is on what might be called "macro-nutrition"—nutrition viewed from a national perspective—requiring socioeconomic analysis and broad preventive treatment rather than the person-to-person diagnostic and curative approach that is characteristic of past efforts to help the malnourished. The benefits of the orthodox, usually medically oriented, approach are widely recognized in the literature.[13] But such measures, despite their good and useful goals, are limited in their outreach. These token efforts of the past are an inadequate and thus unacceptable response to a vast social problem. If governments deem it important to eradicate major nutritional deficiencies, they must take actions of broad consequence. Given a similar commitment, certain deficiencies can be as effectively and rapidly brought under control as malaria and smallpox have been in much of the world.

## CHAPTER TWO

# Malnutrition and Development

The light of curiosity absent from children's eyes. Twelve-year-olds with the physical stature of eight-year-olds. Youngsters who lack the energy to brush aside flies collecting about the sores on their faces. Agonizingly slow reflexes of adults crossing traffic. Thirty-year-old mothers who look sixty. All are common images in developing countries; all reflect inadequate nutrition; all have societal consequences.

## Nutrition and Economic Man

Malnutrition adversely affects mental development, physical development, productivity, the span of working years—all of which significantly influence the economic potential of man.

### Mental Development

Malnutrition during the fetal period and in infancy is associated with intellectual impairment. Although the significance is not fully understood, severely malnourished children have brains smaller than average size[1] and have been found to have 15–20 percent fewer brain cells than well-nourished children (of those who had a low birth weight—implying malnutrition in utero—the deficit was 40 percent).[2] There also is a growing body of literature pointing to malnutrition as a cause of abnormal behavior as well as evidence that suggests that abnormalities in the young may produce chromosomal abnormalities that may persist.[3]

That malnutrition inhibits a child's ability to cope with the requirements

9

of daily existence is apparent. However, whether early inflicted damage leaves a permanent scar is a complex question that is just beginning to be answered. Studies in several countries indicate that once-malnourished youngsters perform less well on mental tests in later years than their well-nourished counterparts.[4] Other unmeasured (perhaps unmeasurable) deprivations—such as lack of stimulus and maternal warmth to the institutionalized child—make it difficult in human tests to isolate the nutrition variable. "It is most probable," according to the pioneers in these measurements, "that both primary abnormality in the nervous system and defective experience are independent and interactive. However, the data leave little doubt that severe malnutrition with hospitalization has a long-term persistent effect not only on measured intelligence but also in learning basic academic skills. Survivors of early severe malnutrition are different from normal children."[5] Furthermore, "the available knowledge leaves no doubts about the strong association between the antecedent of severe malnutrition in infancy and suboptimal performance at the school age."[*][6]

There has been much debate over whether the damage caused by malnutrition is reversible in later life. For some, "the evidence is becoming more and more weighty that malnutrition in infancy permanently affects the minds of the children who have been afflicted."[8] For others, less sure, conclusions about permanent effects of malnutrition seem premature. Unfortunately, the question whether damage brought on by malnutrition is reversible has so dominated the thinking and research on malnutrition that attention has been diverted from the more significant public policy considerations. The tendency is understandable; irreversibility suggests a dramatic difference in kind, with a consequence infinitely less tolerable than a temporary affliction. For many public officials it appears to be imperative to do something quickly about malnutrition if it is irretrievably limiting; if it isn't, it poses a lesser sense of urgency.

From a policy perspective, such a posture is dangerously misleading. Malnutrition interferes with a child's motivation, ability to concentrate, and ability to learn, whatever its ultimate effect on the condition of the brain itself. Learning time is lost during the most critical periods of learning. A malnourished child is listless, lacking in curiosity, and unresponsive

---

* Perhaps because of the difficulty in isolating the nutrition variable, less work has been conducted to measure the effect of moderate malnutrition on later intellectual performance. Studies that have been conducted find that malnutrition does play a role apart from social background factors.[7] More systematic research is needed.

to maternal and other stimulation. Even if he were not so, the maternal stimulation he requires for proper development frequently is unavailable; the mother herself is often a victim of nutritionally induced lethargy.

Whichever the origin of the child's apathy, he is late in reaching the standard development milestones. He slides from the norms, and by the time he enters school he already is behind his adequately nourished classmates. This child is less aware of his world than are his well-nourished counterparts. He is mentally and physically fatigued and thus has difficulty being attentive in class. Frequently he seems detached from the life around him.

If this were not a sufficient competitive disadvantage, the malnourished youngster falls further behind because of his frequent bouts with nutrition-related illnesses. In four Latin American countries, illness caused children to miss more than fifty days of school a year,[9] this constituting as much as one-third of the scheduled school days. In the United States, the average is eight days.

The malnourished child thus falls behind, often until he is unable to cope with the school situation. To the extent duller children fail to advance in grades, they occupy seats others might fill; 26–30 percent of children in Central America, Brazil, and India repeat their first school year at least once, and 17–26 percent repeat the second.[10] The level of instruction must be lowered to accommodate the scope of comprehension of the dull children, thus lowering the returns to education expenditure. Obviously, school performance is affected by a child's home and school environment, and nutritional improvement alone may not significantly better the learning capacity of the child disadvantaged in a multitude of ways. There is little doubt, however, that malnutrition contributes to the poor performance, to the low aspiration to higher education levels, and to the substantial student dropout rate often found among the poorly fed portions of the population. Sixty percent of first graders in Pakistan (1959) and Central America (1961) dropped out before the end of the first year; in Mexico (1966), 67 percent had dropped out.[11] For every thousand rural Guatemalan children entering the first grade in 1962, 327 passed directly to the second grade, 130 to the third, 46 to the fourth, 19 to the fifth, and 16 to the sixth. (An additional 23 of the original thousand finished later as repeaters.)[12] Fewer than 40 percent of the pupils entering Indian primary schools reach the fourth grade, which is regarded as necessary to achieve lasting literacy.[13]

Thus, whatever may or may not happen to his brain development at some future date, the malnourished child is permanently handicapped. He has suffered an irreversible loss of opportunity.

Another and perhaps more compelling policy consideration is the projected availability of nutrients. Those who argue for reversing poor learning and behavior patterns assume that the nutrients now in short supply to these children will be available to them at some future date. However, for a substantial portion of people in developing countries, that future date will not fall within their lifetimes, given family food habits, their present low incomes, and likely rates of income growth. For example, 150 million Indians must at least double their current incomes if they are to be able to buy even the minimum acceptable diets. Unless a new strategy is evolved to short cut the traditional means of providing nutrition, it will be near the turn of the century before the poorest third of India's population can afford a minimum adequate diet.

*Physical Development*

While heredity is the key to the ultimate size a youngster can attain, nutrition largely determines how close he will get to his genetic potential. Studies in Japan, Taiwan, and other countries witnessing nutritional improvement in recent years all point to remarkable increases in stature.[14] In many economically less developed countries, however, large parts of the populations clearly are falling significantly short of their genetic potential because of inadequate nutrition.[15] Almost universally, low-income populations have a smaller body size than the norm;* more than 300 million children suffer "grossly retarded physical growth."[17] It is not uncommon to mistake youngsters whose growth is retarded 20–30 percent for healthy children—the malnourished nine-year-old for a healthy six- or seven-year-old. Ninety percent of a group of three thousand low socioeconomic children examined in India were below the tenth percentile norm of height and weight for healthy youngsters.[18]

Other than for jobs that require more than average physical prowess, physical size in itself generally is not economically significant. But the shortfall in size may be related to a shortfall in performance. Small stature

* J. M. Bengoa, head of the nutrition section of the World Health Organization, has said that "despite genetic differences and other disease factors . . . short stature in a population is now regarded as an indication that malnutrition exists, and plays an important role in physical development in many developing countries."[16]

often reflects other disabilities. Presumably healthy Arab children—alert, of good proportions and good general appearance—camouflaged dwarfing to such an extent that "without knowledge of their exact age they could have been taken for healthy children"; in fact, 70 percent were grossly short for their ages, and their accomplishments and behavior were more in keeping with their size than their age.[19] Experts contend that a six-year-old with the physical development of a three-year-old can be compared in learning and behavior with neither age group; "he is another being altogether, with his own biological and behavioral characteristics."[20]

### Adult Capacities

The nutrition problems of poor countries, so far as food is concerned, are both quantitative and qualitative. The former refer to an inadequate supply of food to meet the energy requirements of the body; the latter are concerned with the body's needs for particular nutrients that are required for growth, repair, and preservation of the body and bodily functions.

Man is subject to the laws of thermodynamics; he must absorb energy to produce energy. Men living on 1,800 calories a day have been shown to lose 30 percent of their muscle strength and 15 percent of their precision of movement. Speed, coordination, and many behavioral characteristics also have been altered.[21] Improvements in clearly inadequate diets have often been found to bring increases in work output[22] and work attendance.[23] The inadequately fed apparently make compensating adjustments in the energy they expend to preserve their internal processes. For the adult worker this means, in effect, living a less than average life as a less than average man. He adjusts for his nutritional shortfall by a mixture of slowly paced work, savings on muscular exertion, opportunities for innovation or extra effort forgone, low body weight, and a moderate departure from a condition of general well-being. In addition, other deficiencies—for instance, iron—also affect his ability to work. His life is further complicated by illnesses that proper nourishment would counteract.

The relationship of nutrition to productivity was well recognized a century ago by slave owners, to whom malnutrition meant depreciation of their capital. In northeast Brazil, sugar plantation owners "soon learned that the energy of the African in their service, when abused or subjected to strain, paid less dividends than when it was well conserved . . . which accounts for the plentiful and nourishing food . . . the owners [passed] out to their slaves. . . . The Negro slave in Brazil appears . . . to have been, with all his alimentary deficiencies, the best-nourished element in society."[24] Some slave owners in the United States too were aware of the close relationship between diet and economic return. A Virginia planter, for instance, advised in the 1837 *Farmers' Register* that the most important subject in slave management was sufficiency of food: "The master who gives his field hands half a pound of meat per day and two quarts of meal, (or something short of this when an allowance of vegetables is made) is better compensated by slave labor, than those who give the ordinary quantity."[25]

### Working Life Span

Though life expectancy in a poor country jumps dramatically once the average person survives the perils of young childhood,* early adult mortality is still substantially greater than in industrialized countries. The average ten-year-old boy in Chad, for example, can expect a life some fourteen years shorter than a ten-year-old Indian, and twenty-eight years shorter than a Taiwanese the same age. The twenty-year-old girl from Guinea looks forward to approximately half as many remaining years as her Swedish counterpart. Clearly, their potential period of productive employment is cut short and the potential return to investments during childhood reduced.

Malnutrition and undernourishment are important associated causes of the high death rates among adults, although not so commanding as among infants and young children. The relative impact of malnourishment as a factor in weakening resistance to otherwise nonfatal diseases (or of childhood malnutrition on later adult health status) has not been carefully studied as a cause of adult mortality. Nor has the relative effectiveness of nutrition been investigated as an alternative to vector control and other such methods of attacking local causes of morbidities and reducing mortality risks. Data on identifiable primary causes of mortality among adults in low-income countries make clear, however, that certain major killers, such as tuberculosis, are less apt to be fatal as the general level of health and resistance improves, and that improved nutrition is a major factor contributing to the greater resistance.[26] Nutritional status is also directly related to the length of an illness and the length of time required for recovery after serious infection, wounds, and surgery.

* See Appendix B, Table B-5.

*Nutritional Deficiencies*

The most severe and widespread nutritional deficiencies, especially among children, are a consequence of protein and calorie malnutrition, resulting both from inadequate intake of food and malabsorption of nutrients that are eaten. With serious deficiencies, children may suffer from marasmus—a gross shortage of both calories and protein—or kwashiorkor—primarily a shortage of protein. Characterized by the shrunken, wizened features and gross physical retardation of the child, marasmus affects 1.2–6.8 percent of preschool-aged children surveyed in low-income countries. Kwashiorkor, with its trademark of bloated bellies and glassy stares, at any given time affects 0.2–1.6 percent. Over a year, however, actual figures probably are six to eight times higher since unhospitalized kwashiorkor victims seldom survive for more than a short time (and approximately one in four of those hospitalized will not survive).[27] In Haiti, 7 percent of one-to-three-year-olds are kwashiorkor victims.

Inadequacies of other nutrients, either directly or in combination with protein or calorie shortages, are well discussed in medical texts, but limited data suggest many vitamin-deficiency diseases no longer are prevalent. Once serious problems such as rickets, scurvy, and beriberi may have, for policy purposes, in most countries become of secondary importance. (In certain areas, under unusual circumstances, this is not true; for instance, rickets still is seen in crowded urban areas where children lack adequate sun or where practice of purdah exists, and goiter is prevalent in some belts.) *

The two prominent exceptions to the rule are vitamin A deficiency and iron-deficiency anemia. The sickness and sluggishness—and the effect of fatigue on physical performance—brought on by anemia are so common in poorer societies that the condition is often accepted as the norm. Pregnant and lactating women are especially vulnerable to nutritional anemia. In Latin American countries, 29–63 percent of expectant mothers have been found to be anemic. In India, 66–80 percent are anemic, and 10 percent of maternal deaths in childbirth are the result of nutritional anemias.[28] (Maternal death rates of developing countries are many times those of more affluent societies; India's is thirteen times that of Sweden.[29])

---

* Just beginning to receive concentrated attention is the possibility of damage caused by deficiencies of such trace minerals as zinc, chromium, copper, manganese, vanadium, and selenium. Recent studies, for example, suggest zinc deficiency impairs growth (perhaps in part because it leads to a loss in taste acuity and thus appetite), and in severe cases leads to dwarfism and the total stunting of sexual development.

The nutritional anemias of mothers extend precarious health to the new-born; stillbirths and premature births are much more common among anemic mothers, and premature children are much more likely to die. (Seventy percent of the Indian deaths studied in a perinatal period were among infants weighing less than 2.5 kilograms at birth.[30]) Anemias are also common among older children—67 percent of preschool-aged youngsters studied in Lebanon were anemic; 68 percent in Indonesia; 70 percent in India; 87 percent in Zambia; and 88 percent in Tanzania.[31] In Guatemala, anemic men do less well on physical exercise tests than others, and correction of the anemia results in improved work performance as measured by these same tests.[32]

The second exception is vitamin A deficiency. Commonly up to half of the children in developing countries have subnormal levels of this vitamin, which affects growth, skin condition, the severity of other nutritionally related illnesses, and vision. Severe vitamin A deprivation can lead to blindness and is the major cause of blindness in low-income countries. In India alone, there are an estimated million cases of blindness that are of nutritional origin and thus preventable.[33] But these figures are a bit misleading, since children blinded from diseases brought on by inadequate vitamin A often will not survive; for every survivor in Indonesia, one child dies, and the survivor's chance for further survival is lower than his age partners'.[34] In addition, for every case of total or near-total blindness, there are many others of mild or moderate visual handicap; 10–15 percent of children in India are said to suffer from night blindness (inability to see in dim light) and more severe ocular manifestations of vitamin A deficiency.[35]

## Nutrition and the National Economy

The mathematically precise economic growth models that have been in vogue since the 1940s seldom take explicit account of the notion of investment in human beings. Increases in tomorrow's income are assumed to result primarily from today's additions to material capital, and since consumption displaces capital investment, it becomes an enemy of growth, not a handmaiden. Consumption in the form of educational services, clothing, and eating of course have an instrumental impact on productivity, but since the effects of such consumption are difficult to identify, all growth in income is imputed to those more easily measurable factors included in the model. Expenditures on health and nutrition are also classified as consumption and thus fail to show up as factors affecting national growth.

Recently, however, the concept of capital has been extended to human beings. Development of the new theory was prompted by the discovery that "increases in national output have been large compared with the increases of land, man-hours, and physical reproducible capital. Investment in human capital is probably the major explanation for this difference."[36] A significant part of economic growth in the United States and Western Europe, for example, has been attributed to education, and any residual growth to "knowledge."[37]

In similar attempts to begin to measure economic returns to health investment,[38] the cost of preventing a death is compared with the worker's future income, had he lived. Or the investment in human capital—the health, food, clothing, housing, education, and other expenditures necessary to enable a person to develop his particular skills—is measured against his loss through death any time prior to retirement. Those costs can also be measured against debility, where death is not a factor.[39] Whether an illness results in temporary loss of work days or some temporary or permanent reduction in work capacity, the estimated loss in output added to the cost of medical care can be compared with proposed expenditures for preventing the occurrence of the illness in the first place.[40]

Similar comparisons can be made of the benefits to be gained from expenditures on nutrition. Improved nutrition that returns an absent worker to the active labor force, or helps lengthen his working life span, or overcomes a debility that is reducing his productive capacity, or that enables a child to return to school or to improve his understanding or retention of things taught, or that enables an adult to absorb more effectively in-service training or the advice of an agricultural extension agent clearly raises the flow of earnings above what it would have been in absence of the improvement in well-being.

Once a person's well-being is stabilized, nutrition costs become a maintenance expenditure. Increments of nutrition no longer lead to increases in productivity. An improvement in nutrition thus can help to improve or maintain the productivity level of an active member of the labor force, or it can take the form of an investment—for example, helping to push up the expected lifetime earnings of a two-year-old child.

*Savings on Medical Costs*

One measure of the benefits of a nutrition program is in the medical costs saved through reduced demand for medical services. In Caribbean hospitals, 20–45 percent of the pediatric beds are filled by nutrition cases; in India, 15 percent; in Guatemala, 80 percent.[41] Nearly half a million hospital in-patients from thirty-seven developing countries were officially registered for malnutrition in 1968[42] (actual numbers may be higher due to classification of nutritional ailments under other diseases). At an average cost of $7.50 a day for ninety days for each case,* costs for treating malnutrition are on the order of $340 million a year to the thirty-seven countries.[43] If treatment were provided to the approximately 10 million preschool-aged children who need it†—without it, severe (third degree) protein-calorie malnutrition is generally fatal—annual costs would be on the order of $6.8 billion.

Clearly it is cheaper to prevent malnutrition than to cure it. However, as long as the elimination of, say, a case of kwashiorkor frees a bed and other medical resources for treatment of some other sick person who was otherwise unable to gain entry into the system, total hospital costs will not go down. Since unsatisfied demand for curative services is typical in low-income countries, reduction of malnutrition is not likely to bring about either a net reduction in medical expenditures or a slowing of the rate of growth in medical system investment. Adequate nutrition, however, would enable the medical system to increase the welfare and restore the productivity of all those persons on the queue who would be able to replace malnutrition patients in the system.

*Reducing Productivity Losses*

Another potentially large nutrition benefit for developing countries is the reduction in productivity losses caused by the debility of a substantial portion of the labor force. Unfortunately, medical data of the kind needed for calculating debility seldom are available for poor countries, and even if clinical data are accessible, they do not include many of the sick who

---

* Cost of hospitalization in Guatemala is $7.31 a day; in Uganda, $7.84 a day. This compares to national per capita health budgets in many countries of between $1 and $2 a year.

† An estimated 3 percent of the 325 million preschool-aged group in developing countries need such treatment; that is twenty times the number of medical facility cots available for children for all diseases.[44]

never enter the statistics because of the excess demand on the medical system. In any case, the synergistic interaction of malnutrition with much prevailing illness makes it difficult to pin down the exact contribution of each factor. Often malnutrition itself does not put sufferers into the queues.

An alternative approach to measuring productivity losses is through use of aggregative data on food supply and the occupational distribution of the labor force. From estimates of daily caloric need in different occupations, shortfalls in work capacity can be calculated for different levels of shortfall in caloric intake. Comparison of a country's average caloric need to average national caloric consumption then yields national working capacity shortfalls. For low-income countries these shortfalls are almost always very substantial, often as high as 50 percent. While this means of linking individual productivity to national productive capacity is conceptually useful, it relies on such aggregative data that its utility in estimating the cost of malnutrition is limited.*

### Extending Working Years

Another cost of malnutrition is the reduced number of working years resulting from early death. For the majority of the developing countries, increases in the life expectancy of adults would add years to the working lives (rather than retirement years) of most adults. In countries where life expectancy at ten or twenty is particularly short, the added working years would be those when healthy adults would be at the peak of their powers and earning capacity.

Other things being equal, a lengthening of working life reduces the country's dependency ratio—the proportion of those in the population (largely the young) who produce no income to those who work. In 1960 for every 100 persons of working age in the typical developing country population, there were an estimated 76 dependents, compared to only

---

* The example given here is based on the work of Hector Correa,[45] who recognizes that because of data limitations many of his assumptions are heroic. A more refined model would offer finer breakdowns of the labor force, adjustment of work factors for local conditions and of caloric requirements by occupation and local conditions, and estimates of daily intake by income level and by season. It would still fail to take account of such important factors as employment opportunities, intrafamily food distribution, the impact of cooking habits on nutrient content, the problems of efficiency of absorption, and the productivity impact of early malnutrition on mental and physical capacity.

about 59 in the typical industrialized country.[46] Lower dependency ratios, of course, increase per capita income and, potentially, per capita savings as family incomes are required to support fewer numbers.

The age structure and life expectancy rates of developing countries indicate that reductions in adult mortality would not only add years to income-generating lives and reduce dependency ratios, but increase the "yield" on education and other investments society makes in workers during their formative years. The advances are only potential, however, because they depend on productive employment being available.

### The Problem of Surplus Labor

Restoring a worker to good health adds nothing to national production if no job exists for him. The apparent slow growth of employment opportunities compared with the growth of the labor force in poor countries is a common source of development economists' skepticism that better health and nutrition will bring economic benefits. Many countries have a substantial labor surplus in the form of seasonal idleness in agriculture, open urban unemployment, and part-time or work-sharing employment which has been called disguised unemployment. Hence the case for seeking productivity benefits from better nutrition, especially for the masses of the unskilled, would seem weak.

Yet, in rural areas of low-income countries, labor is more commonly in short supply than in surplus during harvest and other periods of intense activity.[47] Do farm workers try to feed themselves seasonally to higher capacity, like draft animals? In fact, can they do so during the weeks preceding harvest, when cash income is at the lowest annual point and grain prices are at their peak? What happens to the productivity of workers who undergo alternating periods of well-being and malnourishment?

Open unemployment does not necessarily mean that production problems can be solved merely by hiring additional workers. Many functions impaired by a worker's malnourishment cannot be satisfactorily corrected by added hands. Most machine-paced operations have precisely defined needs for which the human work input cannot be divided among more workers to compensate for inefficiency. If a job is strictly machine paced, the worker would have narrow scope for reducing his performance below the machine's automatic demand. Malnutrition might then be reflected in shoddy output, particularly if the work is dependent on the worker's manual precision or strength. Malnutrition also is reflected in accident rates and poor work attendance. (In numerous instances, factories that have introduced feeding programs have experienced lower accident and absenteeism rates.[48])

In many urban centers the army of the unemployed is not the commonly perceived homogeneous collection of surplus (and impoverished) human energy. Considerable numbers of unskilled laborers are in the pool, but the rate of urban unemployment is sometimes greater among skilled and educated young people. In Malaya in 1965 the urban unemployment rate among males fifteen to twenty-four with secondary education was 30.9 percent; among those with primary education 19.5 percent; and among illiterates 10.4 percent. In urban areas of Venezuela in 1969 the unemployment rate among laborers with secondary education was 10.2 percent; among those with primary education 7 percent; and among illiterate laborers 4.3 percent.[49] The young, who are conspicuous, often volatile, and therefore a problem, often choose to wait for the job in the field for which they are trained and in which they will earn the largest future stream of income. Since the educated unemployed do not normally compete with the unskilled, this type of unemployment is not relevant to the question of whether and how investment in the nourishment of the poor will pay off.

It is worth recalling that in many areas of the developing world, man-to-land ratios are relatively low and there appears to be no substantial "disguised unemployment" problem. Much of southeast Asia was historically what Adam Smith called a "vent for surplus" economy—that is, an economy in which only an increase in export demand was needed to motivate farmers to extend their area of cultivation, trading leisure for additional work to take advantage of a vent or opportunity for exporting the potential surplus. Though an increasing population makes this description less apt for southeast Asia today, it would fit many subsistence agricultural parts of Africa and South America.

*The quality of labor.* Productivity is of course more than a function of human energy, of numbers of workers. Energy loss is a limited basis for calculating the effect of malnutrition on national production. As development proceeds, human energy is replaced by machine energy; human quality becomes more important than sheer physical capacity. Demands on human physical energy ouput decrease as the proportion of the work force in agriculture declines. (Although this may sound like a long-term description of the development process, it is already happening in some developing countries.) In agriculture, timely initiative, physical dexterity, and comprehension of increasingly sophisticated techniques all become critical to the successful exploitation of new technologies. In cultivating the new high-yielding grain varieties, farmers fall short of maximum returns because they fail, in varying degree, to apply the recommended practices. Some constraints, like inaccessibility or high cost of credit, are beyond the farmers' control. But errors of planting depth and timing, pesticide application, and fertilizer application rates and timing are not economic; they may reflect such factors as education, mental performance level, dexterity, and attention.

The small farmer exemplifies the problem. His decision making on the use of his own resources is not divisible. If malnutrition during his childhood limited his learning opportunity and undernourishment as an adult is compounding his disadvantages, his potential efficiency in making decisions is not increased by the presence of unemployed labor in the neighborhood.

Given the gross unemployment picture—and clearly this is one of the major challenges facing many countries—an economic, as distinct from welfare, case cannot be made for special expenditures merely to upgrade the potential productivity of those masses of unskilled, landless, adult workers who have dim prospects of gainful employment. There are, of course, other limiting factors in the picture besides malnutrition—poorly functioning extension and credit services, inadequate transport systems, inadequate equipment (perhaps exacerbated by policies encouraging capital rather than labor intensive technologies), illiteracy, and so on. Any presumption that improvements in nutritional status are a sufficient condition for realizable improvements in productivity would therefore be simplistic.

Yet, it would be equally simplistic to dismiss the productivity value of nutrition because of the existence of idle adults. To do so is to assume that underemployed labor is available (or can be made available) in the vicinity of an activity at the right time, that it possesses required skills, that it can be hired in fact, and that the work is technically capable of being divided among more workers than are currently employed. Often this is not the case. Much of the unemployed and underemployed today turns out to be a diverse and complex group that needs to be sorted out before conclusions are reached about the value of nutritional improvements. Moreover, recognizing the increasing importance of skilled manpower and general labor quality for future national growth, investment in large numbers of malnourished children today can improve the quality of a significant fraction of the future labor force. This is probably the area in which nutrition will prove critical to development in the long run.

Although many of these nutrition investment notions are new in the context of development planning, for some years they have been endorsed and commonly incorporated into the planning of military organizations, which have established special nutrition units and developed special nutritious products. AID Nutrition Director Martin Forman has noted that in some developing countries a sizable portion of the total nutrition research budget is directed to the effectiveness of the fighting man, and his feeding receives priority attention.[50]

### Other Economic Benefits

Nutrition programs promise a number of economic benefits in addition to the direct productivity benefits:

• As the incidence of communicable diseases among the adequately nourished is lowered, the exposure of others to these diseases will be reduced.

• The increased income of well-nourished workers (or well-nourished children when they enter the labor force) should improve the living standards of their dependents, thereby raising both their current consumption and their future productivity.

• Housewives, whose activities are not measured in a market economy, should when better nourished improve performance on a number of economically important functions, not least of which is the quality of care for the young.

• Returns may be raised on other investments closely related to human well-being, particularly education. (Low-income countries now spend nearly 4 percent of their gross national products on education, almost a third more than in 1960. The efficiency of the education systems they support may be reduced as much as 50 percent by the dropout and repeater rates to which malnutrition contributes heavily.[51])

## Benefits Compared with Costs

Even where opportunities for returns to better nutrition appear to be significant, the costs must be weighed. Will the nutrition expenditure be less than the value of the expected increase in production? How will it compare with returns to alternative investments? The answers will depend on whose malnourishment is to be corrected, what increments in their productivity can be expected, how much the program will cost, whether its effects will be immediate or delayed, and what discount rate is applied to determine present value if benefits are delayed.

Productivity payoffs from nutrition investment can be anticipated for workers employed in machine-paced occupations in modern manufacturing sectors, students for whom malnutrition limits the potential joint returns from education and health expenditures, and small farmers facing the more exacting demands of new agricultural technologies. The widest and most lasting impact, however, probably would come from providing adequate nutrition to mothers in the last trimester of pregnancy—the critical period for fetal growth—and to children six months through two or three years of age (most of the needs before six months can be met through breast feeding). The greatest physiological need and greatest growth occur in the early years: 80 percent of eventual brain weight, for example, is reached by age two. During this time children require, relative to body weight, two and one-half times as much protein as adults; without adequate nourishment, they are susceptible to severe consequences of childhood infections such as measles and whooping cough and to diarrheal diseases. Even if a child's diet is fully adequate only in utero and during the critical early years of life, he probably will be brought closer to his growth potential. If, during adulthood, his energy intake level falls short of some desirable norm, his productivity will already have been ratcheted to a higher level—more relevant to a modern economy—than a lifetime at his current nutrition level could achieve.

### Payoff on Child Nutrition Investments

An institutional feeding program designed to meet all nutritional deficiencies of a child from six months through his third year can cost roughly $8 a year or a total of $20.* (This *annual* cost to prevent malnutrition is approximately the same as the *daily* cost to treat it in a number of coun-

* The $8 would meet deficiencies of a diet that currently satisfies three-fourths of a child's protein need and two-thirds of his caloric need. The estimate is based on the production and distribution costs of Bal Ahar, used in India's child feeding programs (the child feeding program is being used here only for illustrative purposes, and is not being suggested as the lowest cost means of achieving the nutrition goal). The average cost of the commodity per child per year is $5.60 (for very young children

tries.) Suppose that the program averts a disability in a child's later performance. Assume also that if the disability were not avoided, the child would be able to produce (or earn) an annual income of $200 over a thirty-five-year period starting at the age of fifteen. How much of an increase above $200 would be required to make the nutrition investment break even?

Of course, returns beginning twelve years after an investment is made are remote, and they should be adjusted to account for the long waiting period. If a discount rate of 10 percent is used to convert future benefits to present value, an improvement of only 4 percent ($8) in annual earning capacity is needed to break even—the annual productivity increase is about the same as the annual cost of the feeding. Both the time stream and the discount rate are on the conservative side, however. In developing societies a child often turns worker at eight or ten. Though a discount rate of 10 percent is commonly used for developing countries, it is probably too high for important irreversibilities—for assets or opportunities that once forgone can never be restored.[52] The irreversibility of the human condition or opportunity resulting from malnutrition would place nutrition investments at the lower end of any discount range, increasing their competitive strength as investments.

Nonetheless, an increase in future productivity of 4 percent is a modest reflection of higher levels of performance. The actual rate of return will depend on a number of factors. The higher the initial income of the worker, the smaller proportionately need be the break-even increase in productivity. The larger his shortfall in working capacity due to malnutrition, the greater will be the increase in his performance from better nutrition. If his improvement in performance can move him upward in occupational groups, the gains may be more significant. Increased productivity ought also to include side benefits and enhanced returns to other investments. In a study that compared nutrition levels and IQ differences of Chilean children with IQ and productivity (or wages) of Chilean workers, the potential increase in earnings from child feeding that would offset protein-calorie deficiencies during the critical periods of early growth was estimated to range from 19 percent to 25 percent.[53] Those rates are quite

who receive smaller portions, probably less). Administration cost of the program is 65 cents per child. The remaining $1.75 is largely a notional figure to cover costs, often difficult to measure directly, such as fuel, cooking equipment, and the time teachers and health center officials devote to the program at the expense of their other duties (see Chapter 10).

competitive with returns to education; in India, for example, education returns have been estimated in the range of 9 percent to 16 percent.[54]

It would be hard to find a more favorable investment opportunity than avoidance of vitamin A blindness. Poverty-stricken societies where such blindness is considerable have few facilities for training the blind for productive occupations. The upkeep of the blind, minimal as it is, represents a total burden to their families or the society. Assuming that the average blind person could be sustained at a subsistence cost as low as $25 a year, the cost is 1,250 times the annual ingredient cost of the vitamin A needed for prevention. If vitamin delivery techniques should raise the cost several times, the arithmetic would still be highly favorable. The average blind person need only be in position, if sight loss were avoided, to produce a modest fraction of this annual consumption for the investment in his sight to yield an enormous return. For India the consumption burden (at $25 a year per person) of one million people blind from vitamin A deficiency will cumulate to $1 billion over their lifetimes. Similar returns can be made from investments to prevent what are in some places common cases of irreversible cretinism and deaf-mutism linked to endemic goiter. In parts of Bolivia, for example, 40–50 percent of the population is goiterous and 5–10 percent of these suffer from cretinism and deaf-mutism. Cost of the iodate to prevent goiter (and the equipment necessary to add the nutrient to salt) is one-sixth of a cent a year per person covered.*[55]

Many of the links between diet, performance potential, and economic returns are poorly understood and may remain so, given the complexities of human development and behavior. Little is known, for example, about the relative damage caused by different degrees of malnutrition at different ages and of varying durations. The major benchmark provided by medical science is the concept of "minimum daily requirements" of specified nutrients. Any sustained diet below the minimum daily requirement implies damage, especially in environments where widespread diarrhea and other ailments lead to heavy nutrient losses. Although it is known that the extent

---

* Another documented and highly productive nutrition investment is the fluoridation of water. Dental caries are reduced 60–70 percent where water is fluoridated. The $13 million (about 10 cents per person) it would take to fluoridate the unfortified water supplies in the United States would save an estimated $700 million a year in dental bills.[56] Fluoridation is less significant to national development, both because of the lack of centralized water supplies in many places and because of the lesser importance of tooth decay compared to consequences of other nutrient deficiencies. There are, however, preliminary signs that fluoride, at least in animals, may also be important to the rate of growth.

of damage increases as the level of nutritional deprivation falls—as a child moves from first to third degree malnutrition—the shape of the curve relating deprivation to loss of physical, motor, and mental development, and to the severity of nutrition-related diseases, is unknown. The threshold beyond which the extent of loss becomes serious cannot be defined, nor can the degree of mental or physical shortfall or other resulting damage that separates the serious from the inconsequential be calculated.

Although it may never be possible to separate the mass of the world's malnourished children into neat groups whose potential performance can be forecast from specific investments in varying nutritional supplements, a clear line can be drawn between those who will live and the significant number of those who will die of malnutrition or related causes. Before children born today in developing countries reach their fifth birthdays, approximately 75 million youngsters will die of malnourishment and associated illnesses. The known numbers of those whose lives will be marked by illnesses that seriously strike the malnourished are so great, and the effects of malnutrition on educational and productive capacity so apparent, that investment in nutrition programs can almost be undertaken as an act of faith.

Even though much information is lacking—and priority should be given to obtaining it—the lack of exacting data on which to base policy is not a dilemma confined to the nutrition field. In many sectors, substantial resources have been allocated to programs whose returns were long run and difficult to calculate with anything approaching precision. The contribution of gradations of education to individual productivity and to national economic growth, for instance, is difficult to analyze and less easy to identify as the numbers of educated unemployed continue to rise. Yet, the overall importance of education to long-run economic progress has been demonstrated beyond dispute.

Often the economic and engineering precision of projections in other sectors proves to be illusory, victim of the same real-life complexities that make the study of malnutrition's impact so difficult. In the case of rice, for example, conditions on the farm have turned out to be so substantially different from conditions under controlled research that costly mistakes have been made along the road generally recognized as the right one to higher rice production.

Nutritional guidelines can be established to help define policy and direct the use of limited resources—for example, big deficiencies are more serious than small, very young children (including the last few months in utero) are more critical to reach than older children and adults, low-income portions of the population are usually more vulnerable than other portions, and so on. But governments interested in attacking malnutrition will have to operate in gross terms. Remedies will have to be as imprecise as the diagnoses.

In sum, much is still unknown about the developmental effects of malnutrition—reflecting partly the relative youth of the field, partly the enormous complexity of measuring human growth and performance. Yet, governments should not insist on more rigorous measurement of the impact of malnutrition than of other problems to which large sums are commonly allocated. While further research—especially longitudinal studies—is needed, it seems reasonable to assume that the return from improvement in the performance and well-being of a substantial fraction of the population can be an important stimulant to national growth. Economic judgment recommends that even while these implications are being explored, developmental plans be shaped to take account of nutrition objectives.

### Beyond Standard Economic Benefits

In economic terms the life of agricultural laborers and their families often would be categorized as "very poor" or "destitute." Yet, for all their economic privation, these rural families have the potential for enjoying a wide range of noneconomic goods—nature, love, friends, good talk at the coffee or tea stall, the joy of children. These enjoyments, independent of economic status, include some of the major sources of satisfaction in life, satisfactions which by their nature are not marketable services and are not quantifiable in the national accounts when the economist totes up the per capita availability of goods and services for personal "consumption." But those who are apathetic and physically drained by nutritional anemia or debilitated by the seemingly constant bouts with nutritionally related diarrheas cannot really savor these satisfactions. It is well-being, not income, that determines whether a man, rich or poor, has the capacity to enjoy these most fundamental sources of human satisfaction. Well-being is the primary requisite, the sine qua non, that determines the utility men derive from all other forms of consumption, whether measurable or not. The developing economies are not likely in the near future to provide a very much wider range of material goods to those in lower income levels. But it may be within the power of public policy to improve the level of nutrition, which in turn can increase the capability for a substantial portion of the population to enjoy whatever sources of consumption are available.

For societies whose prevailing philosophy places a premium on egalitarianism, the intellectual loss that is caused by malnutrition may be a strong obstacle to attaining this social goal. Nutrition is not, of course, a cure-all; educational barriers, for example, are immense. However, a malnourished child's chances for social mobility are greatly restricted no matter what is offered in education or other avenues designed by policy makers to facilitate upward movement within a society. Adequate mental development, hence adequate nutrition, would seem to be a prerequisite to other programs for mobility that are being developed as a matter of social policy. If a child lacks curiosity and mental energy—to say nothing of the possibility of mental capacity—the other opportunities are not significant.

Even more difficult to quantify than the costs of widespread malnutrition among the working masses—but no less real—is the loss to society of potentially outstanding individuals. Since the origin of so many superior people in the middle and upper class is a result of opportunity rather than genetic potential, it seems appropriate to ask how many potentially superior minds are lost because of malnutrition. If nutritional risk is as high as studies now indicate—affecting as much as half of some populations—a substantial number of potentially superior people will never come forward. They are not only the Tagores and the Gandhis but also the one-in-a-thousand or ten-thousand who can organize large resources, who is innovative, an entrepreneur, a mover of men. Considering how very thin in most countries is the leadership elite on whom rests the burden of the nation's success or failure, such losses would seem to inhibit the chances for economic development.

The purpose of national development—of forgoing consumption today in favor of more investment—is to generate a higher level of human well-being tomorrow for more people. To most people in low-income countries, that mostly means a better diet. Food is a major, perhaps the major, problem of their lives. It is central to both their consumption and their production activities. For a person living at the income level that characterizes the malnourished, typically 65–80 percent of income goes for food. As his income rises, the proportion devoted to buying more food declines, but generally the proportion remains high. The inadequacy and uncertain availability of food from year to year represents the condition of underdevelopment at its most immediate and palpable and dangerous level.

Thus nutrition-cum-food represents the thin margin between mere survival and adequate growth and well-being. For governments to be concerned with food as a commodity but not with nutrition—which is food analyzed into its nutritional constituents, as it reaches and affects people —reflects a double vision. Yet economic distinction commonly is made between food and nutrition—ranking food "high," nutrition "low"; or food "essential," nutrition "welfare." Food has obvious tangibility features that nutrition lacks. Food costs and supplies can be measured, subjected to economic analysis, and entered into the national accounts. Nutrition in contrast often is invisible and dimly understood, and it seldom commands a price, especially among those who need it most. Even when food quantity is sufficient, there are instances in which the individual's effective demand for nutrients is inefficient for meeting his needs. Eating is a complex activity that satisfies several wants besides nutrition—aesthetic preferences, religious proscriptions, social customs. Some of these demands may be mutually inconsistent (for example, aesthetics and nutrition). As the consumer chooses among them, the demand for needed nutrients may be distorted. The consumer is least capable of evaluating the nutritional component and of recognizing the degree to which meeting the other objectives, within his tight income constraint, may deprive him of the health he assumes he is acquiring. Such considerations argue strongly for government intervention. Moreover, new techniques and technologies are now available to governments to provide shortcuts to substantially better nutrition and well-being for people of much lower incomes and at an earlier time than previously was possible.

## CHAPTER THREE

# Improved Nutrition and the Population Dilemma

The notion of improving nutrition sometimes prompts the uncomfortable question: Why go to such efforts to keep people alive when the basic problem is too many people? Moral considerations aside, it may be that better nutrition is one of the important ingredients necessary for an effective family planning program. Although other essential factors are also involved, an important precondition for bringing down the birthrate may be to keep more children alive, and improved nutrition is one of the keys to achieving this. There is no question but that the immediate effect of reducing child mortality will be a population spurt. But against this certainty is the hope that a lowering of child mortality rates now will have an important effect in later years on reducing the population growth rate. The evidence of a causal relationship is suggestive enough and the problem important enough to merit pursuing.

## The Population Problem

With the apparent success of the agricultural revolution in many of the poorer areas, the problem most critical to development in a number of countries is the unbridled growth of population, a growth that has partly offset other development achievements. World population is increasing by about 75 million people a year. More than 80 percent of this increase is in low-income countries, where commonly there is little prospect for reducing the level of growth in the near future. At present rates of increase,

31

India's 1967 population will double—to a billion—by the turn of the century. Assuming the family planning program is extremely effective, the smallest population that can be expected is 900 million.[1]

Such an assumption, of course, cannot be made. Family planning efforts are plagued by the same kind of program and administrative difficulties that infect any large new activity, and these are not easy or inexpensive to overcome. Nor does the assumption even begin to address a major obstacle to success in such programs—the lack of reversible contraceptives that are both effective and acceptable. Each of the contraceptives now in use has limitations. The condom requires discipline and a comprehensive marketing and distribution system. So with the pill, which, in addition, requires a consumer regimen often lacking even among women from the most educated environments. The loop presupposes physiological acceptability and professional follow-ups often out of easy reach; 65 percent of Indian women express fear of the loop because of anticipated bleeding and other problems.[2] Sterilization operations require a motivation strong enough to overcome apprehensions of pain and impotence and to induce the decision to chance ending fertility permanently.

Eventually an effective, easy, inexpensive, reversible, aesthetically acceptable, and easily understood contraceptive may be available. But before it can be an effective part of a family planning effort, there will be a time lag for development, testing, obtaining acceptability, communicating to the ultimate user, and generating the necessary bureaucratic momentum to carry out the program.

## The Need for Children

Even greatly improved and acceptable contraceptives would solve only part of the population problem. Insufficient motivation to practice birth control is increasingly recognized as a large and more difficult obstacle.

The chief premise of much of the early family planning effort has been that either ignorance, inadequacy, or nonavailability of contraceptives is the cause of the burgeoning population. Reexamination of that premise now suggests that in much of the developing world most births would occur anyway, that parents consciously want many children.[3]

The wish is a reflection of a need that the typical family history in today's poor countries makes apparent. The average family wants at least two adult sons. The reasons vary: a mark of success, of good fortune, of religious favor, of maintaining the family name and property, of ceremonial duty, of economic necessity—and always of security. In many countries the villager commonly expresses his need for sons "to take care of me when I get old."

In most poor countries, sons provide the only effective form of social security. The premium placed on male offspring is confirmed by an Indian study of vasectomized fathers, who had an average of more than three times as many sons as daughters.[4] Another study concluded that "only as reduced mortality and morbidity provide some physical security can concepts such as planning, saving, or investing for the future have meaning, whether they are applied to one's family or to the whole society."[5]

Of course, child mortality in the low-income countries has started to fall. The declining death rates that have brought on the population explosion apply not only to those who survive to adulthood. Yet child mortality rates remain high. Most families experience the loss of one or more infants or young children, and the uncertainty of their children's survival hangs over most couples. In many poor areas, where large percentages of children die before reaching a productive age, uncertainty and the overcompensation it induces are major factors in the common bearing of seven or eight offspring to assure two male survivors. A village study in India's western state of Gujarat concluded "families continued to have children until they were reasonably certain that at least one boy would survive. Once they had this number, they attempted to stop having more."[6] Even in the Punjab, which includes India's best nourished people (they consume nearly 50 percent more food per capita than people in states like Bihar and West Bengal), wives in their mid-forties had given birth to an average of 7.5 live-born children, of whom 34–44 percent died.[7] Nearly half the women over forty years of age had lost at least three live-born children; only one in seven had lost none.[8] A study using computer simulation indicates that with current estimated infant and adult death rates in India, a couple must bear 6.3 children to be 95 percent certain one son will be surviving at the father's sixty-fifth birthday. The average number of births in India per couple is 6.5.[9]

The combined desire for adult sons and recognition of high child mortality are among the contributors to the population dilemma. This suggests paradoxically that keeping more children alive, although it inevitably will increase population in the short run, may be a powerful contribution toward lowering the population growth rate in the long run. Experience in the Western world is not inconsistent with the notion that reduction of the death rate may be a prerequisite to reduction of the birthrate.* The same seems to be true among countries such as Taiwan and Korea that are now increasing in affluence. Demographic trends in Mauritius, Ceylon, and British Guiana also suggest that as death rates decline, birthrates begin to fall.[11] A study of population dynamics in rural Punjab concluded that "until they have good assurance that live-born sons, and daughters, will survive, couples in the Khanna area are unlikely to be interested in restricting the numbers of their children beyond their present practice."[12]

Such assurance means creation of a climate in which, among other things, parents realize there is no longer need to bear many more children than are really wanted. This will take time, and while conscious efforts are under way to drive down child mortality, there clearly will be a period when numbers will grow before it could be hoped that they will begin to stabilize. The lag between decline in infant mortality and that in birthrate was an estimated twenty years in Puerto Rico (1930 to 1950) and Chile (1909 to 1929); in Sweden, fifteen years (1873–77 to 1888–92); and in the United Kingdom, ten years (1901 to 1911).[13]

Family size, of course, is determined by a number of very complex behavioral phenomena. What are the key factors—income, education, urbanization, and other elements of "modernization"—that govern the lag between declining mortality and fertility rates and that eventually convince people to have fewer children? What is the relative importance of lower infant mortality, the rate at which it declines, its relation to other determinants of population size at any particular rate? How powerfully, and under what conditions, could a deliberate program to drive infant mortality down to low levels contribute to an overall population policy? Many questions are still to be answered, but it does appear a reasonable hypothesis that at least a substantial further reduction of child mortality, although not a sufficient condition of itself, may be a necessary precondition to induce a large fraction of the present population to lower the number of desired births.

If this is so, the sooner action is taken to reduce child mortality rates the better. The longer action is delayed, the larger will be the population base from which the future generations will be reared.

---

* Noted, for instance, in seventeenth-century England, when twenty-two (of the thirty-two) children of British royalty died before reaching the age of twenty-one. The result of the high death rate was repeated royal pregnancies to assure survivors. The royal birthrate declined dramatically as life expectancy increased.[10]

## Reducing Mortality Rates

Reducing child mortality in developing countries means primarily two things: decreasing the incidence and spread of disease and increasing the individual's ability to withstand illness. The first is largely a matter of public health, and in most countries measures to deal with it have been extensive and effective. In many areas in recent years, malaria, plague, smallpox, and cholera have been controlled. While there is still much to be done, many basic, and in some ways the easiest and least costly, steps in disease control have been taken.

In contrast, relatively little has been done to strengthen the resistance to illness. The bulk of childhood deaths in developing countries are attributable to otherwise minor childhood infections that are aggravated by the malnourished state of the child. A minor illness such as measles or chicken pox or even a cold cannot be overcome because the child's resistance has been lowered by nutritional deficiency. Diarrhea occurs and more nutrients are lost. Commonly the prescribed remedy is to withhold solid foods when the only hope is more and better food. All too often the child's malnutrition begins in the womb with the mother's own anemia and other nutrient deficiencies. Pregnancy wastage—miscarriage, stillbirth, birth abnormality—is common among malnourished women. And the live babies they do bear are often premature and underweight, both increasing the risk of early death.[14] All this suggests that improved nutrition among those cohorts in the population experiencing high child mortality may be an important condition for reducing child death rates—and eventually birthrates.

## Operational Relationships

Not only may nutritional well-being help in the long run to curb family size, but nutrition programs can serve immediately in an operationally direct way as a mechanism to encourage family planning. The mother whose child makes a quick and dramatic recovery from malnutrition is a prime prospect for further help. The sight of a child on the verge of life-long blindness can, for example, virtually be saved overnight by sufficient intake of vitamin A. Similarly, appropriate nutritious foods can revive a child near death in a matter of weeks. A mother's receptivity to advice from the person who thus saved her child is also dramatically enhanced;

that advice can quite logically include family planning. In India's Punjab, a Johns Hopkins University rural health research project found that with nutrition services "the dramatic improvement in a child with marasmus has more impact on general rapport and relationships with village families than anything else which we have tried to do in active medical care. The change in the children is so obvious, and the whole process is so readily understood, that such efforts do lend considerable credibility to what our village workers say on other matters."*[15]

Other nutrition activities also provide means of reaching young mothers. Through child feeding programs, for example, millions of preschool children are being fed institutionally, and most of them are brought to feeding stations by their mothers. These young mothers of childbearing age constitute a large, voluntary, generally appreciative, and readily accessible audience for family planning instruction. Nutrition programs, of course, are but one means of winning confidence and instructing mothers on family planning needs. Whether they are the most cost-effective means under given conditions is open to empirical examination.

The provision of child health and nutrition programs—and the demonstration of government care and concern for the child—is likely to provide a better climate for governments to operate family planning activities. A citizenry suspicious and perhaps resentful of a government population program can be a drag on family planning acceptance. India's Planning Secretary Asok Mitra reports differences arising "over suspicions, real or imagined, that politics is being imported into eugenics."[17] Although ethnic suspicions are relatively minor, religious and caste groups in the rural countryside sometimes watch each other's family planning performance out of concern that their relative strength not be reduced. A political leader from Madras publicly voiced concern that his state stood to lose seats in Parliament because family planning had disproportionately lowered its population. In Ceylon, Singhalese extremists and a section of the Buddhist clergy publicized the bogey of potential Tamil domination if the Singhalese stopped multiplying at their current rate. In Kenya, attendance by members of the Kikuyu tribe at family planning clinics dropped 90

---

* The notion of using food and nutrition as an incentive for family planning is sometimes criticized as an inducement not dissimilar to missionaries' occasional use of feeding programs as a come-on to salvation. The analog is not farfetched, as proselytization in foreign societies was often facilitated by missionaries' offering health services.[16] Free will in family planning practice should be maintained, but there is large opportunity for use of incentives in the context of free will.

percent in 1970 after an eruption of tribal antagonisms. (The country's return to normalcy was partly measured by the return of tribe members to family planning clinics.) Such disruptions of family planning programs were once singled out by an AID-appointed expert committee as "a serious threat to the future commitment of the government to the program."*[18]

## Other Nutrition–Family Planning Relationships

Several other relationships between nutrition and family planning merit mention.

### Nutrition and Family Size

Just as alleviation of childhood and maternal malnutrition could encourage smaller families, so the limitation of family size could in itself contribute to improved nutrition and infant survival. Simple arithmetic from Indian diet surveys demonstrates that protein availability per child in families with one or two siblings would be 22 percent higher (some 13 grams per head) than in those with four or five siblings. In most cases this additional amount would be enough to meet current protein deficits. The Indian National Institute of Nutrition has observed that youngsters with three or more older brothers or sisters constitute 34 percent of the child population but account for 61 percent of all cases of protein-calorie malnutrition in its clinic.[19] During the Bihar famine relief program in 1966–67, the most severe cases of malnutrition were invariably children from large families. Nearly four times as much serious hunger and nearly five times as much protein-calorie malnutrition were found among the younger children of large families. The number of children also has a direct bearing on the nutritional well-being of the mother. Nutritional anemia, a major cause of illness and death during pregnancy, gets more virulent as a mother has more babies. Three times as many pregnant women with four or more children suffer from severe anemia in India as those mothers

---

* In parts of Africa, family planning efforts have been interpreted as means of keeping the nonwhite populations of the world in check. Sometimes, shifts in foreign assistance emphasis have fueled distrust. The major thrust in AID's family planning assistance, for instance, came at a time when other health funds were being eliminated or cut back and when the traditionally liberal food transfer programs were being tightened.

with smaller families. It is the mother who bears the sickly child with mini-mal chances of survival who has little interest in practicing contraception.

### Nutrition and Fertility

Better maternal nutrition could result in more births rather than less where contraception is not practiced. Improved nutrition reduces preg-nancy wastage and lengthens the reproductive period, both because pu-berty occurs earlier in healthier young women and a healthier, longer life can mean more years to conceive.[20] The demographic history of indus-trially developed countries is evidence that the positive effects of good maternal health on the population growth rate are insignificant compared with the eventual decline in birthrate which results from a decline of child mortality (to a large degree a child's health and chances of survival seem related to his mother's nutritional condition while she is pregnant) and other factors in modernization that tend to induce couples to limit family size. In the short run, however, maternal nutrition programs in isolation might well result in increased fertility.

### Nutrition and Contraceptives

Possibilities for successful contraceptive programs may be enhanced if women's nutrition is improved. For example, nutritional anemias, so com-mon among women in poor countries, may be a cause of the high removal rate of intrauterine devices.[21] If so, iron supplements could be an impor-tant ingredient of a successful IUD program. Where the loop is used, it commonly causes excessive vaginal bleeding and related iron loss, exac-erbating anemias. Excessive bleeding, it has been noted, is more deleteri-ous to poorly nourished than adequately nourished women, and poor nutri-tional status may be an added stimulant to bleeding.[22] This may be why a quarter of the women using the loop in two Indian studies reported weak-ness as a side effect.[23] Improved nutrition could counter the nutritional losses caused by nausea and vomiting sometimes associated with birth control pills and compensate for the apparent increased requirement of vitamin A in women on oral contraceptives.[24] The pill itself is a potential carrier of iron and other needed nutrients.

Contraceptives sometimes affect nursing and thus the nutritional well-being of infants. The intrauterine loop appears to stimulate lactation while certain oral contraceptives high in estrogen appear to inhibit it.[25] If the high estrogen pill is taken soon after the baby's birth, suppression of lactation may be 50–100 percent.[26] Contraceptive pills low in estrogen apparently have no effect on ability to breast-feed.

### Lactation and Fecundity

Not only is his mother's milk the most important form of nutrition to the young child, but physiological changes of the mother during the months she is nursing significantly reduce her fecundity. Although maternal nursing does not have the effect of a perfect contraceptive, sufficient evidence is now available to give some credence to the long-held, universal wives' tale that breast feeding does reduce the chances of conception (see Chapter 7).

POPULATION STABILITY in the past was maintained by high rates of both births and deaths. With mortality declining in the developing countries, clearly the only acceptable route to reestablishment of stability (or much slower population growth) is a lowering of birthrates. Although a substantial lowering of child mortality as a means of influencing birthrates is not sufficient of itself—many other factors, varying in importance with social and economic circumstances, are involved—fertility is unlikely to come down to acceptable levels without it. The evidence of a relationship is suggestive enough to encourage major research and trial.

If lowered child mortality is a precondition for lowering birthrates and malnutrition is the major factor affecting child mortality, then the improvement of child nutrition, although exacerbating the population problem in the short run, has enough potential for improving the situation over the longer term to deserve development priority.

## CHAPTER FOUR

# Economic Growth, Income, and Nutrition

In the development business the most commonly heard answer to the question of how to provide better diets to children in poor societies is "economic growth." With economic growth and related increased incomes, nutrition problems, according to this view, will solve themselves. Money, of course, does affect diet—the poorest fed children are usually found in families with the lowest incomes. In developing countries, where the poor spend a high proportion of their income on food (in south India the poorest families spend 80 percent of their budgets on food, the affluent only 45 percent[1]), more money generally means a better diet. As the poor enjoy some increase in income, they usually devote a big fraction of that increase to additional food expenditures. In rural India when the very poor have another rupee to spend, 76 pais (or 76 percent) of it goes for food. This percentage declines as total income increases; upper income rural Indians spend only 34 pais of each additional rupee on food (see Table 1).

Income levels also establish a pattern for what foods are purchased with that additional rupee. The poor spend most of it on food grains, the rich much less so. The allocation for cereals declines and that for milk products increases as families move into the middle-income levels. Also, the higher the income, the larger is the percentage of the increase spent on fruits, vegetables, and other variety food items.

This pattern of food expenditures among poor and rich classes is mirrored in the spending habits of rich and poor nations (see Table 2). In the poorer countries a larger portion of expenditures is allocated to food. And much of any increase goes for food. As a nation's per capita income increases, so does the importance of high protein foods in the diet.

Thus, income is a major determinant of diet quantity and quality. Yet,

40

TABLE 1. *Allocation of Additional Rupee Expenditure by Rural Indians, by Income Group, 1964–65*

In percent

| Expenditure category | Average monthly per capita expenditure, in rupees | | | | | | |
|---|---|---|---|---|---|---|---|
| | 8.93 | 13.14 | 17.80 | 24.13 | 30.71 | 41.89 | 85.84 |
| Food grains[a] | 55 | 36 | 24 | 15 | 10 | 7 | 2 |
| Milk and milk products | 8 | 11 | 13 | 13 | 12 | 12 | 9 |
| Meat, eggs, fish | 2 | 3 | 3 | 3 | 3 | 3 | 3 |
| Oils | 5 | 6 | 5 | 5 | 4 | 4 | 2 |
| Sweeteners | 4 | 5 | 5 | 4 | 3 | 3 | 1 |
| Other foods[b] | 2 | 6 | 8 | 9 | 10 | 12 | 17 |
| Total food items | 76 | 67 | 58 | 49 | 42 | 41 | 34 |
| Nonfood items | 24 | 33 | 42 | 51 | 58 | 59 | 66 |

Source: John W. Mellor and Uma J. Lele, "Growth Linkages of the New Foodgrain Production Technologies," Occasional Paper No. 50 (Cornell University and U.S. Agency for International Development, Employment and Income Distribution Project, May 1972; processed), p. 11.
a. Includes pulses.
b. Includes vegetables, fruits, nuts, beverages, and condiments.

while it is clear that these beneficial relationships between income and nutrition—reinforced by the beneficial effects of rising income on improved health and other family circumstances that interact with nutritional status —hold almost universally over broad ranges of increases in income, it is equally clear that incomes rise slowly for the poor, and that even increased

TABLE 2. *Allocation of Income for Food Expenditure, by Selected Countries, Mid-1960s*

| Country | Per capita GNP, in dollars[a] | Percent of expenditures allocated to food | Percent of increment of expenditures allocated to food | Animal protein as percent of total protein |
|---|---|---|---|---|
| Ghana | 170 | 64 | 76 | 17 |
| Ceylon | 180 | 56 | 79 | 18 |
| Honduras | 260 | 47 | 40 | 27 |
| Malaysia | 330 | 49 | 37 | 30 |
| Sweden | 2,620 | 32 | 20 | 69 |
| United States | 3,980 | 23 | 20 | 72 |

Sources: Expenditures data from UN, *Yearbook of National Accounts Statistics, 1967*, Vol. 2; protein data from UN Food and Agriculture Organization, *Production Yearbook, 1970*.
a. Gross national products are for 1971.

purchasing power often cannot overcome certain food habits and practices that stand in the way of effective nutritional improvement, especially for small children.

There are many exceptions to the commonly accepted rules. In fact, the theory that national economic growth leads to better nutrition rests on a series of often questionable assumptions:

• A national increase in per capita income means an increase large and rapid enough in the income of the poor to be of nutritional significance.

• Increased income of the poor leads to an immediate and automatic increase in the amount the family spends on food.

• Increases in food expenditures by the poor family lead to an improvement in nutrition.

• Improved nutrition in the family means an improvement for the nutritionally vulnerable members of that family.

## Inadequacy of Income Increments

For nutritional planning, the role of income and dietary improvement within a society must be judged in relation to specific target populations and viewed in the context of their base incomes, income trends, and existing diets. The important question is how much dietary improvement will flow "automatically" to a nutritionally needy population from likely changes in their incomes over a given time period.

For many of the nutritionally needy, incomes are not rising or are barely rising at all. From 1960 to 1970, per capita incomes in countries representing two-thirds of the world's population grew only 1.5 percent yearly. And this was average. In some countries the increments in income were distributed in such a way that the poorer segments of the population received even less than the average share. In Brazil, the poorest 40 percent of the population saw their share of national income decline during the period by 20 percent. In Mexico, the income share of the poorest 40 percent fell from 14 percent in 1950 to 11 percent in 1969; the already low share of the poorest 20 percent of the population dropped by a third—to 4 percent of the national income. In short, the nutritionally needy portions of the population often have not benefited from their country's income growth, and in some cases their living standards may even have deteriorated.[2]

Even when income increases at an average rate at the lower levels, improvements come slowly. A composite of 220 surveys of Indian diets,[3] coupled with national economic projections, indicates that unless a new nutrition strategy is adopted and implemented, many of the present generation of Indians will never be able to afford an adequate diet. Per capita disposable income must reach $4 to $5 a month to support an acceptable diet, but 60–70 percent of India's urban dwellers, and even more of the rural population, fall below this line. One-third of India's families would need at least twice their current incomes to attain adequate diets on the basis of rising earnings alone. Even on the optimistic assumption of a 3 percent annual per capita real income rise, it would take about twenty-five years before the lowest third of India's population could afford a minimum diet.

These calculations assume that income distribution will not change over the twenty-five years or, put another way, that Indian growth will be proportionately the same at different income levels. In fact, incomes may not move upward for large numbers of those most in need of help; for example, the fruits of development of the agricultural revolution in India may not be adequately reaching some poorer groups of the society.

In terms of current distribution trends, Max Millikan has calculated that $100-per-capita-income populations would have to realize an eightfold increase in income to afford adequate amounts of animal protein at an annual income growth rate of 2 percent—a hundred-year process.[4] Clearly, reliance on income improvement is too slow for the needy.

## Nonfood Expenditures

Even for those now or soon to be realizing an increased income, more money will not automatically be translated into a larger expenditure for food. The traditionally accepted principle that bigger and better diet is a function of increased income undoubtedly applies over time and over broad increases in income and general living standards. However, the broad data on food expenditures may at times be misleading. When income increases are modest and start from a low base, there may be transitional periods of inverse correlation between income and nutrition. For example, where a subsistence farmer switches from growing a variety of foods for his family's own consumption to cultivating a crop for the market, such items as ballpoint pens and transistor radios compete, for the first time, with what had been largely a fixed food income. In Mysore, a substantial portion of the cash received from home grown vegetables and milk from the family cow was spent on clothes and other nonfood items. The villagers were compensated monetarily, but not nutritionally. Per capita milk consumption in the urban areas of Tamil Nadu is now two and a half times that in rural areas where the milk is produced.[5]

## Expenditures for Nonnutritious Food

But even when expenditures for food are increased, which is commonly the case, additional income does not always lead to improved diet. People spending more for food may eat more, but not necessarily better. In south Asia the common shift with the first increment of income is from sorghum or millet to rice, then from home-pounded rice to the convenience of commercially polished rice; the shifts are aesthetically pleasing but nutritionally costly.* In western India a statistically significant drop in protein intake has been discerned as incomes rise and cereal diets are "upgraded."[6]

Aesthetic pleasure and social prestige appear to be more important instigators of change in food habits than the level of vitamin A or the level of methionine: white corn replaces the more nutritious yellow, white bread the *tortilla;* coffee is taken instead of the corn-based *atole,* tea instead of buttermilk. As consumption of manufactured foods—especially sugar-containing foods—increases, meat and fruit are pushed out of the diet. The deleterious effect in urban slums of popular soft drinks is legend.[7]

Often with increased income, certain items that are identified as foods of the poor are discarded from the diet. Quinoa, an excellent cereal of the Bolivian altiplano, is associated with low social status, and Bolivians invariably choose a more costly but less nutritious substitute when they can afford it. In much of India, greens and papaya are regarded with disdain because they are plentiful and inexpensive. In Calcutta, sea fish is scorned in favor of more costly fresh water fish. In El Salvador there is an abundance of yellow corn to satisfy vitamin A needs, but to get people to eat it over the white is another matter. In some countries, dark bread is still regarded as poor man's food, as are legumes; in several societies, the commonly used phrase to describe someone who has grown rich is "now he doesn't eat lentils anymore."† In India, as low-ranked, meat-consuming

---

* The same is true when increased income makes it possible to "buy up" from *jaggery* (unrefined sugar) to the less beneficial refined sugar.

† The locution appears in Aristophanes' play *Plutus* and probably has an even more ancient origin.

castes begin to rise in income, they sometimes imitate the vegetarian orthodox way of life of more highly regarded castes.[8]

While milk purchases increase substantially in proportion to rises in income,* breast feeding declines radically. Sixty percent of lower income Gujarati women (under $2 per capita per month) continue to breast-feed their children beyond six months. The percentage drops sharply as incomes rise, and only 8 percent of higher income mothers (above $9) offer the breast at the same period.[9] The nursing Indian mother produces approximately one-half liter of milk a day.† An adequate quantity of commercial milk would cost more than $2 a month, a substantial portion of income. Mothers moving up the medium income ladder probably purchase only one-third as much milk (most of which is used in tea) as is lost due to early weaning.

### Illusions of Monetary Income Increases

In many instances, increased income is a reflection of the flow of people from farms and small towns to large cities. These immigrants have more money than the rural poor, but they need more for rent, clothing, transportation, and other necessities of city life. Their food costs more in the big city, and they no longer have access to the free wild foods (leaves, fruits, vegetables, insects, small game, seeds, and berries) of their village days. Among Congolese it was found that those who abandoned village life for Brazzaville made more money and spent more for their traditional cassava flour; but they developed pellagra because they could not buy the familiar niacin-rich cassava leaves in town. Beriberi was found in former rice-eating Senegalese villagers who migrated to Dakar.[11] The same pattern appeared in the transition from a rural to an industrialized society in more affluent countries; in nineteenth century England the diet of the working class probably deteriorated although food supplies increased.[12]

The shift from a subsistence crop to a cash crop normally involves an increase in income. But even if a peasant earns more by growing cotton, tobacco, cocoa, or copra, or working for a man who does, will he eat as well as he did when he grew his own dinner?

---

* But even a manifold increase in the small milk expenditures of the poor may not be nutritionally significant.

† Inadequate nourishment of poor mothers, unlike cows, does not reduce milk output. This leads to the unusual circumstance that the typical low-income Indian mother produces as much milk in a day as the average milk cow of the area.[10]

## Increased Income and the Nutritionally Vulnerable

Even if better quality food does come into a household, there is no assurance it will reach those in the family who most need improved nutrition—the young child, the pregnant woman, or the nursing mother.

### The Young Child

Surveys in Central America, Colombia, Ghana, India, Ivory Coast, Nigeria, and Tunisia show that even when income levels allow older family members to have satisfactory diets, children's diets commonly are 20–30 percent inadequate.[13] This is especially true of the infant; parents often do not recognize the importance of supplementing breast milk at the appropriate age.

In many areas, nutritious foods are withheld from children for fear of adverse consequences. In a Peruvian fishing village, where adult consumption of fish protein is high, fish is not fed to children because parents fear it will make them ill. In parts of Malaysia and Indonesia fish is forbidden to children because it is believed to cause worms, bad eyes, or skin disease. Elsewhere, protein-rich beans and lentils are frequently not fed to children because of concern for flatulence they produce.[14]

In parts of India, eggs are feared to cause jaundice and swelling; in Lebanon and Syria, indigestion; among Yorubas in Nigeria, a child that grows up to become a thief. Eggs are blamed for mental retardation in parts of East Africa, and for late speech development in Korea. In a number of African countries, eggs are not fed to girls for fears ranging from infertility to increased fertility and licentiousness. In Bolivia, some believe cheese will make a small child mute. In Malawi, fish and chicken are feared to cause sterility.[15]

An Indian child may be forbidden to eat curds and fruit because they are "cold," and bananas because they cause convulsions. Some West Africans say oranges make a child "soft"; some East Africans say they cause heartburn.[16]

Besides supposed dangers of certain foods, family feeding order and other general customs also limit the possibility of youngsters' benefiting from an increased family food budget. In Fiji an increasing amount of money is spent on canned beef and other popular European foods, but custom demands that adults eat first, and little of these fancy foods is left for the child. His diet, as a result, is often white bread, tea, and sugar. African families, sitting around stew pots, dip cassava into the pot; the small child, who cannot reach that far, eats only the cassava. Coastal Arabs of Morocco, as a matter of family tradition, do not feed their children milk, eggs, fish, or meat for the first few years of life.[17]

### The Pregnant Woman

Similarly, the introduction of additional food into a household is no assurance that the additional nutrition needs of an expectant mother will be met. The notion of a pregnant woman eating for two is a Western concept; in most Asian countries, in fact, women consciously undereat during pregnancy, with the objective of a small baby and an easy delivery.[18]

Moreover, commonly practiced food taboos during pregnancy further detract from a normal diet. Many Indian women fear papaya or eggs lead to abortion and thus do not eat them ("there's already an egg in the womb"); fearing "one-child sterility," they do not eat plantains. Green vegetables are taboo for expectant Burmese mothers because of concern for flatulence. Many in Malawi believe an animal's traits are transferred to the child when a pregnant woman eats the meat. A study of poor pregnant women in South Carolina discovered nearly half held some deleterious food belief such as milk drunk during pregnancy causes cancer, pork rots the uterus, eggs harm the child's brain, fish is poisonous, leafy vegetables mark the baby, and cheese causes the baby's head to stick to the womb during delivery.[19]

### The Nursing Mother

Neither are the extra food needs of the nursing mother guaranteed by increased family food purchases. In some countries, women consciously attempt to eat less after bearing a child. A study of Malays found that many new mothers had severely restricted diets for forty days following delivery; fruits and vegetables were forbidden. In Indonesia, many women take less food after childbirth to regain their shape. In some Asian countries, many mothers believe that a diet containing animal proteins makes breast milk toxic to the baby. In Java, eggs are taboo during lactation; they supposedly lead to hemorrhaging. In East Africa, eating of mutton by the mother allegedly leads to dimness of baby's vision and eating of groundnuts is believed to cut down the supply of breast milk. In Viet Nam, nursing mothers often avoid certain foods, notably fish. In western India, curds, fruits, leaf greens, and pulses are avoided by the nursing mother. Custom in south India encourages eating some of these same foods during nursing but forbids others like maize and eggplant for fear of paralysis.[20]

All this suggests there is no guarantee that increased food intake by a family benefits the three most nutritionally vulnerable groups.*

PLAINLY, economic growth that entails increases in consumer incomes is a powerful nutrition weapon and one of the primary determinants of nutritional status; for many of the world's malnourished, the basic problem simply is that they do not have enough to eat and lack the purchasing power to buy more. The income picture for the poor, however, has not been bright, even when national growth is moving well—nor is the future promising. Moreover, the relationship between income growth and improved nutrition rests on a series of assumptions that may not hold up in some income ranges and circumstances.

For many low-income groups, malnutrition cannot automatically be solved by development, for the effects of income growth may not be efficient, quick in coming, or equitably distributed. One of the keys to a country's nutritional status is the nature of its income distribution. Mexico, for example, with an average per capita income of $530 a year, very unevenly distributed, is a scene of considerable malnutrition, whereas Taiwan, with a much more evenly distributed per capita income of $270 a year, is not. Although some nutrition problems can be attacked in the absence of income growth, in most poor countries, mass improvement in protein-calorie malnutrition cannot be expected in the near future unless governments undertake policies and development strategies that redistribute income or channel income increases toward the poor. Clearly, social transformations brought about by income redistribution measures go beyond considerations of nutrition; they are only part of the nutrition solution in any case. The important point, however, is that the way development is carried out has powerful effects on the needy—effects more powerful in determining nutritional status than much that normally goes under the rubric of "nutrition improvement programs."

Shifting the nutritional problem into the broader context of development means considering nutrition among the important concerns of public policy and systematically evaluating nutritional impact in the formulation of economic growth policies and strategies. It should be remembered that the rate of national growth is not tied to one special mix of development investment—rarely is there anything magic about the current combination

---

* Food beliefs and folklore of various cultures are not ipso facto in error. Customs that appear quaint or naïve may have evolved over the ages in response to local conditions that bear respectful scrutiny.

of policies and programs. Injecting nutrition into the list of considerations may raise opportunities for changes of the mix that would yield a higher nutritional dividend without lowering the immediate returns to investment in national income growth.

Increased income is not, of itself, a sufficient condition for adequate nutrition, particularly in cases where food beliefs and practices deleteriously affect the nutritional status of the young. Explicit steps such as the establishment of special food distribution mechanisms and supportive measures in education will be required to reinforce the dietary benefits from higher income. Moreover, in some instances, direct methods to improve diets can be effectively employed in absence of increased income.

## CHAPTER FIVE

# Nutritional Effects of Agricultural Advances

Increased attention to agricultural production is often pointed to in development circles as the key to better nutrition. Clearly, agriculture has a strong influence on a nation's nutritional status. But the exact nature of that influence is not clear. Seldom do agricultural policies flow from specifically stated and analyzed nutrition objectives. Rather, the goals of agricultural production are to reduce dependence on foreign suppliers for major staples, expand exports, produce raw materials for industrial goods, and provide consumers with adequate food supplies that will maintain stable prices and avoid pressures on industrial wages and prices.

Plainly, a sector that accounts for one-third to one-half of a developing country's total domestic output of goods and services, as well as the bulk of its exports, and provides the livelihood of two-thirds of the population has an importance that goes far beyond concerns of food and nutrition. But the supply of commodities produced in pursuit of such worthwhile economic goals can affect the nutritional status of needy groups in a variety of ways—ranging from highly beneficial to perverse.

## Nutrient Sources

Currently, economically less developed countries typically depend heavily on cereals for their major nutrients. Several of the nations included in Tables 3 and 4 obtain from cereals more than half of both their calories and protein, the south Asian nations two-thirds. Cereals are prominent suppliers of protein not because they are rich in it, but because they are

TABLE 3. *Sources of Calories in Food Supply of Selected Countries, Late 1960s*

| Country | Total calories available per capita per day | Cereals | Starchy roots and plantains | Sugars | Pulses, nuts, and seeds | Fruits and vegetables | Meat, poultry, eggs, and fish | Milk and milk products | Fats and oils |
|---|---|---|---|---|---|---|---|---|---|
| Brazil | 2,520 | 33 | 17 | 16 | 12 | 2 | 9 | 5 | 5 |
| India | 1,940 | 69 | 2 | 9 | 9 | 1 | * | 5 | 4 |
| Pakistan | 2,350 | 72 | 1 | 8 | 2 | 3 | 1 | 7 | 5 |
| Ghana | 2,070 | 33 | 48 | 5 | 6 | 1 | 2 | 1 | 4 |
| Kenya | 2,240 | 60 | 13 | 6 | 11 | 1 | 5 | 3 | 2 |
| United States | 3,290 | 20 | 3 | 17 | 3 | 5 | 24 | 11 | 17 |
| World | n.a. | 52 | 10 | 7 | * | 10 | 11 | 1 | 9 |

Source: Based on food balance sheets, UN Food and Agriculture Organization, *Production Yearbook, 1970*; FAO data are for various years between 1964 and 1969. Percentages may not add to 100 because of rounding.

n.a. Not available.
* Less than 0.5 percent.

TABLE 4. *Sources of Protein in Food Supplies of Selected Countries, Late 1960s*

| Country | Total grams of protein available per capita per day | Cereals | Starchy roots and plantains | Pulses, nuts, and seeds | Fruits and vegetables | Meat and poultry | Eggs | Fish | Milk and milk products | Miscellaneous, including fats and oils, sugars |
|---|---|---|---|---|---|---|---|---|---|---|
| Brazil | 63 | 28 | 6 | 30 | 2 | 18 | 2 | 2 | 11 | 1 |
| India | 48 | 65 | 1 | 20 | 1 | 1 | * | 1 | 9 | 2 |
| Pakistan | 54 | 70 | 1 | 7 | 2 | 3 | * | 2 | 14 | 1 |
| Ghana | 43 | 42 | 32 | 7 | 1 | 5 | * | 10 | 2 | 1 |
| Kenya | 68 | 52 | 5 | 22 | 1 | 12 | * | 2 | 6 | * |
| United States | 97 | 16 | 4 | 2 | 4 | 39 | 6 | 3 | 24 | 2 |
| World | n.a. | 50 | 5 | 13 | 3 | 13 | 2 | 3 | 11 | * |

Source: Based on food balance sheets, FAO, *Production Yearbook, 1970*; FAO data are for various years between 1964 and 1969. Percentages may not add to 100 because of rounding.

n.a. Not available.
* Less than 0.5 percent.

consumed in such enormous proportions compared to other foods. For the same reason they are a major source of iron in the diets of many people in low-income countries. Pulses are a prominent secondary source for protein, while the traditional protein products—meat, poultry, eggs, fish, and dairy items—account for only a minor portion of the protein in the diets of developing countries. For low-income members of the population, staple crops would usually constitute a higher than average portion of the diet.

Though most common foods contain protein, both the proportion and quality of the protein vary widely. Of the most popularly consumed foods, wheat has about 12 percent protein, millet 11 percent, corn 10 percent, milled rice 8 percent, and cassava, potatoes, and plantains under 2 percent. The quality of the protein is determined by a series of chemical units known as essential amino acids.* The value of protein in a food is only as great as the smallest of these. If the amino acids in a food are envisioned as a series of bars depicting the food's profile, the height of the bars will vary, the protein value being only as great as the shortest bar. The rest is wasted. In wheat, the limiting amino acid is lysine; in corn, lysine and tryptophan lock in the usefulness of the other amino acids; in rice, lysine and threonine are low.

The limiting amino acid can be raised by increased consumption of a staple cereal, forcing quantity to largely compensate for insufficient quality (in cassava and most other roots and tubers the proportion of protein is so low that improvement must come from other sources). Or, the mix of foods may be changed so that those amino acids in short supply in the cereal staple are increased by adding foods high in the same amino acids (for example, pulses); the final amino acid mix of the overall diet, not the individual food, is important. The protein quality of the diet also may be upgraded through genetic improvement of the seed of the staple,

---

* At least eight of the essential amino acids must be supplied for man. The nonessential amino acids are those that can be synthesized in the body. Other factors besides the amino acid balance that affect the value of the protein in a food are availability of certain vitamins and minerals needed for protein utilization; the damage done to protein in the processing or cooking of food; the level of digestion or absorption of the protein in the body, due to other health factors; and the level of caloric intake. (It was assumed that unless a person had a minimum caloric base, added protein would be burned for energy; thus any special protein supplement would be an expensive source of calories. Indications now are that at least a portion of the protein will be utilized.[1]) There are several techniques that attempt to measure protein quality—net protein utilization (NPU), protein efficiency ratio (PER), biological value, and chemical score, among others—none totally satisfactory to the full scientific nutrition community.

or nutrients may be added through cereal fortification and new formulated foods.

## Impact of the Green Revolution

Given the dominance of cereals in providing the major nutrients, the recent remarkable advances in cereal production, especially in south and southeast Asia, have important nutritional implications. (Fortunately, the so-called green revolution first centered on countries in greatest food need.) The significant trends of the 1960s are noted in Table 5. West Pakistan's 1971 wheat production was up 76 percent from its 1961–65 average, Latin American corn production up more than 50 percent, and Indonesian rice production up a third. The Indian wheat crop of 1971 doubled its 12-million-ton record of six years earlier.

Such achievements are all the more remarkable given the somber agriculture projections common in the mid-1960s. Concerns were then expressed about exhausted soil, primitive tools, lack of capital, traditionalism, unskilled farmers, apathy, and the population rise that was out-pacing food production. In high quarters, mass famine was thought to be inevitable throughout the developing world by the mid-1970s. The fact that the 1972 harvest was respectable despite unusually bad weather conditions reflects the enormous advances made.[2]

Key to the dramatic turnabout was the development and spread of new high-yielding seeds of wheat and rice and of the technologies necessary to service them. The new seeds, along with fertilizer, irrigation, and pesticides, provide greater yield per harvest, often doubling traditional output per acre. They also permit two, and sometimes three (often varied), crops a year where formerly there was one.* These achievements have taken place on only a small portion of the land devoted to cereal crops.[3] Although significant problems must be overcome for the full potential of the new technologies to be felt, the prospects for cereal production expansion in many countries are much more promising than they were in the mid-1960s.

---

* The new plants mature more quickly than traditional varieties. One of the new rices matures in 120 days, 30 to 60 days earlier than traditional rices. Varieties less sensitive to daylight mature in a predictable number of days, a great help in planning crop rotations. New dwarf and semidwarf varieties of wheat and rice are less likely to be blown over (to lodge), and are generally highly yield responsive to fertilizer.

TABLE 5. *Cereal Production in Countries Using New Seed Varieties, 1960–70*

| Country and commodity | Production, thousands of tons | | | | Production increase 1960–70, percent | Change in imports 1960–69, percent |
|---|---|---|---|---|---|---|
| | 1960 | 1966 | 1968 | 1970 | | |
| India | | | | | | |
| Wheat | 10,324 | 10,424 | 16,540 | 20,093 | 95 | −29 |
| Paddy rice | 51,297 | 45,657 | 60,645 | 62,500 | 22 | −30 |
| All cereals | 84,600 | 80,163 | 102,445 | 111,209 | 31 | −23 |
| West Pakistan | | | | | | |
| Wheat | 3,909 | 3,916 | 6,418 | 7,294 | 87 | −53 |
| Paddy rice | 1,030 | 2,048 | 3,051 | 3,248 | 215 | −95 |
| Corn | 439 | 587 | 626 | 717 | 63 | a |
| All cereals | 6,043 | 7,287 | 10,795 | 12,059 | 100 | −61 |
| Bangladesh | | | | | | |
| Paddy rice | 9,672 | 14,362 | 17,033 | 16,714 | 73 | b |
| All cereals | 9,720 | 14,413 | 17,111 | 16,841 | 73 | b |
| Iran | | | | | | |
| Wheat | 2,279 | 3,964 | 4,977 | 4,000 | 76 | n.a. |
| All cereals | 3,914 | 6,143 | 6,908 | 6,204 | 59 | n.a. |
| Ceylon | | | | | | |
| Paddy rice | 897 | 955 | 1,347 | 1,514 | 69 | −48 |
| All cereals | 927 | 986 | 1,374 | 1,648 | 67 | n.a. |
| Malaysia | | | | | | |
| Paddy rice | 975 | 1,041 | 1,218 | 1,430 | 47 | −65 |
| All cereals | 979 | 1,048 | 1,225 | 1,437 | 47 | 42 |
| Philippines | | | | | | |
| Paddy rice | 3,705 | 4,094 | 4,445 | 5,659 | 53 | 0 |
| All cereals | 4,915 | 5,584 | 6,178 | 8,059 | 64 | 76 |

Sources: Data compiled from FAO, *Production Yearbook, 1963* and *1970;* Dana G. Dalrymple, *Imports and Plantings of High Yielding Varieties of Wheat and Rice in the Less Developed Nations,* Foreign Economic Development Report 14 (U.S. Department of Agriculture [USDA], 1972); FAO, *Trade Yearbook, 1963* and *1970;* Sheldon K. Tsu, *High Yielding Varieties of Wheat in Developing Countries* (USDA, Economic Research Service [ERS], 1971); *Indices of Agricultural Production for East Asia, South Asia and Oceania* (USDA, ERS, 1972); and interview, John Parker, April 26, 1972.

n.a. Not available.

a. No corn imported in 1960; 28 million tons imported in 1969.

b. Included in West Pakistan data.

## Increased Cereal Production

The nutrient composition of the new seed varieties probably is basically the same as that of traditional varieties.* Apparently the protein level may

* It is difficult to make precise statements about the nutrient levels of grain seeds because of the complex interplay of genetic makeup, of both quantity and timing of nitrogen fertilizer applications, and environmental factors such as temperature and

vary sharply between regions and change from year to year, like wine, depending on growing conditions. The increased yields mean not only more calories but also more protein, vitamins, and minerals. In 1971, 50 million acres in developing countries, principally in Asia, were planted with high-yielding varieties of wheat and rice. If, as a rule of thumb, high-yielding varieties are assumed to have increased wheat yields 100 percent and rice yields 25 percent, about 13 million extra tons of grain were produced: this translates into roughly 2 million tons of protein. These quantities are equivalent to the total protein requirements of the combined populations of Egypt and Nigeria.

The production increases in green revolution countries in terms of the individual's nutrient intake are shown in Table 6. This takes into account population rise during the same period. In Pakistan, average per capita annual wheat production was up 44 percent between 1960 and 1970; in India, 50 percent. Rice moved up 33 percent in Ceylon during the same period. The increased per capita amounts of protein, calories, and iron available to individuals often constituted a not insignificant portion of nutrient requirements.

Thus a successful policy for increasing the supply of cereal staples can be a powerful tool for nutritional betterment. But a successful production strategy may not, of itself, assure an improvement in the nutritional levels of those in need. As the supply of staples rises and their prices fall, the real incomes of those who buy the staples will rise, enabling them to buy more staples, as well as other foods, with the same amount of money. While the effect of such a process is clear for the consumer, it is less clear for small producers of the staples. The impact of production policies can vary considerably, depending on the nature of the policies, the social and economic structure of the rural society, and whether the producer is a large or small commercial farmer, a tenant or owner, a subsistence farmer or a landless laborer.

In some areas the principal beneficiaries of profits from the new high-yielding seed varieties have been larger farmers;[5] their profit margin makes grain production remain attractive even when supplies rise more rapidly than demand and farmers' wholesale prices are allowed to fall. But the

---

length of growing season. Protein quality is an even more complex matter. In this discussion it is assumed that the nutritional values in the various varieties of wheat and rice are roughly comparable. (For a discussion of protein levels, see Dana Dalrymple's analysis.[4] Little is known about the relative value of other nutrients.)

TABLE 6. *Average Per Capita Grain Production Increases in Countries Using New Seeds, 1960–70*

| Country and commodity | Population increase, percent | Total production increase, percent | Per capita production increase, percent[a] | Daily per capita increase in | | | |
|---|---|---|---|---|---|---|---|
| | | | | Commodity, grams[b] | Calories | Protein, grams | Iron, milligrams |
| India, wheat | 27 | 95 | 50 | 33 | 114 | 3.8 | 1.2 |
| West Pakistan, wheat | 29 | 69 | 44 | 104 | 358 | 12.0 | 3.6 |
| Bangladesh, milled rice | 31 | 73 | 32 | 104 | 368 | 8.3 | 2.1 |
| Malaysia, milled rice | 32 | 47 | 11 | 28 | 99 | 2.2 | 0.6 |
| Iran, wheat | 32 | 76 | 33 | 96 | 330 | 11.0 | 3.4 |
| Ceylon, milled rice | 27 | 69 | 33 | 54 | 191 | 4.3 | 1.1 |
| Philippines, milled rice | 39 | 53 | 10 | 25 | 189 | 3.0 | 0.5 |

Sources: Data compiled from FAO, *Production Yearbook, 1963* and *1970*; Dalrymple, *Imports and Plantings of High Yielding Varieties*; UN, *Demographic Yearbook, 1970*; FAO, *Agricultural Commodity Projections 1970–1980*; and Michael Latham, *Human Nutrition in Tropical Africa* (FAO, 1965).

a. Net trade, changes in stocks, and losses are not accounted for in these figures.

b. One hundred grams of wheat contain an estimated 344 calories, 11.5 grams of protein, and 3.5 milligrams of iron; 100 grams of milled rice contain an estimated 354 calories, 8.0 grams of protein, and 2.0 milligrams of iron. Daily requirements for an adult male 22–35 years old, according to the U.S. National Academy of Sciences, Food and Nutrition Board (1968), are 2,800 calories, 65 grams of protein, and 10 milligrams of iron.

small farmer without irrigation whose output and costs change little may find both his income and his nutritional level reduced. His marketable crop now earns lower returns. If he sells only the surplus after his needs have been met, his cereal consumption may not be affected; but his purchases of other goods—including foodstuffs he does not produce himself—will decline, with possibly adverse impact on his family's nutrition.

The small farmer's ability to adopt the miracle seed technologies depends on such factors as his access to credit, the effort the government's extension service makes to reach and communicate with the poorer cultivators, and the tenurial arrangements that determine the tenant farmer's risks and potential returns from investing in small-scale irrigation or other inputs, and from borrowing to make such investments.

In subsistence economies, where scope for exchange is limited by commodity and by geography, a family's income and its own production often are virtually the same thing. Low income and inadequate supply are merely different names for the same localized problem of low productivity, and a supply policy that helps such farmers increase food output helps directly to alleviate nutritional deficits. Similarly, programs to help monetized small farmers raise a "back yard" of vegetables, poultry, and so on, can conceivably contribute directly to the family's nutrition (in practice such programs have fallen short of expectations).[6]

Some countries employing the new rice and wheat technologies have maintained high price supports (for what can only be a transitional period), often well above world prices, to promote self-sufficiency in food grains. Such policies benefit the grain producer who owns his own land. They may benefit the tenant farmer and the landless laborer less, depending on tenurial relationships, the extent of unemployment, and the arrangements for distributing harvest proceeds.[7] Price supports designed to increase production may result in higher retail grain prices, hurting urban consumers and landless laborers, unless the government subsidizes those groups by selling grain below support levels and absorbing the loss in the national budget.

The nutrition of landless agricultural laborers can be affected in other ways by a country's agricultural development strategy. Between the heavier volumes of food, the greater requirements of agricultural inputs and work per acre, and more frequent plantings as well as multiple cropping, the new cereals technology generates both greater demand for rural labor during peak work periods and more frequent demand for labor throughout the year. Higher wages and more working days mean higher incomes and better nutrition for the landless laborers, who are usually at the bottom of the income ladder. The mechanization that follows on the heels of production increases can, however, result in labor displacement. Whether the kind of mechanization adopted is more or less labor intensive depends heavily on the price of agricultural machinery, and its operating and maintenance costs, in relation to agricultural wages. Both the supply and the price of sophisticated equipment are affected by tariffs on imported machinery, the cost of agricultural investment credit, and other trade, investment, and financial factors.

In other words, what might appear to be simply technical questions of a production supply policy turn out to have important effects on who participates in the development process, who has access to productive inputs, to whose income the increased supply accrues, and thus the impact on the nutritionally deficient groups. In the near euphoria surrounding the green revolution such considerations often have been slighted.

### Declining Pulse Availability

The green revolution has had a number of indirect consequences. One of the most disturbing is the decline in the production of food legumes or pulses, the family of food crops that includes peas, lentils, beans, chickpeas, mung beans, pigeon peas, and broad beans.

In some areas of the cereal revolution, pulse consumption has declined markedly. While the per capita wheat yield in India was increasing 25 percent between 1961 and 1972 (from 31.9 to 40 kilos per person), the per capita yield in pulses dropped 38 percent (from 29 to 18 kilos per person). The relationship is not clear, since even before the introduction of the high-yielding cereal seed varieties, the pulse decline had begun. The cereals push in the late 1960s probably accentuated the per capita pulse production decline, and in some areas, there was direct crop substitution. The Khanna study, which took place in the heart of India's green revolution area, reported that while acreage for wheat and corn doubled from 1960 to 1969, cultivation of lentils "virtually disappeared."[8] While land for growing wheat increased by 1.03 million hectares in Punjab and Haryana, land for pulses declined by 1.2 million hectares. The remarkable 44 percent decline in area devoted to pulse production was not made up elsewhere in India; throughout the country, land used to produce pulses declined 11 percent in the 1960s. In 1965, pulses constituted 16 percent of all food grain production in India, five years later 11 percent.[9]

Much the same thing occurred in West Pakistan in the 1960s. Per capita wheat production was up 44 percent, per capita chickpea production (the major pulse) down 31 percent. Availability of all pulses in Pakistan dropped from 30 pounds a year for each person in 1963 to 18 pounds in 1970.*[10]

In most low-income countries, pulses are widely accepted staples of the diet, per capita daily consumption ranging from 30 to 70 grams, five times as high as that in wealthier countries. Since the pulses are 18–25 percent protein, they are particularly important to low-income diets. The protein content is double that of wheat, triple that of milled rice, and some twenty-five times that of cassava. Thus, though the quantity of pulses produced per hectare is low, pulse yields in terms of protein are often highest of a nation's major crops (see Table 7). In addition, the quality of the pulse protein is better than that of cereals. (Moreover, the amino acid balance of pulses makes them a nutritional complement of cereals; the nutritional value of the two combined is greater than the total of the two eaten at different times.) The effectiveness of pulses in overcoming protein deficiencies has been widely reported.[11] Pulses are one of the best sources of iron; an average serving of beans, for example, provides six to twelve times the iron of a slice of unenriched bread. Their riboflavin content is five times greater than most cereals, their thiamine content ten times greater. For these reasons, pulses are frequently called "the poor man's meat."

Because of the dominance of cereals and pulses in low-income diets, the dramatic production shifts in the two in developing countries should be weighed in nutritional terms. Since wheat and pulses contain about the same number of calories per kilogram, the increase of per capita average wheat consumption far offsets the calorie loss due to a smaller intake of pulses. However, since the protein content of pulses is approximately double that of wheat, the protein change is much less dramatic, perhaps in some places resulting in a slight decline, when taking into account that pulse protein is of higher quality than cereal protein. Because pulses contain two to three times as much iron as wheat, some slight decline in iron intake may take place. Whatever the adverse effects of the shift, they would be more pronounced for the already disadvantaged portions of the population than for the average citizen.

The net nutritional effect of a shift to wheat from pulse also depends on

* Figures are based on per capita availability because per capita consumption data are not available. Aside from waste, availability and consumption are not the same since pulses are sometimes used as animal feed.

TABLE 7. *Protein Yield of Important Crops in Brazil, Zaire, the Philippines, and India, 1970*

| Crop | Average yield, kilograms per hectare[a] | | | | Protein content, percent | Protein yield, kilograms per hectare[a] | | | |
|---|---|---|---|---|---|---|---|---|---|
| | Brazil | Zaire | Philippines | India | | Brazil | Zaire | Philippines | India |
| Wheat | 1,010 | 1,000 | n.a. | 1,210[b] | 11.5 | 116 | 115 | n.a. | 139[b] |
| Milled rice[c] | 1,093 | 693 | 1,187[d] | 1,107 | 8.0 | 87 | 55 | 95 | 89 |
| Corn | 1,470 | 1,060 | 980 | 1,080 | 10.0 | 147 | 106 | 98 | 108 |
| Cassava | 14,800 | 14,300 | 5,800 | 12,900 | 0.7 | 104 | 100 | 41 | 90 |
| Pulses[e] | 620 | 620 | 770 | 720 | 20.0–24.5 | 133 | 152 | 165 | 144 |

Sources: Compiled from data in FAO, *Production Yearbook, 1970*; and Tsu, *High Yielding Varieties of Wheat.*

n.a. Not available.

a. One kilogram per hectare is about 0.9 pound per acre.

b. Average yield of traditional and new varieties. Latter was planted on 37 percent of Indian wheat land.

c. For the purpose of comparison, milled rice, rather than the usual paddy rice, figures are used here. In the process of milling, paddy rice is reduced by one-third, losing its hull and its protein-rich bran.

d. Average yield of both traditional and new varieties. Latter was planted on 50 percent of Philippine rice area.

e. In the case of India, chickpea with 20.0 percent protein; Brazil and Philippines, dry beans with 21.4 percent protein; Zaire, dry peas with 24.5 percent protein.

60

how much additional wheat the individual can consume to offset the protein and iron advantages of pulses (a child's capacity is limited); whether added calories are reducing an existing deficit and thus increasing the efficiency of protein utilization; and whether the economic influences of the crop shift are causing other changes in the diet.

It is unclear what pulse production would have been in absence of the cereals revolution. The decline, as noted, apparently began prior to the introduction of the seed varieties. Moreover, had cereal needs become more critical, grain prices probably would have risen, adding to the attractiveness of cereal production.

In any case, pulses were neglected as research and resources concentrated on high yielding cereal grain varieties.* Cereal not pulse crops were stressed in foreign assistance programs, and rightly so, given total food needs. In part, the neglect of pulses in favor of cereals may reflect the complexity of dealing with pulses—some twenty varieties are consumed in sizable amounts—and the relative unfamiliarity of pulses in aid-giving countries from which much of the impetus of seed development has come.

Clearly, the need exists for pulse varieties with higher yields, shorter growing periods (so that they can be used as short season crops between major cereal crops), and more resistance to insects and diseases that now take a major toll. In addition to improving production efficiency, attention should be given to improving marketing techniques. In some cases, a government price support and purchase program may be desirable to make pulses more attractive to both producers and consumers.†

### Breeding for Nutritional Improvements

Breeding can improve quality as well as increase quantity; in fact, the nutritional impact of both cereals and pulses could probably be increased substantially. One of the most dramatic and potentially significant agricultural breakthroughs for nutrition was the 1963 identification and subsequent development of a strain of corn with protein value triple that of

* The compound growth rate for pulse yield from 1950 to 1971 in India was 0.03 percent.[12]

† Just as pulses are displaced by cereals, so are cereals sometimes displaced by lower protein foods when it is economically attractive for the farmer to do so. In Uganda, when cassava production increased from two tons an acre to seven, it displaced millet which has a protein value a dozen times as great. Millet cultivation also is frequently displaced in Africa by the low protein plantain. In Peru nearly two-thirds of the quinoa crop, with its 17 percent protein, has given way to potatoes.

standard corn. Instead of the 500 grams normally required to satisfy 75 percent of a child's daily protein needs, half that quantity of the new corn could meet 90 percent. Providing nearly the same protein quality as milk, the new opaque 2 corn can cure a child with kwashiorkor, even when the corn is the only source of protein in the diet.[13]

The high protein corn varieties have already been multiplied in quantity for commercial production. A small portion of the yield is used as an ingredient in the Latin American blended cereal food Duryea; most is used in animal feed, reducing the amount of oilseed protein needed in the feed.

By the late 1960s, similar breeding principles were being applied to other basic cereal grains. Thousands of varieties of each grain were being collected throughout the world in an attempt to identify those with desirable nutritional traits that genetic engineering could then transfer to other strains.*

At this early stage of development, some of the new high-protein varieties are more susceptible to plant disease and to pests than standard varieties;[15] there is some concern whether, because of the softness of the kernel and unfamiliar appearance, they are suitable for processing, including home grinding, and whether they will be acceptable to the consumer. Most important, many of the high protein seeds tend to produce yields lower than other varieties. Unless these failings can be overcome, or unless economic incentives such as a preferential pricing system to encourage production of high protein grains are adopted, farmers may be unwilling to plant the new high protein seeds.†

Plant geneticists are confident that disease-resistant strains can be developed with characteristics that satisfy processing and consumer requirements. The major issue is whether seed can be produced that is competitive in yield. The tradeoff between caloric volume and utilizable protein volume per acre is a problem not only for the producer, who has no incentive to substitute quality for volume (since protein value does not presently influence market value), but also for the consumer who suffers from a caloric insufficiency as well as a protein deficit. A lower rate of growth in

---

* It is also possible by genetic means to develop totally new food crops. One manmade crop is triticale, a high-protein cross of wheat and rye first marketed in 1970.[14]

† Pricing in the United States within wheat classes is based on protein content, but primarily because baking characteristics vary with protein level. For many years, preferential pricing, keyed to butterfat content, was employed for milk quality.

Price policies favoring a higher nutrient content may also have certain nutrition education features, in that farmers will want to know why they are being paid more for higher nutrient varieties.

total supply would mean relatively higher prices, raising the question of what would happen if the calorie-protein ratio in the diet were changed in favor of protein at the expense of daily caloric intake.

Although a number of years may be required to develop and successfully multiply cereal grain seeds to satisfy all these needs, breeding clearly offers long-range promise for nutritional improvement. In the interim, other means of upgrading cereal products, such as fortification, must be sought. Improved seed and fortification need not be competitive approaches; at certain points it may be economically advantageous to improve the quality of a food via breeding, at others via fortification.[16]

Pulses also can be bred for better nutrient content. Until 1972, when an international pulse research project was organized, only modest and inconsistent efforts had been put into pulse research; there was little of the systematic screening of germ plasm that has helped determine the genetic range of cereals, or the intensive experimental programs applied to adapt cereals to local conditions. However, one preliminary screening of 1,800 strains of pigeon peas in India found a protein range of 18–32 percent, suggesting that there is good potential for genetic improvement.[17]

If the plant geneticist should succeed in producing strains of cereals and pulses that differ from existing high-yielding strains only in their protein content—if the strains have the same yield, respond the same way to fertilizer, produce the same income for the farmer as lower protein strains, and have exactly the same cooking qualities and taste as existing strains— the effect would be akin to waving a magic wand over the production-income-diet complex, and protein intake could be improved at a very small cost. The approach deserves major support—for pulses as well as cereals, and for other important nutrients as well as protein.

## A Look at Traditionally Regarded Sources of Protein

Meat, milk, eggs, and fish—traditionally regarded as the source of proteins—play a small and sometimes insignificant role in the diets of low-income portions of the population. For most of the world's malnourished the price of such proteins is out of reach, so that meat consumption, for example, is only a few pounds a year (compared to per capita meat consumption in the United States of 186 pounds).* It is unlikely that the poor

* There are exceptions, such as Brazil where about one-fourth of the protein of the diet of low-income portions of the population comes from animal sources.

TABLE 8. *Cost of Various Foods Supplying Protein in South Indian Diet, 1972*

| Food | Retail price, dollars per kilogram | Protein, percent | Protein cost Dollars per kilogram[a] | As percent of laborers' daily wage[b] |
|---|---|---|---|---|
| Meat | 0.39 | 24.0 | 1.49 | 373 |
| Eggs | 0.67[c] | 12.8 | 5.05 | 1,263 |
| Fish | 0.66 | 25.0 | 2.55 | 638 |
| Fresh milk | 0.20[d] | 3.5 | 5.34 | 1,335 |
| Whole wheat flour | 0.24 | 11.0 | 1.49 | 373 |
| Milled rice | 0.26 | 8.0 | 2.24 | 560 |
| Corn meal | 0.17 | 9.5 | 0.66 | 165 |
| Pulses | 0.20 | 24.0 | 0.58 | 145 |

Sources: Protein data from Benjamin T. Burton (ed.), *Heinz Book of Nutrition* (2nd ed., McGraw-Hill, 1965); prices supplied by Kalmann Schaefer, Tamil Nadu Nutrition Project. All costs are given in U.S. dollars.
a. Cost of product containing 1 kilogram of protein minus cost of carbohydrates and fats in product (see F. R. Senti, "The Case for Plant Proteins" [paper presented at American Society of Animal Science Meeting, Cornell University, June 28, 1967; processed]). Cost is based on weight of proteins because reliable data based on qualitative measures such as net utilizable protein are not available.
b. Wage estimated at 40 cents.
c. One dozen eggs weigh about 0.7 kilogram.
d. Liter.

in most low-income countries will soon be able to afford nutritionally significant quantities of these foods. The price of animal protein is such a disproportionately large share of the daily earnings of laborers (see Table 8) that one may question the appropriateness of investment by governments and foreign aid agencies in such products as a means of improving nutrition. Such an investment may be reasonable to parlay a comparative advantage in meat exports. But the allocation of national resources to promote exports should not be viewed as a nutrition policy, except in the broad sense that general increases in national income, properly directed, can be beneficial to nutritional status of a population.* The following once-

* Also, a limited segment of livestock production—especially dairying and meat processing—is labor intensive, thereby sometimes increasing employment and income among the poor. It has been suggested that governments can adjust price policies to get more animal protein to the poor, just as has been proposed for vegetable protein. Although hypothetically possible, subsidies of this type would be an expensive means for an already financially hard-pressed government to deal with the nutrition problem. (For an approach to measure the nutritional possibilities of livestock projects, see Appendix D.)

over-lightly treatment of several of the more commonly considered sources of high quality protein stresses the nutritional implications of production emphasis in these fields.

## Beef

A government policy consciously aimed at increasing the availability of animal protein may even have a perverse nutritional impact. Under some circumstances, land and other resources may be taken away from production of grain for human consumption. Or the grain itself could be diverted to livestock production. It takes five pounds of grain to produce one pound of meat, an allocation few developing countries can afford, even given the dramatic increases in cereal production. Many countries are barely able to meet direct human consumption needs. A relatively low amount of grain is fed to animals in the developing countries. India uses only 0.5 percent of its total cereal supply for animal feed; the United States uses 80 percent.[18]

Although more meat can be produced, it is another question whether it will be available for domestic consumption or whether the nutritionally needy can afford it. More meat is being raised in Central America than ever before; it seems, however, to be ending up not in Latin American stomachs but in franchised restaurant hamburgers in the United States (see the contrast in production and consumption in Table 9). A 75 percent increase in meat production in Nicaragua was accompanied by only

TABLE 9. *Production and Consumption of Beef in Central America, 1961–65—1970*

| Country | Production, thousands of tons | | Produc-tion change, percent | Per capita consumption, kilograms | | Con-sump-tion change, percent |
|---|---|---|---|---|---|---|
| | *1961–65 average* | *1970* | | *1961–65 average* | *1970* | |
| Costa Rica | 21.4 | 41.1 | +92 | 12.3 | 9.1 | −26 |
| El Salvador | 21.0 | 20.0 | −5 | 7.7 | 5.9 | −23 |
| Guatemala | 41.0 | 57.4 | +40 | 8.2 | 7.7 | −6 |
| Honduras | 16.7 | 29.6 | +77 | 5.5 | 5.0 | −9 |
| Panama | 24.7 | 32.0 | +30 | 20.9 | 21.8 | +4 |
| Nicaragua | 32.2 | 56.4 | +75 | 12.3 | 12.7 | +3 |
| Mexico | 475.0 | 605.3 | +27 | 10.9 | 10.9 | 0 |

Source: Compiled from *World Agricultural Production and Trade* (USDA, 1971).

a 3 percent increase in average consumption; a 40 percent increase in Guatemala by a 6 percent decrease in average consumption; and a 92 percent increase in Costa Rica by a 26 percent decline in per capita consumption.

Brazil—with 97 million head of cattle, the third largest herd in the world after the United States and the Soviet Union—experiences regular beef shortages that send meat prices soaring and reduce per capita consumption among the poor.[19] When meat is brought into a poor home, most of it is eaten by the adults, usually the males; it is seldom included in diets of the young in developing countries.[20]

Livestock production may of course be encouraged for export reasons. It is often appropriate in regions where land is unsuitable for other agricultural uses. Some areas that cannot produce grain do grow grass. Nevertheless, investment in livestock production may sometimes have the effect of benefiting the better off at the nutritional expense of the poor.

### Milk

Although milk has a higher rate of protein conversion than meat, it is still an expensive form of protein; in many developing countries a liter of milk costs half of a laborer's daily wage. Per capita milk consumption consequently is low and in some places is declining. In India, despite major dairy programs, milk production increased less than 1 percent from the mid-1950s to the mid-1960s, actually a decrease in per capita terms because of population growth.[21] Unlike Europe and North America, where milk constitutes 25 percent of the protein in protein-rich diets, in the Philippines milk constitutes an average of 6 percent of the dietary protein and in Ceylon 2 percent. Even the already low averages of per capita consumption are misleading since consumption patterns are heavily skewed against low-income groups. Middle and lower middle income groups, however, often can usefully benefit from milk production increases.

One reason for the short supply of milk is the pathetic yield; the typical south Asian cow produces a tenth as much as the European cow. With improved breeding practices, better feed, and disease control—and their attendant costs—the mass of nondescript animals could yield substantially more milk. Even with efficient dairying, however, milk would be costly for nutritionally needy families. Although investment in milk yield may lead to economically viable projects, in many instances it will, under conventional dairying, marketing, and pricing, be a long time before the urban poor will benefit. For rural families owning cows, a cost-effective improvement in milk yield could have direct nutritional benefits. However, in many rural areas, milk is sold rather than consumed on the farm because of its relatively high price. Milk consumption in the producing areas may thus be lower than elsewhere. In some West Bengal villages, milk is curdled and sold in Calcutta where it is used in the preparation of popular Bengali sweets. In Kerala, 90 percent of the milk produced in villages is sold in the towns, where 14 percent of the Kerala population live, despite pronounced protein malnutrition in the villages.[22] The effect of such sales on nutrition will depend on how the added income is used.*

*Poultry and Pork*

In comparison with other animals, the chicken is an efficient converter of plant protein to animal protein. Here, too, however, differences in yield are dramatic. The average American chicken is several times as large as the typical south Asian chicken—80 percent of which are scavengers—and produces three to four times as many eggs.

Few other than the affluent in developing countries consume poultry meat and eggs, except possibly on special occasions. In 1969, per capita egg consumption in the United States was 314; in India it was 8, and for young children of disadvantaged families, the number was surely less than the national average.

Though beliefs widely held in poor countries that eating eggs is bad for young children, girls, and pregnant women may limit consumption, the primary constraint is price. Eggs in developing countries commonly sell for 40 cents to 70 cents a dozen. Even in the unlikely event that the figure could be halved, prices would (in part because of transport and keeping quality problems) still be beyond the reach of the typical laborer.

Families in many developing countries keep a small number of poultry, whose feed comes solely from scavenging. They involve no investment of any significance and the practice no doubt should be encouraged, to achieve whatever modest nutritional or economic contribution is provided. In countries where more elaborate back yard and community poultry proj-

---

* Recent studies suggest that some racial groups, particularly non-Caucasian populations, may not be able to consume normal quantities of milk without diarrhea and abdominal discomfort. This probably results from a lactose intolerance in otherwise healthy groups. There is still much that needs to be known about the relationship of milk intolerance and lactose, but because of the wide-reaching implications, the matter clearly calls for full examination.[23]

ects have been promoted, the eggs produced have commonly found their way into the city and thus have had little direct nutritional impact on the families of the producers.[24] Such egg production, like meat and milk production, should not be regarded as a nutrition project except in the sense in which the income increase can be nutritionally useful.

Pork production is in many ways like poultry production. Backyard pigs, common in many developing countries, frequently are scavengers or, if penned, are fed on waste. Under such circumstances, there is little cost involved in this form of production of animal protein.

### Fish

The potential of fish as an important but relatively neglected nutrient source is a matter of some controversy. One school holds that the unexploited oceans could provide several times the 62 million tons caught in 1971,* another that a sustained catch could not much exceed 100 million tons annually, and yet another that the seas are not inexhaustible and that because of ecological problems the catch may decline. Most marine biologists agree that for traditional table fish, the maximum level of sustainable catch has almost been reached.[25]

While 71 percent of the earth's surface is covered by oceans, only 1 percent of the world calorie consumption—and 3 percent of protein consumption—comes from fish. In low-income countries, fish consumption is proportionately smaller; in the Middle East, fish accounts for only 1 percent of total protein intake. (By contrast, 17 percent of the protein in the Japanese diet is in the form of fish.) If fish, either traditional or nontraditional, were to play a significant role in world nutrition—meeting, say, 20 percent of the protein need in low-income countries—a more than sixfold increase in catch would be necessary. To achieve this would require a revolution in the primitive fishing techniques practiced in most countries, and the building of tens of thousands of mechanized fishing boats capable of longer range and larger load than the traditional craft.† Also, major steps would

---

* Approximately two-thirds of this is consumed by humans, the remainder used for animal feed. The largest national catch by far—12.6 million tons—is by Peru, a country with significant malnutrition. Much of the Peruvian catch is exported for poultry feed.

† The Food and Agriculture Organization's indicative world plan estimates that to meet an expected demand for 69 million tons of fish for human consumption by 1985 (plus more than half again as much for animal feed) will require an investment of $8.5 billion.[26]

be required for better preservation. Fish spoil more rapidly than other foods and, unless dried, require costly storage and handling. Fish consumption among the poor is now usually limited to those who live within a few miles of the sea or lake where the fish are caught.

Thus, major investments in ocean fishing as nutrition moves seem inappropriate, although some countries may make them to exploit comparative advantages in international trade. Again, as with investment in meat production, this should not be mistaken for a nutrition investment. Except for those living near the water—and this is not always an inconsiderable number—it is unlikely that fresh sea fish will offer major benefits to the poor.

Other types of fishing projects such as pond culture, where fish are multiplied under controlled conditions—particularly in paddy rice areas— deserve further exploration as a possible means of making fish available at varied locales and at lower cost. Remarkable yields with pond culture have been demonstrated—up to five tons an acre under ideal conditions. Also, there is the potential for large-scale use of fish in new, processed forms— like the fish sausages and hams now popular in Japan (fish protein concentrate is one of the ingredients for the new foods discussed in Chapter 8).

## Whither Horticultural Crops?

Should the green revolution at some point reduce the amount of land necessary to satisfy cereal needs, former cereal acreage might be used for cultivation of vegetables, fruits, and other crops.* No such shift has yet been apparent. Although the amount of land devoted to fruit and vegetable production increased markedly during the 1960s in certain rapidly developing countries (in Mexico by 29 percent and in Taiwan by 59 percent), land use for cereals also increased.

A more likely short-term effect of the cereals revolution on vegetables and some fruits is that, with multiple cropping of the faster maturing cereal varieties, horticultural crops can be squeezed into the regular cropping sequence—or, as the case may be, squeezed out in favor of an additional cereal crop. (Unfortunately, the available data offer little indication of what, in fact, is happening; because a large portion of fruit and vegetable production takes place in back yards, much goes unreported.)

* Or used for nonfood crops or nonagricultural purposes.

Vegetables and fruits are excellent sources of vitamins and minerals, but increased demand for them, like animal products, is closely tied to income. Demand for many products starts well up in the income brackets of developing countries, often because problems of bulk, perishability, and transport lead to high prices.

Governments could, as with other crops, encourage expanded horticultural production through research, extension education, and price policies. But expansion programs should be tied to specific nutrition need; cultivation of crops identified as necessary to meet local nutrient deficiencies should be encouraged. Such has seldom been the case.

## Reducing Food Waste

Discussion of nutrient availability would be incomplete without some mention of food waste. Although losses are difficult to compute, and estimates vary widely,[27] there is little question that large portions of food produced in low-income countries are lost either in the field, in storage, or in handling and processing. The Food and Agriculture Organization (FAO) estimates world food losses at between $24 billion and $48 billion a year. In Latin America annual losses are believed to be about 40 percent of the total crop, in tropical Africa over 30 percent. It has been estimated that if half of the world's storage losses were prevented, enough calories would be saved to satisfy the diets of half a billion people. And disinfecting cereal grain alone would net an estimated extra 9 million tons of protein a year,[28] equivalent to the protein needs of 375 million people. In many countries, combined losses due to rodents, insects, and fungi are double or triple the food deficits.*

Given this picture, a country looking for ways to provide better nutrition might conclude that a promising area for investment was better storage facilities, modern rodenticides, chemical fumigants, improved milling and processing equipment, and other means to prevent loss of nutrients.

It is tempting to assign high priority to programs designed to reduce waste—a problem made all the more poignant by the malnutrition caused by large food deficiencies. But reduction of food waste requires changes of

---

* Food spoilage is more than a problem of quantitative loss; infection, infestation, and contamination all pose health hazards.

practices and substantial capital investments that are not easily achieved. Also, waste in agricultural production, processing, and distribution is economically the same as waste in inefficient industrial, power, or other branches of the economy. In any area, such waste can be considered a cost of production, one of the inputs needed for the final product, arising from the inefficiencies of economic activity along the way. Will the largest increases in supply be obtained by reducing destruction by pests in the field, by reducing losses in storage and transport, by increasing production through greater investment in seeds, fertilizers, pesticides, or irrigation, by increasing recovery from the milling process, or by some combination of these? How does the economic return from the most productive of these measures compare with the return on investments elsewhere in the economy? Any country that focuses its solutions on waste alone may be committing the error of nutrient autarchy—sole reliance on domestic production of nutrients. As long as external trade is possible, the question of agricultural waste becomes part of the supply problem generally—how best to exploit an area's comparative advantages to meet the population's needs.

IN A NUMBER of developing countries, agricultural growth—sparked by the new seed varieties—has been very encouraging. By almost any measure, the recent transformation of countries with heavy cereal deficits into self-sufficient or nearly self-sufficient nations is remarkable, especially in view of the food and population trends that prompted famine projections in the mid-1960s. Problems will arise that may impede the advance of the green revolution, problems of plant disease, insects, pests, institutional rigidities, and so on. But these will be problems arising from progress, not barriers to breaking out of agricultural stagnation. The new seeds may affect the well-being of more people in a shorter period of time than any previous technical advance in history.[29]

Agricultural self-sufficiency, however, does not mean nutritional self-sufficiency; what the market will clear is quite different from what is required to satisfy nutritional need. Although agriculture clearly plays a major role in determination of nutritional status, even substantial increases in food production cannot fulfill the nutrition needs of all groups of consumers, and in some cases the effect on nutrition of agricultural progress may not even be positive.

Many of the nutritional consequences of agricultural policies occur by happenstance. Targets for food production programs are usually based on aggregate projections of demand, growth in per capita income, elasticities of demand of specific products, and population rise. Agricultural production is also shaped by export considerations, desire to minimize dependence on imports, industrial requirements for raw materials, and concern for price stability.

In the formulation of supply strategies, the relation between food supply increases and the circumstances of the malnourished is seldom explicitly taken into account. Calculation of aggregate (and potentially misleading) national per capita availability of specific foods or nutrients is ordinarily the closest attempt at consideration of nutritional need. Explicit measures are almost never taken to raise the effective demand of the poor. Nor are agricultural research efforts usually designed with an acknowledged concern for the nutritional content of output—especially of foods largely eaten by the poor.

The supply of nutrients emanating from common economically oriented agricultural activities does not of itself result in satisfactory nutrition conditions. Although many millions have benefited, serious problems of undernutrition and malnutrition remain, even in countries boasting rapid agricultural modernization. Mexico, for example, world-famed as the source and a large producer of the new miracle wheat and corn varieties, continues to be plagued by malnutrition in the low-income regions, even though it is now an exporter of cereals. Nutrition of the vulnerable very young children in India's Punjab reportedly shows no demonstrable improvement, although the Punjab in many ways is a model of economic and agricultural development.[30]

None of this is to sugggest that development specialists should diminish their pursuit of increased cereal yields. They must, however, begin to consider the nutritional quality of foods and means of distributing them. The nutritional implications of changes must be weighed in new agricultural policies and programs. Introduction of a high-yielding cereal variety need not be turned down simply because the grain is low in protein or may displace other nutritionally important but less profitable crops. But in the government's decision to support an agricultural improvement, nutritional effects should be included among the costs and the tradeoffs involved. Beyond that, price supports, research policies, qualitative grading of crops, infrastructure investments, extension coverage, and so on, can be used as specific means for bettering nutrition via agriculture.

Even then, however, the resulting foodstuffs cannot alone assure that the needs of the malnourished will be effectively met. Many other factors are responsible for much of the malnutrition, especially among small children, in low-income countries. Often food practices—withholding of solid foods at an age when they are needed (even when family food supply is not a constraint) and insufficient breast feeding—are at the root of high mortality and morbidity in the young. Similarly, nutritional deficiencies often persist despite adequate food supplies because of distribution mechanisms that are incapable of reaching those in need. Thus deliberate attention should be given to supportive measures in education, distribution, and so on.

## CHAPTER SIX

# Educating for
# Better Nutrition

An important part of the nutrition gap is the information gap. Although lack of purchasing power is a major constraint, many nutritional deficiencies would be moderated if people knew how better to use the resources already at hand. Cicely Williams, who first identified and described kwashiorkor, reports that in West Africa "malnutrition is due not to economic poverty, but to a poverty in knowledge of the nutritional needs of a child."[1] In Brazil, ignorance and a lack of trained personnel on nutrition have been called "the major factors responsible for . . . protein malnutrition."[2] Likewise in Zambia, nutrition problems have been described as "due to a lack of knowledge."[3] And in Kenya, reportedly, "practically every case of malnutrition is due to ignorance, and only some are due to ignorance combined with poverty."[4]

Malnutrition raged among the Bangladesh youngsters crowded in Indian refugee camps in 1971, even when adequate foodstuffs were available to their families. The Bengali mother's traditional treatment for her child's diarrhea is to give barley water and withhold solids, a sure-fire prescription for protein-calorie malnutrition.

One of the few foods accepted throughout south Asia is *dal,* cooked pulses that are high in protein. But weaning infants often are not fed *dal* out of fear it will produce flatulence and illness. It is commonly eaten only by adults, even though the infant's protein requirements are proportionately two and one-half times as great as his elder's. Vitamin A deficiency prevails in Java, even though vegetables are commonly available to low-income families. The young, however, seldom consume vegetables, especially boys since vegetables are not regarded as suitable food for men.[5] In general, there is little recognition of the special needs of children, especially at the time of weaning, and rarely does the child's diet receive special attention.

Because they seem so obvious, changes in food habits are tempting solutions to dietary problems. Abetted by their own childhood experiences, and memories of being told that eating some things would be better for them than eating others, government officials commonly are attracted to nutrition solutions based on food habit change.[6] The appeal of nutrition education is in its seemingly lighter demand on resources than other types of nutrition programs. Also among its attractions is the presumably one-shot investment it requires—once habits are changed, they are expected to remain changed—without the recurring expense of, say, a fortification project or a school feeding program.

Thus, nutrition education—the process of acquainting people with the value of resources already available to them and persuading them to change existing practices—deserves thoughtful consideration as an element in an overall nutrition strategy. Unfortunately, such consideration is not easy. Surprisingly little good information is available on nutrition education, despite the vast number of undertakings over the years. Evaluation may have been neglected on the unquestioned assumption that nutrition education is worthwhile, or it may have been scheduled to take place after the end of a nutrition education campaign, and many projects never get that far. Commonly, programs that have been analyzed have been measured in numbers of pamphlets printed or numbers of people reached, rather than by how many of the needy were reached, how their diets were changed, and how their nutritional status was improved. To evaluate its potential impact as a component of a national nutrition strategy requires starting anew in asking those basic questions that underlie the suggestion that investment in nutrition education is a valid means of bringing about nutritional improvement.

## Planning Nutrition Education: The Questions

Although nutrition education clearly is important, how much nutritional improvement can actually be obtained in a specific setting merely from specific changes in decisions made by the food buyer and preparer? Assuming that nutrition education will be totally effective, how far can it go toward achieving nutritional objectives, given the constraints that are imposed by income, ecology, and local supplies? Clearly, diets cannot improve if the recommended foods are not available or if they require reducing expenditures on staple caloric foods when caloric deficiency is also a threat.

If the message successfully educated people to realize the benefits that could be obtained by change—no easy achievement—how powerful would that realization be as a behavioral determinant? Many factors—biological, geographical, psychological, sociological, religious, economic, technical—govern food practices. In short, what would be the effect on the "irrational rigidity" of the human diet?[7] There is perhaps no aspect of personal life less flexible than eating patterns. Tunisian immigrants to France, for instance, changed their food habits long after they had accepted the dress, language, and newspapers of their adopted country.[8] Even among the most sophisticated elements of society, change comes hard: many are the doctors whose breakfasts still include eggs, butter, cream, and sugar despite health warnings circulated in recent years. Frequently the educational effort clashes head-on with well-ensconced, sometimes deleterious, food practice.

Another important question in an education effort is the length of time it will take—months, years, or generations—to achieve the objective. That depends first on how long it takes to reach the target audiences, then how lengthy and vigorous the educational effort must be to bring about the desired change. For example, face-to-face nutrition education as now generally employed—in applied nutrition programs, mothercraft and rehabilitation centers, health center education and other extension activities —could take many years to cover a population, depending on the size of the country and the education effort.

What does a nutrition education effort cost in comparison with alternative means of achieving the same nutritional objective? The standard of measurement must not be campaign costs, since nutrition education is more than a transfer of information, but the cost over time of bringing about an actual change in food practice. (Cost analysis of conventional nutrition education typically fails to account for planning personnel, material preparation, training, and a variety of indirect administrative costs.) If the education is given at schools, the cost seldom takes into account the subject-matter time that is preempted by nutrition. Similarly, the projection of nationwide costs from successful pilot projects often ignores the difficulties entailed in large-scale replication of a person-to-person effort. The initial success is often the result of the personality and enthusiasm of the initiator, and the same level of performance can rarely be reached once his or her charisma has been replaced by the routine of a formalized bureaucracy.

Changes in food behavior may also impose costs that, although negligible in an economic sense, are substantial in an aesthetic or psychic sense. Particular food practices are among the few satisfactions available to people living in poverty. The values other than nutrition that food expresses —refreshment, security, prestige, the fulfillment of religious proscriptions —are not frivolous. They will be important determinants of whether an effort to stimulate change is practical.

Beyond comes the task of choosing the best means of motivating people to adopt proposed behavioral changes, selecting the instruments to be used and the messages to be communicated.

## Standard Nutrition Education Techniques

Nearly all the nutrition education activities undertaken to date in poor countries have relied on face-to-face communication techniques. Another common characteristic is their limited outreach, and thus their limited success, if measured in scope of impact.*

Applied nutrition programs are an integrated approach to village-level nutrition. They include education on food practices as well as on local production of nutritious foods (the latter via school and community gardens, fish ponds, poultry units, and so on).

The Indian applied nutrition program was declared in 1971, after twelve years of practice, to have made no significant difference in general dietary practices, "particularly in respect to nutritionally desirable commodities which are promoted under the program."[9] Similarly, villagers' understanding of nutritional needs was no greater than that of villagers outside the program. The production portion of the program failed to enlarge the supply of vegetables, fish, and eggs; and the feeding portion—the education component—"nowhere was conducted in the spirit of an education activity." The general failure of the program was attributed more to "the conceptualization behind the program" than to shortcomings in its organization. Similar conclusions have been reached in studies of programs in Indonesia and the Philippines.[10]

---

* This is true even though nutrition education sometimes constitutes a large portion of whatever nutrition budget is available, usually second to local support of institutional feeding programs.

In one community in south India that was part of the applied nutrition program, a prize-winning garden with impressive papaya and vegetable production had been worked by professional *malis* (gardeners). There was virtually no community participation, nor any educational exposure to horticultural practices, which was the intent of the program.

At a school that had won the blue ribbon for the best school garden in its state, the headmaster estimated that a third of the boys participated in the gardening after school. They were the students who could afford to bring a midday snack to school. Most of the others went without food and had to rush home immediately afterwards for sustenance. No thought had been given to using the garden's production as a midday feeding for all the students; the produce was divided among those who worked in the garden.

The idea of the applied nutrition program is attractive; in practice, it is less attractive.

Nutrition rehabilitation or mothercraft centers are village efforts to educate mothers in feeding and child care through practical demonstration in treating their malnourished children. Unlike hospital cures, whose techniques are foreign to the mother, the centers' treatment allows the mother to see her child's nutritional rehabilitation in an environment and under circumstances familiar to her. Initiators of these projects often claim successes in changing habits[11] although, by their own figures, the per capita cost is excessive for local budgets. Some, however, feel that while the effect on children in the centers is favorable, very few benefits are being carried into the home.[12] Although the rehabilitation centers are less expensive than hospitals as treatment facilities, they are nonetheless expensive as a nutrition education device. Conceivably, the amount spent on the centers could better be spent in ways that would lessen the need for rehabilitation.

Maternal-child health centers offer conventional village health care, including education through posters, growth charts (in more progressive centers), and so on. The nutrition education provided has been limited, primarily because of a preoccupation with curative health practice. Generally, the physician in the rural health center is not equipped, educationally or temperamentally, to become involved in nutrition education. "In generating health consciousness as a part of the way of life of the people, he has clearly not succeeded."[13] Traveling health personnel, including auxiliary nurses, have the same kinds of limitations in their work.

Nutrition extension agents, usually female field workers, attempt to communicate better food practices to local women, either individually or in small groups. In some countries, touring nutrition education vans offer food demonstrations. No serious evaluations of the impact of extension workers seem to have been made. However, in India, extension workers often seem to lack enthusiasm, knowledge, or understanding of program objectives;[14] rarely do girls who train in home science colleges go on to do extension work.

Women's clubs—locally organized efforts to institutionalize community involvement, especially of mothers—often include lectures and demonstrations on food practices in their programs. The clubs sometimes are tied to participation in local child feeding programs. Day care centers theoretically offer similar opportunities for maternal education on nutrition. Little analysis has been made of the nutritional impact of clubs or day care centers in low-income countries.

### Outreach and Cost

The personal transfer of information obviously has merit. But even assuming that person-to-person nutrition education translated to a large-scale effort can sustain accuracy in its instruction and enthusiasm in its workers, it cannot overcome the basic limitation of person-to-person communication: the size of the audience. The number of persons in the lower socioeconomic groups that can be reached varies by country but is seldom great, especially in larger countries. The needy ordinarily do not participate in—and often are not aware of—activities from which they might benefit. To reach them would require an army of field workers—in some cases diverted from other priorities—and an army-like budget, requirements unlikely to be met by the already strained resources of most developing countries.

To conduct a comprehensive nutrition education program in rural India, for example, would require reaching 65 million farm families in 567,000 mostly isolated villages.

• To provide a single visit by a mobile audiovisual unit to each village would take eight years if each district had its own van (twenty times the seventeen vans the Indian government had in 1970).

• In the last ten years the applied nutrition program, the largest of the nutrition education undertakings, has reached fewer people than the population growth during the same period.

• The education portion of the applied nutrition program carried on through the *balwadi,* the community facility for preschool-aged children, reached a small fraction of the target group—less than 2 percent in Tamil

Nadu, one of the most nutritionally conscious states. At the rate of increase planned by the government—200 new *balwadis* a year—it would take more than 150 years to cover the target population, assuming population size did not increase.*

• Based on the cost figures of the Haitian mothercraft center program, a nutrition education and rehabilitation program undertaken in India on a comprehensive scale would cost $1.5 billion.[16]

### Prospects for Change

The basic issue remains whether nutrition education can successfully prompt diet change in poor societies, and whether the change will last. There is little evidence to support this notion. Traditional nutrition education activities in low-income countries have been sufficiently disappointing to raise the question whether food habits can be changed by education; perhaps we are idealizing in assuming that without income increases and associated cultural changes, the human being can be induced to alter his centuries-old regimen.

Yet, nutrition education techniques aside, recent experience in many parts of the world suggests that existing food habits are not immutable. Despite dietary conservatism, substantial numbers of people have changed their eating habits in the last decade, and not always as the result of income increase. Foods that were totally foreign to millions are now regarded as dietary staples. Corn and wheat are now consumed in many parts of India, and rice in Africa. Although little is known about why these changes took place, they may have occurred in some regions in part because of foods made available by the new agricultural technology, the adoption of which, in itself, explodes the myth of the intractable nature of the tradition-bound peasant. (It is worth recalling that a decade ago the aim of introducing new seed varieties seemed as formidable as the idea of changing food habits does today.) The agricultural changes brought a shift of cropping patterns and a different mix of products, and diets were affected accordingly even when income went unchanged.

Another influence on diets of some has been mass communications, especially commercial advertising and sales promotion. In recent years a marked increase has occurred in low-income countries in consumption of bread, confections, soft drinks, and so on. The increasing sales of many

* This also assumes the *balwadi* would be restricted to those in the lower 50 percent of the income scale. In fact, the poor seldom participate in *balwadi* programs.[15]

items new to large population groups demonstrate that if the consumer perceives product value (bread for convenience; glucose confections for pleasant taste and energy; soft drinks for refreshment and status) his diet will change.

## Mass Communications Techniques

Can the same instruments that have sometimes been directed in ways that affect diets negatively—pushing the consumption of soft drinks, for example—now be used to improve them? On the surface, the limitations of mass media appear formidable.

The role of mass media in selling social change is unlike its conventional function—selling nutrition is not like selling soap, but like the much more difficult and abstract job of selling the concept of cleanliness. It is not merely a matter of curing a headache by selling an aspirin; people must first be convinced that they have a headache.

Most orthodox mass media in low-income areas seem not to reach the masses as they do in more affluent countries; target groups—especially the rural poor—are frequently outside the range of conventional forms of coverage. In India, for example, newspapers reach only 1 percent of the population. Television reaches only token numbers of the very affluent; less than 5 million of the 250 million television sets in the world are in south Asia, Africa, and the Arab Middle East. In some Asian and Latin American countries, statistics are less stark, but coverage limitations nonetheless exist.

Audience characteristics further hamper communication via the mass media. Most of the nearly 800 million illiterate adults in the world are from low-income countries. In Nigeria, 20 percent of the total population can read; in Ethiopia, 10 percent (probably a lower percentage of women and those in rural areas, especially the nutritionally needy). In some countries, language differences raise additional problems. India has fourteen basic languages, many as different from one another as French is from Chinese, and seven hundred dialects. Some African countries have more than a hundred languages apiece. There are also broad differences in standards and styles of living, values, aspirations, religious proscriptions, ethnic backgrounds, climate and geography, and the varying cultural patterns that these imply—all of which affect the messages as well as the media of an effective mass communications program.

The market-research techniques that industrialized countries rely on are commonly more difficult to apply in less advantaged countries. Basic statistics are often unavailable or unreliable. Original data from surveys are usually difficult to obtain; there are few survey organizations of high quality with extensive coverage. Moreover, people from conservative societies often do not willingly communicate their attitudes to the market researcher.

Not only is there little experience on which to base mass media campaigns, but the value of communication in development projects has yet to be accepted in most developing countries. Even when its value is recognized, the use of mass communications to bring about change sometimes is regarded with suspicion.

Yet, for all their limitations, the mass media suggest unusual opportunities for nutrition education.[17] The orthodox mass media may have limitations of outreach, but devices exist in all societies for reaching large numbers of people with information about a mass problem. Only a small fraction of the numbers of "educators" needed for a conventional face-to-face program are necessary for a mass media nutrition education campaign. Mass media can reach people more quickly and at greater distances. And since mass media materials are prepared and produced centrally, the message may be communicated with less distortion and a greater sense of urgency than the person-to-person message transmitted through a series of administrative layers down to the village worker and ultimately the target audience. New notions that are received with suspicion in face-to-face communication take on an aura of authority with mass media, challenging the individual's tendency to accept himself as his own food expert.

Because mass media reach everyone in the same form, they offer a common experience that, properly nurtured, is capable of conveying a sense that something of significance is happening. The momentum may lead to greater consciousness of nutrition than might be possible through isolated conventional techniques.

A high rate of illiteracy does not rule out use of the printed word for purposes of nutrition betterment. Even where illiteracy is prevalent, materials can be directed to the school child or to those lettered village leaders who play important roles in influencing transfer of new ideas. At any rate, the need for change in food practices is not restricted to the poor, illiterate villager. Significant nutritional deficiencies are often found among families who can afford better.

A mass media campaign cannot be expected to offer a cure-all that would eliminate the need for alternate forms of nutrition education. It should be designed, as it was in Zambia, to complement rather than compete with conventional techniques. In some instances, mass media can only create interest and receptivity—the agent of change may still be the local worker.[18]

### The Audiences

The success of a nutrition education campaign is dependent on more than media contact with the nutritionally needy target group. First, political leaders and officials of government agencies (and foreign assistance agencies) who have a potential role in the nutrition effort must be educated. Until they appreciate the magnitude and implications of malnutrition, no significant effort to combat the problem can be mounted. In India a special education program, developed by the Protein Foods Association, was specifically directed to the decision and opinion makers. One advertisement in the New Delhi press read: "There is a shadow looming over us today that could frustrate many of our national goals." Another was headlined, "A generation condemned . . . because we don't care enough?" The sponsors also planned for billboard space directly across from the Parliament to remind legislators of the nutrition issue.

Medical and paramedical personnel also need better nutrition education. Medical schools usually teach a good deal about basic nutrient metabolism, but little attention is given to the application of this information.[19] Medical schools often regard nutrition as a field for dieticians, and thus not very dignified, or as a field for specialists rather than one every practicing physician should learn. (The implied criticism is equally valid for those studying public health in more affluent countries.[20]) "It is possible to take the course in maternal and child health . . . at . . . leading schools of public health without hearing the word 'nutrition' mentioned."[21] The results are apparent. For example, in most tropical pediatric wards little if any effort is made at nutrition education. The mother usually takes the child home to the "same regime as precipitated admission in the first place."[22]

Another vehicle of change in some societies is the school child (and the preschool-aged child when he can be reached). Though his home consumption is primarily dictated by family practices, the child is an important audience for a nutrition education campaign because he forms dietary habits early in life, he is more receptive to change, he is a future parent (in many developing countries at an early age), and in some instances he can influence family behavior, at least by exposure to new ways. The exposure of the child to nutrition education in school has been cited as the most important influence in the introduction of new foods in Israel.[23] The formal education system is itself a kind of mass medium. Nutrition, however, is usually relegated to home economics classes rather than being woven into such broader courses as science, mathematics, or reading, or treated as a special subject. Nutrition should be incorporated into the curriculum of teachers' training colleges, and special manuals and refresher courses should be made available to teachers.[24]

Other audiences providing selective opportunities for nutritional education include members of the armed forces, agricultural university faculty and students, religious leaders, mass communication figures, government bureaucrats, hospitalized children, children participating in institutional feeding programs, and participants in adult functional literacy courses.

### Media and Messages

The manner of transmitting the message depends not only on the audiences selected but the means of communication available. Techniques that may have long since disappeared from use in more industrialized countries may be appropriate. For a prototype program designed to promote Bal Ahar in India, the communication devices recommended were messages printed on school workbook covers and slates, signs on bicycle rickshaws, comic books, religious calendar art, and the like.[25] In remote villages in Ecuador, Ghana, and India, pictorial calendars are often the only art available; homes often have a dozen or more as their major source of interior decoration. In India's Kulu Valley, there are few large boulders that do not carry a message about malaria eradication, and few villages throughout India are without family planning symbols printed on prominently visible walls. The advent of the transistor makes the radio an especially attractive medium for social programs at the less-affluent levels. In Thailand, 77 percent of the farmers are regular radio listeners, even though actual numbers of radios are relatively small. Farmers in north India who have taken to the new high-yielding strains of wheat sometimes refer to them as "the radio seeds."[26] Increasingly, commercial films are produced in developing countries; India now makes twice as many feature films a year as the United States. These widely attended movies offer obvious opportunity for mass exposure to nutrition messages.

Themes for nutrition education campaigns include encouragement of breast feeding, provision of food supplements to nursing infants at the appropriate age (many mothers do not begin feeding solid foods until after ten months, though they should before six months), family food budgeting, avoidance of waste, and better food distribution within the family. People must see reason to change. This means the campaign, in its communication, must identify the problem (often the target individual is unaware of the nutritional need), engage the emotions, explain the cure, and demonstrate the results. Potential causes of hidden resistance to change must be identified so the message can be designed to address such obstacles as economic resistance ("I can't afford it"), social status resistance ("Everyone else eats this way, and they can't all be wrong"), and uncontrollable forces-of-fate resistance ("We have been eating this way for generations").[27]

There must be understanding of cultural food imagery, such as the "hot" and "cold" classification of foods that is widespread in poor countries.* One needs also to distinguish between food beliefs and food habits. The former involves emotionalism, usually with a religious or other cultural value. (Interestingly, food taboos, the negative form of food beliefs, most often relate to protein foods. Also worth noting—and worth speculating upon—is that food taboos seem to apply least often to the adult male.) The food belief is not as amenable to change as the food habit which is ordinary behavior—the way things have always been—without moral judgment attached.[29]

Experience suggests it is doubtful whether changes in food habits can be achieved by teaching nutrition as nutrition. Much of the existing nutrition education effort now starts with the assumption that basic facts of the science of nutrition must be included. More effective, it seems, would be identification of the benefits to the potential adopters and the emotional play on universally expressed human needs, such as survival and the minimization of suffering—including suffering due to loss of child. The theme

---

* Some foods are considered "hot," and others "cold"; these designators have nothing to do with the temperature of the foods when served or the spiciness, but perceived built-in characteristics of the food itself. Eggs, milk, and gram generally are considered to cause burning and thus are withheld during "hot" illnesses and during hot seasons. Green vegetables often are regarded as "cold" and not served during cold seasons. There is no universal "hot/cold" classification. What is regarded as "hot" in some places is "cold" in others. In Thailand eggs are considered "cooling" and in Bangladesh eggs are considered among the "hottest" foods. In Malaysia, differences of interpretation have been noted from one village to another.[28]

of a nutrition education campaign designed for use in India was "Mother, love is not enough." Emotional themes include: *love* ("Feed your child better"), *ambition* ("What do you want of your child's future?") and *fear* ("If you don't feed a child correctly, he will be dull").[30] Vitasoy, the soy-based soft drink in Hong Kong, was at first unsuccessful as a health food, but was extraordinarily successful when it began advertising "Vitasoy will make you grow taller, stronger, prettier."

Efforts to encourage new food preparations must be made with appreciation of the expense and scarcity of fuel, the lack of storage, and the absence of all but the most basic cooking utensils. Advice requiring precise measurement or sterilization of feeding bottles is "unreal, impractical, and impossible."[31] In short, the prescribed solution must be doable in local circumstances. In the same vein, it is important that whatever message is communicated cannot be misinterpreted. The Ghanaian Farmers Council once encouraged its members to switch from rice production to much less nutritious cassava and yams because it was under the impression from reading nutrition materials that eating rice caused beriberi.[32]

Although the nutrition message need not be transmitted to the same audience ad infinitum, it must be sustained for a sufficient period to achieve the objective. During this period the message must be frequent and consistent. There should be a common theme and a common look and, in audio materials, a common sound. There must be coordination of all agencies involved in the education endeavor. Moreover, communications encouraging change must relate to other links in the marketing chain. To create demand for an unavailable product would be a waste of education and source of dissatisfaction and lessened receptivity in the future. To create increased demand without accompanying adequate supply would have the effect of increasing prices which would, in turn, lower the demand.*

* Among the shortcomings of conventional nutrition education materials are: (1) A tendency to overload the message; more effective is reinforcement of a single theme. (2) Commonly used messages often lack specificity. Generalized concepts are dimly perceived. Directions must be simple and very specific as to what actions are to be undertaken. (3) The message often is not relevant to local needs. Comprehension is directly related to familiarity of and access to problem solutions—points often missed in existing materials. (4) To be understood, the message must be interesting; it often is not. Margaret Mead has termed standard nutrition education immensely boring, full of exhortations and admonitions. Similarly, the physical materials themselves usually are uninteresting. (5) The message often is too abstract. Unsophisticated villagers have difficulty dealing with abstractions, their perception being restricted to experience. A case in point occurred in connection with the devel-

*Gauging Effectiveness*

Too often, feedback is a neglected aspect of activities of this sort. Without some idea of audience response, there is no valid way of knowing the usefulness of the investment in nutrition education. After a one-year, $97,500 mass media nutrition education campaign in the western Indian state of Maharastra, the portion of the population familiar with campaign specifics, the amount of message recall, and the shifts in knowledge (based on benchmark data) brought about by the campaign were all measured. Effectiveness was judged by the ability of the contacted person to recall important elements of the message and his projection of a favorable attitude toward dietary improvement. In these limited terms, cost per effective contact was about 4 cents.[35]

NUTRITION education—a commonly employed device for trying to upgrade diets in developing countries—appears not to have brought about large-scale changes in eating habits. Whether the emphasis on education should be increased, or even be continued at current levels, depends on the comparative effectiveness and cost of this means of combating malnutrition.

Scant evidence is available on the value of past programs; both the scope of the programs and the methodology for evaluating them have been limited. The isolated instances of success in pilot projects have often been heavily dependent on the initiator's personality; none has demonstrated any likelihood that it could be extended to statistically significant portions of the needy population.

If nutrition education is to be pursued as part of a nutrition strategy, substantial changes are necessary. A better understanding is needed of why people change their habits, how best to communicate with them, and what messages to communicate. Social scientists should have a part in de-

---

opment of the trademark for Bal Ahar, the blended food produced for India's child feeding program. After a field survey to determine reactions to various personalities considered for use as a product emblem, it was learned that of all the many types of people considered—political figures, movie stars, businessmen, and so on—children in eastern India most admired the local wrestlers. Hence, a symbol in the form of a bust of a healthy child flexing the muscles of his right arm was proposed. When this symbol was tested in Bihar, a common response was, "Isn't it a shame this child has only one arm."[33] Advertising of Incaparina in Colombia initially was based on a before-and-after effect of the product on severely malnourished youngsters. The parents did not identify (or preferred to tune out the ugliness of the images) and sales reflected this.[34]

signing and directing nutrition education efforts; food habits should be studied from a policy or program point of view so that the voluminous literature on food beliefs and practices can be put to operational use.

The most important change is one of conceptual orientation; nutrition education to date has been treated primarily as a nutrition problem, not an education or communication problem. Most of the practitioners have been professional nutritionists or home economists, not professional communicators.

Since malnutrition is a mass problem, it probably ought to be addressed through mass communications instead of the face-to-face contact that has dominated nutrition education. Mass media, however, have their shortcomings, and little is known of their effectiveness in the field of nutrition. But the fact that mass media have helped in bringing about change in other social, political, and commercial activities, including the change of food practices through commercial promotion, offers considerable promise.

Conventional forms of nutrition education need not be abolished. Needs vary by locale; what may work in a small island will not necessarily work in a country of continental proportions. Conventional forms and mass techniques may prove to be mutually supportive or complementary approaches.

Finally, nutrition education should not be regarded as sacrosanct. Although the principle of involving the consumer in a conscious voluntary change offers obvious attractions, other techniques are available that can bring about positive dietary change without direct individual involvement. No conscious consumer participation is needed, for example, in improvement of the diet by upgrading of the nutritive quality of seeds or fortification of consumer staples. Similarly, better nutrition can result from price policies and other market actions intended to favor better-quality foods for disadvantaged portions of the population. However, just as alternate nutrition education techniques need not be mutually exclusive, the idea of nutrition education itself need not be viewed independently from—but as a complement to—other nutrition intervention programs.

## CHAPTER SEVEN

# The Crisis in Infant Feeding Practices

An unusual depletion in the crude oil reserves of an oil-producing country of Asia or Latin America would be termed a crisis. Its economic and social implications would be so apparent that actions to reverse the trend would be awarded high priority. Yet a comparable crisis, involving a valuable natural resource and losses in the hundreds of millions of dollars, is going virtually unnoticed in many of the poor countries of the world. The resource is human breast milk, and the loss is caused by the dramatic and steady decline of maternal nursing in recent decades. Already substantial in both economic and human terms, the costs and the probable major consequences suggest that methods aimed at arresting or decelerating this trend should be a prime concern in any effort to combat malnutrition.

## The Economics of Breast Feeding

Breast feeding is the traditional and ideal form of infant nutrition, usually capable of meeting a child's nutritional needs for his first four to six months of life. Even after the essential introduction of supplemental foods, human milk can serve as an important continuing source of a child's nutritional well-being. From the sixth to the twelfth month it can supply up to three-quarters of a child's protein needs and a significant portion for some months beyond.[1]

For most infants in low-income countries, prolonged breast feeding is vitally necessary to growth and, quite often, survival, as it represents the only easily available source of protein of good quality containing all the essential amino acids.

*Monetary Value*

The child who is nursed through the first two years of its life receives an average of 375 liters (396 quarts) of breast milk.[2] That is nutritionally equal to 437 liters of cow's milk, which cost about $65, a not insubstantial portion of most family incomes in developing countries.* (A laborer in Uganda may need to spend as much as 33 percent of his daily wage to feed his baby milk;[3] in Chile, 20 percent; in Tanzania, 50 percent.) For packaged dried milk formulas, which increasingly are finding their way into food stalls of local bazaars, the cost would be close to $140. These costs for commercial milk do not take account of any waste or of diversion to other members of the family. Nor do they reflect the bottle-fed baby's need for bottles and nipples, cooking utensils, refrigeration for fresh milk, fuel, and, perhaps most important, medical care, which is frequently ten times greater than for breast-fed babies.

*Costs of the Decline in Breast Feeding*

Yet, in many developing countries, mothers are abandoning breast feeding. Twenty years ago, 95 percent of Chilean mothers breast-fed their children beyond the first year; by 1969, only 6 percent did so, and only 20 percent of the babies were being nursed for as long as two months.[4] Potential breast milk production in Chile in 1950 was 57,700 tons, of which all but 2,900 tons, or 5 percent, were realized. By 1970, 78,600 tons (or 84 percent) of 93,200 potential tons were unrealized. The milk of 32,000 Chilean cows would be required to compensate for that loss. In Kenya, where the decline in breast feeding is less dramatic, the estimated $11.5 million annual loss in breast milk is equivalent to two-thirds of the national health budget or one-fifth of the average annual economic aid.†

In the few developing countries where surveys of breast feeding have been conducted over the years, the common pattern is one of significant decline, as shown in Figure 1. In Singapore, between 1951 and 1960 there was a decrease from 71 percent to 42 percent of children in low-income families breast-fed at least three months (the decline took place during a period when the number of babies born, and thus the potential for breast

---

* The method used in calculating the relative value of breast milk is explained in Appendix C.

† These calculations are not designed to suggest that breast milk can be replaced by expenditures for health or by aid, but rather to establish estimated values of breast milk that can be judged in relation to the resources of a country.

FIGURE 1. *Extent of Breast Feeding in Selected Countries and Years, 1946–71*

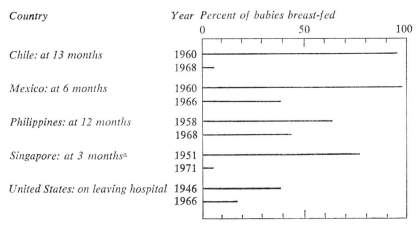

Sources: Diva M. Sanjur and others, "Infant Feeding and Weaning Practices in a Rural Pre-industrial Setting," *Acta Paediatrica Scandinavica,* Supplement 200 (1970), p. 15; Ma[ria] Linda Gabucan-Dulay, "Current Feeding Patterns as Observed among 1,000 Filipino Infants," *Philippine Journal of Pediatrics,* Vol. 19 (April 1970), p. 101; F. B. Mönckeberg, "The Effect of Malnutrition and Environment on Mental Development," *Proceedings of Western Hemisphere Nutrition Congress II, San Juan, Puerto Rico, August 1968* (Chicago: American Medical Association, 1969), pp. 216–20; Wong Hock Boon, *Breastfeeding in Singapore* (Singapore: J. L. Morison Son and Jones [F. E.] Pte, 1971); and Herman F. Meyer, "Breast Feeding in the United States," *Clinical Pediatrics,* Vol. 7 (December 1968), p. 709.
a. Low socioeconomic class only.

milk, increased 28 percent). The implied loss in the rejection of mother's milk for babies under a year old was $1.8 million. By 1971 only 5 percent of the babies were not weaned by age three months.[5] In the Philippines, 31 percent fewer mothers nursed their babies in 1968 than a decade earlier;[6] the $33 million waste for that year is nearly double the $17 million waste of 1958. In Colombia, as breast feeding of babies from birth to eleven months declined, milk imports increased rapidly; in 1968, they were seven times greater than the 1964–67 average.[7]

The estimated costs of breast milk losses would be lower if the additional calories recommended for a lactating mother were taken into account.[8] But poor women in poor countries seldom get an enlarged or special diet during lactation. (Nearly three-quarters of low-income women studied in Gujarat and two-thirds in Maharastra reported taking no special foods during the nursing period.[9]) When extra food is consumed, it is usually much less than is recommended. (The average intake by lactating women in India is 1,425 calories, half the recommended allowance.[10]) If a mother were to eat all the additive calories recommended during nursing —and efforts should be made to encourage this—the cost would still be less than a third of that necessary to provide artificial feeding to the infant. Generally, breast feeding is satisfactory for the infant even without extra food for the mother, but the child's need is met at the expense of the mother's tissue, a very real health cost.[11]

### Losses in Urban Areas

In most low-income countries, breast feeding is the general rule in rural areas. Its abandonment is primarily an urban phenomenon, often not so much because urban mothers work as because bottle feeding is one of the sophistications of city life the urban migrant adopts.[12]

Three-quarters of all mothers in the rural Punjab still breast-feed twenty months after delivery, half at twenty-six months, and a quarter at thirty-three months. In major Indian cities, however, approximately a third of the mothers either do not begin nursing or discontinue it within a year.

The rural-urban pattern is consistent throughout the poor countries of the world. In Guatemala, 98 percent of rural Indian babies continue to be nursed after their first birthday, compared with 57 percent of urban children. In Indonesia the comparable figures are 90 percent and 70 percent. In Taiwan, 97 percent of rural mothers breast-feed their offspring for six months compared with 61 percent of their urban counterparts. In Gambian cities, breast feeding usually ends between six and nine months after delivery; in rural areas, weaning comes between twelve and twenty-four months.[13]

The concentration of the loss of breast feeding in urban environments is especially alarming because cities in developing countries are undergoing mammoth growth. In addition, as communications techniques become more effective, city habits and life styles will have an increasing influence on rural societies. In rural Mexico the decline in breast feeding is already being felt; between 1960 and 1966 the percentage of babies under six months of age who were fed only by breast milk in one rural Mexican community declined from 95 to 73.[14]

An estimated 87 percent of the world's babies are born in the developing countries, about a quarter of them in urban areas. If 20 percent of the estimated 27 million mothers in urban areas do not breast-feed, the loss in breast milk is $365 million. If half of the other 80 percent do not continue to breast-feed after the first six months, the total loss reaches $780 million. These estimates, however, clearly understate the situation; losses to developing countries more likely are in the billions.

### Breast Feeding as Birth Control

In terms of national development, lactation has another major economic asset—its link to family planning. As a key to child survival, better nutrition through breast feeding may be an important precondition for reducing birthrates. Another benefit of breast feeding is its role in limiting conception; in some societies, in fact, it may constitute a major form of contraception. There is little doubt that breast feeding offers better protection against pregnancy for up to ten to twelve months than does the sort of haphazard and ineffective contraception practiced in many places.[15]

The pregnancy-preventing effect of lactation is firmly rooted in the folklore of unsophisticated societies. Recent studies have lent credence to the notion. One investigation reported that the incidence of pregnancy in the first nine months after childbirth of nonnursing mothers was twice that of mothers who breast-fed, including those who simultaneously used other foods. Others confirm that although breast feeding does not serve as a perfect contraceptive, the risk of pregnancy is relatively small for mothers whose babies receive only breast milk.[16]

The contraceptive value of lactation is most effective if in the first four to six months the infant receives only human milk, for the sucking stimulus appears to inhibit ovulation.[17] In the lactating mother, menstruation and ovulation are delayed from ten weeks to as long as twenty-six months. In Taiwan it was estimated that lactation prevented as many as 20 percent of the births that would have occurred otherwise.[18] In India the same ratio would mean prevention of approximately five million births each year.

In some areas of the world where breast feeding is regarded as essential to a baby's survival, social custom limits sexual intercourse for lactating women, thus reinforcing the link between breast feeding and contraception. Intercourse is avoided as long as one year after giving birth in parts of India, for two years in New Guinea, and twenty-seven months in Nigeria. In some societies the taboo reflects the belief that intercourse will dry up the milk flow and in others that it will poison the milk. In parts of South Africa, if a baby dies, it is assumed the mother has ignored the taboo, thus killing her baby with "bad milk."[19]

### Costs in Infant Health

Just as breast milk can be the major source of nutrition, the failure to provide breast milk is a major cause of infant malnutrition and mortality. (And just as premature weaning is harmful, human milk unsupplemented with other foods is, after four to six months, inadequate both in protein and calories.[20] A child fed breast milk only until the age of twelve or eighteen months becomes "breast starved.") Discontinuance of nursing implies an alternative source of food, which in the early months is often in the form of a nutritionally inadequate substitute, such as barley water or cornstarch and water.[21] Milk "formulas," when used, usually are mixed with contaminated water and offered in an unclean bottle with a crusty nipple. (One investigation, for example, found that 80 percent of bottles examined had a high bacterial contamination.[22]) The reasons are clear. Poor parents usually cannot afford sustained purchases of commercial milk and as a result commonly dilute it (in Lebanon, by two or three to one[23]) or substitute for it (in Indonesia, with rice fluid costing a half cent per kilogram[24]). Their lack of education prevents them from reading or understanding the instructions for preparation and, together with ignorance of sanitary requirements, fosters a high incidence of illness. Even mothers aware of hygienic needs often find it difficult to meet them with limited and unclean water, inadequate fuel, poor storage, and a single bottle and nipple. In Chile half the mothers receiving milk from the National Health Service were found to be using it incorrectly.[25] For these reasons, bottle-fed infants have illnesses, especially diarrhea, more frequently, more severely, and earlier than breast-fed babies.[26]

Diarrhea occurred ten times more frequently in a group of nonbreast-fed Mexican children than in a group of breast-fed children. In Liverpool, England, in 1943 the rate of gastroenteritis among bottle-fed babies was more than twelve times that among breast-fed infants.[27]

Bottle-fed infants also have a much higher mortality rate than those exclusively breast-fed. According to a 1970 study in San Salvador, three-quarters of the infants who died from the end of the first through fifth month had been breast-fed less than thirty days, if at all; of those who died in the last half of the first year of life, slightly over half had been breast-fed less than a month. A similar study in Recife makes the point even more dramatically: 79 percent of the children who died in the second through fifth month had been breast-fed less than a month; 70 percent of those who died in the ensuing six months, and 60 percent in the following four years, had been nursed for less than a month or not at all. Deaths of children from diarrheal diseases (which are usually nutrition related) in Recife, where only 22 percent of the children were breast-fed at least one month, were nearly three times the rate in Kingston, where the corresponding figure is 73 percent.[28]

As breast feeding has decreased over the past two decades, the average age of youngsters suffering from severe forms of malnutrition has also dropped—from eighteen to eight months.[29] Generally in India, severe protein-calorie malnutrition is found less frequently among those under one year than those between one and two. However, among Indian immigrants in south Trinidad, protein-calorie malnutrition is much higher in the first year than in the second, and the decline in breast feeding of infants in this age group is believed to be responsible.[30] Since malnutrition in the early months of life is most critical to brain development, this lowering of the average age of incidence of severe nutritional deficiencies takes on special significance.

## Policy Implications

Such concerns have received virtually no attention from national planners. In the increasingly broad spectrum of nutrition options that national ministries examine—food fortification, genetic seed improvement, processed foods employing new protein technologies, dairying and agricultural projects, even (interestingly, in this context) food waste prevention—programs that address this most fundamental determinant of infant nutrition are conspicuously absent. Whence this neglect? Few officials seem to have given it any thought. One Indian planner who had paid fleeting attention to the value of breast milk dismissed it as a "commodity I could do nothing about." He admitted being frightened off by the intimate nature of the subject. Breast milk plays such a dominant role in infant nutrition that inaction in face of this trend casts a touch of irony on the current efforts to promote other, less consequential, nutrition activities.

## The Practice of Breast Feeding

Historically, human milk has been universally recognized and revered as the only means of infant feeding. Frequent references to it are found in religion, folklore, and value systems. The Koran prescribes that "mothers shall suckle their children for two whole years." In ancient Egypt, nursing was commonly continued for three years, and in biblical Israel for two years. In Babylonia, the mother goddess Ishtar was often depicted nursing her baby. A Spartan royal law of the fourth century B.C. required mothers to breast-feed their babies, and Caesar ridiculed Roman mothers who retained nurses for their children.

"The sap of immortal life divine" is the way breast milk was described in the ancient Indian ayurvedic writings. The glorification of breast milk was reflected in the prayers the physician recited as he worked a charm over the mother to promote lactation during the first feeding: "May four oceans, full of milk, constantly abide in both your breasts. . . . Drinking of the milk whose sap is the sap of immortal life divine, may your boy gain long life, as do the gods by feeding on the beverage of immortality."[31] Even today in north India, village women often demand similar ritual ceremonies, the timing of which is influenced by a particular star or an "auspicious" time.[32] Usually the rites require a symbolic washing of the breast with buttermilk and grass by the sister-in-law; if she lives at a distance, the initiation of breast feeding may be held up two or three days.

Early Indian belief held that the longer the child received breast milk, the longer would be his life, and it was not uncommon therefore for children to be breast-fed up to the ages of seven and nine years.[33] But prolonged breast feeding practices are not confined to antiquity. Forty years ago, Chinese and Japanese mothers nursed their children up to five and six years, Caroline Islanders up to ten years, and Eskimos up to fifteen years. In 1943, children in Burma reportedly were nursed from three to four years, and in 1950 in Kenya sometimes for five years.[34] A 1969 study near Hyderabad found nearly 30 percent of youngsters breast-fed between ages three and four, and 10 percent between ages four and five.[35] In south Asia in the 1950s, breast feeding up to age three was typical.[36]

### The Merits of Breast Milk

Human milk is in many ways the perfect food.* In the words of Oliver Wendell Holmes, "the breasts were more skillful at compounding a feeding mixture than the hemispheres of the most learned professor's brain."[41]

---

* In the second century A.D. the Greek pediatrician Soranus prescribed a technique for determining the quality of breast milk that was used for the next fifteen hundred years: a drop of good milk placed on a fingernail, laurel leaf, or other smooth surface would, when shaken, retain its shape.[37] In India the ancient *Sarira*

Breast milk is healthful; it meets most of the metabolic needs of the baby; it contributes to good growth; it is clean, thus lowering the risk of intestinal illness and general infection. Furthermore, it provides a host of protective factors. Breast-fed babies are more resistant to malaria and to infection caused by bacteria or viruses (including the polio virus). And they are less likely to suffer from rickets and iron-deficiency anemia.[42]

Breast milk, unlike many substitute foods, is easily digestible. Also, the baby generally is receptive (a study of West Bengali women who stopped breast feeding revealed that in only one case was this because the baby refused the breast).[43] Breast milk is readily available and requires no preparation of any kind. The rural West African mother commonly conducts her business—even striding along, carrying a basket on her head—while the youngster perched on her back feeds from her long pendulum-shaped breasts stretched to the side. Moreover, the quantity of breast milk for the infant's first half year is relatively satisfactory, even though the mother's diet may be inadequate.

Although nursing makes physiological demands on the mother with an inadequate diet, breast feeding is in some ways beneficial to the health of the mother. The nursing woman, because she does not usually menstruate, conserves her iron stores—an important consideration in poor countries where many women are anemic. Breast feeding is pleasurable, offering the mother the contentment of contributing very immediately to her baby's well-being.[44] Also, of course, it greatly reduces the cost of child rearing. For the affluent, milk purchases may not pose a financial burden, but their purchases for early weaning from a stable local supply increase demand and therefore price, thus reducing the ability of the poor to purchase milk for their families.

### The Decline

The current trend away from extended nursing in most of the poorer countries apparently has been strongly influenced by the wealthier ones. A

---

*Sthana* said that milk should have "natural color, smell, taste and touch and when poured into a pot of water, it should mix at once and perfectly with the water, being of a natural kind."[38] In China a milk drop on the table must be round and raised and not capable of being blown into smaller drops. A sample is weighed on the gold scale and when the pan is full, the milk should weigh two *chien* and eight *li*.[39] In Pakistan, milk is dropped on a beetle, which supposedly will die if the milk is not good. If milk dropped on a wall runs down, it is too heavy and harmful according to the Telegus in south India, but if it is quickly absorbed, it is regarded as good for the infant.[40] In at least one society, the test of good milk is its ability to attract flies.

continuing nationwide study of 2.5 million babies in the United States found that the number of mothers who were breast feeding at the time they left the maternity hospital had declined by nearly half in only ten years; the national average, which had dropped from 38 percent to 21 percent from 1946 to 1956, slid again to 18 percent in the following decade. The decline is most pronounced in the poorest states. In Arkansas, 84 percent of infants were totally or partially breast-fed in 1946; by 1966, only 22 percent. The analogous figures for California are 60 percent and 38 percent.[45]

Although there has been a resurgence of interest in breast feeding in the United States, it has been concentrated among the college-trained and well-to-do.[46] In the Boston area, breast feeding was found to be nearly twice as prevalent among upper income families as among lower income families.[47] Middle income mothers in New York and San Francisco were six times more likely to breast-feed their babies than lower income mothers.[48] In a circumscribed poverty area in Chicago, only 5.9 percent of infants under one month old were being breast-fed.[49] Nationwide surveys in 1971 showed that 32 percent of college-educated mothers breast-fed compared with 8 percent of grade-school educated mothers.[50]

Declines in breast feeding similar to that in the United States have been noted in Great Britain, Australia, Sweden, and Poland.[51] The stigma against nursing, with its unfortunate consequences, is one of the values unwittingly communicated to the less industralized world. In developing countries, artificial feeding—fashionable at first only among mothers of higher income with an awareness of hygienic needs—has penetrated to middle and even lower income families, especially in urban settings with their fully developed advertising and other communications and their premium on sophistication.[52] A 1970 Brazilian study of 879 public maternity centers reported that after their first day, only 44 percent of the babies were fully breast-fed.[53] In urbanized southeast Asia, it was not unusual for mothers-to-be to arrive at the hospital carrying canned formula.[54]

Although children can thrive on artificial feeding under ideal conditions, the income, education, and sanitation levels are rarely adequate in developing countries. Women who do not have the purchasing power to sustain proper artificial feeding, once begun, and who do not recognize possible dangers, are apt to dilute milk and baby foods heavily. In Latin America, mothers use a popular corn starch as a baby food, assuming it is like milk because, when mixed with water, it looks like milk.

*Why the Decline?*

What are the causes for the dramatic decline in breast feeding? Encroaching urbanization and modernization and new social values are significant influences. Breast feeding is often viewed as an old-fashioned or backward custom and, by some, as a vulgar peasant practice. Indeed, anthropologists, struck by the relationship of artificial feeding to societal change, have used the duration of nursing as an inverse measure of acculturation for some countries. In most developing countries, the greater the sophistication, the worse the lactation: the bottle has become a status symbol.[55]

Failure of lactation is one of the responses to the stress of modernization. Among the tensions in a changing environment is the mother's anxiety about her capacity to breast feed. Her failure to initiate or to continue breast feeding is rarely traced to a physical cause* but often to psychophysiological causes that interfere with the key "let-down reflex." In a study of Indian women, over 80 percent of the highly educated in the highest socioeconomic group were unable to breast-feed their infants for as long as six months, while among the lowest socioeconomic classes, failure to breast-feed the infants for at least six months "was practically unknown." "Social and cultural factors and their psychological and emotional accompaniments were far more important determinants of lactation performance than dietary and nutritional factors."[57]    *158565*

Changing social attitudes regarding the body reinforce the trend. Some women fear that breast feeding will ruin the shape of their breasts, a crucial concern in the increasing number of societies that emphasize their role in sexual attractiveness.†[58] In parts of Africa, where less than a generation ago women rarely wore upper garments, photographs of bare-bosomed women are now banned. Nursing in public, a common sight a decade ago in most parts of the developing world, is rapidly disappearing, as the modesty accompanying the changes in attitude grows.

Convenience also is a factor in the abandonment of breast feeding. Women no longer bound by tradition and now enabled by the changing

---

* It is conservatively estimated that 85 percent of all women have the capacity to breast feed for six months or longer.[56] Physiological difficulties, such as breast engorgement, mastitis, and inverted nipples, rarely occur, and even then do not prevent breast feeding.

† The effect is equally deleterious among Chinese women in Singapore who "despise the normal female figure and thus wear tight bodices which produce atrophy of the breasts and depressed nipples.[59]

pattern of home life to take advantage of an increasing number of diversions have turned to artificial feeding to free themselves from the constraints of motherhood. Although this is especially true of those who wish to join the organized work force, they are only a small part of the women who have abandoned breast feeding.[60] In Latin American countries, less than a fourth of women of child-bearing age hold jobs, and in Egypt only 6 percent. Only 15 percent of the nonnursers in the West Indies and 10 percent of those in Singapore are employed (in jobs recorded in labor statistics; others, of course, work at odd jobs).

For many women, improved communication has brought knowledge of the alternatives to breast feeding. A leading Latin American nutritionist reports an immediate decrease in breast feeding as the unsophisticated Chilean mother learns of the existence of infant formulas via alluring advertising claims.[61] In some countries, aggressive sales promotion tactics persuade the new mother to succumb to the blandishments of the processed food companies. In the West Indies, competitive representatives of baby food manufacturers visit the homes of new mothers and give free product samples.[62] And in Nigeria, women from commercial firms make the rounds of maternity clinics, distributing free samples (doctors are given supplies for their own children[63]). "The pediatric nutritionist is left increasingly frustrated by the well financed, steam roller, marketing techniques of the food industry to sell totally unaffordable and inappropriate infant foods in impoverished communities, while mouthing sanctimonious platitudes about their world role in improving child nutrition."[64]

The easy availability of free skim milk through institutional feeding programs also has been blamed for the wholesale defections from breast feeding. Distribution of free powdered milk—including that sponsored by the National Health Service—has been partly responsible for the radical decline of breast feeding among Chilean mothers.[65]

## A Conservation Policy

Given societal sensitivities and the highly personal nature of the subject, is it possible to intervene to reverse this trend? The potential for success of any organized effort is by no means clear. Yet, even modest improvements—an increase by a few percentage points of the proportions of mothers who elect to breast-feed, or extension of nursing by a few weeks or months for those who already do—could be translated into millions of dollars and, more importantly, probably millions of lives.

The idea of a government campaign to encourage maternal nursing is not new. The high infant mortality related to an eighteenth century vogue against breast feeding led the French government to print posters encouraging mothers to nurse.*[66] Finland reportedly went further; by royal proclamation, penalties were assessed on nonnursing mothers whose children died in the first six months of their lives.[68] After the decline in weight and height of British infantry recruits forced the minimum height requirement down from 5 feet 6 inches to 5 feet 3 inches in 1883 and to 5 feet in 1900, questions in Parliament led to a committee investigation and ultimately to a campaign to encourage breast feeding.[69] In the mid-1960s the government of Uganda made a conscious effort to convince mothers that breast feeding is not a backward custom. And in the United States, sixteen years after it was formed in 1956, the La Leche League had 1,220 groups promoting maternal nursing.

To design a single campaign that would be applicable to the many and diverse cultures in developing countries would be impossible. Some societies may be ready for a confrontation with the problem employing all the resources of the mass media while in others public mores would demand, at least at the outset, a more discreet form of intervention. Moreover, a campaign properly designed to meet cultural constraints may find political and economic obstacles impeding its success. Yet, recognizing these inherent difficulties, the costs and potential obstacles of such a campaign may be less imposing than those of alternate nutrition intervention programs designed to achieve the same ends.

### Improve Understanding

The most essential objective of a campaign to counter the current trend is improved understanding of the benefits of breast feeding and of the dangers of forgoing it. (Linked with this should be an effort to encourage added caloric intake for the mother during the nursing period and adequate food supplements to the child in the second six months of life.) A

---

* According to Walter Harris, the outstanding pediatrician of the late seventeenth and early eighteenth centuries, "Ladies of quality did not breast feed so they could have more time to dress, receive and pay visits, attend public shews and spend the night at their beloved cards."[67]

conscious campaign apparently can make a dramatic difference: An educational effort in Minneapolis designed to increase breast feeding in 1920 had the result that 93 percent of mothers nursed for at least three months, 80 percent for at least seven months, and 72 percent for at least nine months. Infant deaths, which had averaged 772 a year in the previous three years (and were higher before that), dropped to 65 in the first year of the campaign.[70] The work was replicated in Nassau County, New York, with comparable results.[71]

The stark facts about illness and death among nonbreast-fed babies in low-income countries must be convincingly communicated. Where feasible, the message that human milk is a safe, ready-made, simple, and inexpensive form of nutrition should be carried via mass media because of their apparent effectiveness in changing food habits. The same advertising techniques that partly are responsible for the increase in artificial feeding can be used to counter the trend.

Even in societies liberated from tradition, some will be uneasy about attracting public attention to breast feeding. Here, family planning is an encouraging forerunner. Not too long ago, contraception was a subject fit for discussion primarily in medical circles. In India, concern arose when large billboards promoting family planning were first erected in the mid-1960s. Letters to the editor about them reflected embarrassment, repugnance, and, as could be expected, amusement. Since then, however, the country has been blanketed with family planning propaganda and its discussion, if not its practice, has become an accepted part of Indian life.

India also has begun to create awareness of the need for breast feeding. In 1970 a photograph of a mother nursing her child appeared in a four-column advertisement in a number of national periodicals. Although care was taken to insure that the picture would be inoffensive, criticism was anticipated. None materialized. In fact, the public response to the offer of a free nutrition booklet was reported to be among the highest to a single advertisement in the history of Indian advertising. Posters declaring "Breast Feeding Is Best for Baby" also have had wide distribution in Zambia and in South Africa.

In countries where cultural inhibitions about breast feeding rule out the use of billboards or other media designed to reach the general public, efforts should be made to direct the campaign selectively to the easily identifiable audience of young mothers-to-be. Magazines and daytime radio programs directed specifically to women can serve as channels. Places where women congregate—the city bazaar, the village well—are obvious dissemination points. The package containing special women's products can carry the message, and health clinics and maternity hospitals can easily reach women at the critical time. Home science classes for girls are only the most obvious of the many opportunities the school system offers.

In creating awareness, rehabilitation of the social acceptability of breast feeding should not be neglected. The objective must be not only to remove the stigma of backwardness associated with nursing, but to defuse the sexual association. Perhaps there is no better technique to achieve these ends than the testimonial. In Uganda, Mrs. Milton Obote, wife of the former president, appealed on television for breast feeding among her people. Cinema stars and other public figures could do much to upgrade the acceptability of breast feeding and to remove its recently acquired taint of embarrassment. Experience in Israel and the Soviet Union demonstrates that, with proper societal attitudes, the decline in breast feeding need not be an inevitable consequence of urbanization.

### Regulation of Advertising and Sales Techniques

A more forceful step toward halting the undesirable trend away from breast feeding is government action to control the advertising that might best be described as "antinutrition education." At a minimum, advertisers should be required to abandon the misleading claims of some patented baby foods, both explicit and implicit—the Latin American advertisement for corn starch that, making no overt claims to being a baby food, nevertheless prominently features the picture of a robust infant.* But these are obvious cases for action. Even honest advertising presents problems. In India, one of the honored trade names advertises its baby food: "Use [our formula] as a substitute for breast milk . . . right from the first week." Intrusion on an existing commercial activity is, of course, difficult. Advertising means revenue for the media and sales to the manufacturers, benefits they will not relinquish without battle. Food firms are large and their markets extensive, and they are not without their influence on government. If political realities make regulatory action impossible, informal

---

* A more palatable but administratively awkward method would be to require that the products be advertised in the context of the alternatives. Rather than boast of "superior quality," an ad might read: "Next to mother's milk, $X$ is best"; or "If your baby can't have mother's milk, $X$ will give him the nutrients he needs." Governments can also insist that producers of packaged baby foods include highly simplified instructions for safe preparation.

pressures should be applied to make food companies aware of the harm their products can do and to encourage voluntary compliance to some standards.

Just as advertising needs control, so do the product promotion techniques that food firms employ. The young mother, frequently uneducated, is ill equipped to reject persuasive arguments and, besides, once having weaned her child, is in need of commercial products. (For those women who cannot or should not nurse their children, milk substitutes are, of course, extremely useful.) Those who artificially create this need for their own profit are obvious candidates for control and even penalty. Governments should prohibit in their health facilities the commercial posters, calendars, and other sales media promoting products inappropriate for local usage. Representatives of such products should be denied access to government facilities (especially hospitals, health centers, and schools) for product demonstration and distribution of free samples.

### Facilities and Incentives for Breast Feeding

Governments can encourage breast feeding by making it more convenient. In urban areas where privacy is virtually nonexistent, inexpensive facilities can be provided. Just as governments build bus stands and public restrooms, so might they provide small structures in crowded downtown areas for nursing mothers. Similarly, special rooms for nursing could be set aside in factories and other places of employment.

Mothers who breast-feed might be given incentives. For the working mother, this may mean government regulations requiring that she be allowed nursing time. In the Soviet Union a four-month maternity leave is granted to make sure that the mother establishes a breast-feeding routine before she returns to work; when she does return, the baby is put in a nursery at the place of employment, and every three hours the mother is given a nursing break.[72] Monetary and material bonuses may also serve as inducements for mothers who nurse their youngsters. Early in the century, British mothers were offered free or very inexpensive meals during lactation.[73]

In Switzerland, monetary incentives are provided to mothers who nurse their children at least ten weeks; the system began in 1911 when only 43 percent of Swiss women nursed their young and the mortality rate for nonbreast-fed children was double that of those being nursed.* The incentives apparently had the desired effects until the last decade when, amidst Swiss affluence, "the breast feeding allowance (raised most recently in 1964) is no longer able to fight against the present trend which consists in not breast feeding."[75]

### Recognizing Problems of Free Milk Distribution

It is the responsibility of those who plan free milk programs to recognize the problems they may raise. Such activities—especially the distribution of dry skim milk, which often is directed to the infant—must not be allowed to act as a disincentive to breast feeding. The Chilean government during the last ten years has increased twelvefold the free milk available for infants, but the decline in breast feeding has been even greater and, perhaps relatedly, the infant mortality rate in urban areas has increased.[76]

### Influencing the Professionals

Obstetricians, pediatricians, general practitioners, midwives, medical students, nurses, auxiliaries, and other government health workers should be indoctrinated in the importance of breast feeding and breast-feeding methods. Medical education generally gives little attention to nursing and often emphasizes the importance of artificial feeding. Of the sixteen hundred pages in the major U.S. textbook on pediatrics, only one and a half concern breast feeding, with no mention of the "let-down reflex."[77] A number of observers have suggested that the indifference of the health profession is at least partly responsible for the decline in breast feeding.[78] Health workers must be educated to the importance of breast feeding and both before and immediately after birth make every effort to counsel new mothers accordingly.

### Preventing Failure of Lactation

Finally, efforts must be undertaken to prevent lactation failure, which has become increasingly common under stress of modernization. A program should include information not only on the "why" of breast feeding,

* Unsuccessful efforts were made by special commissions in both 1945 and 1954 to increase the period to six months.[74]

but also its "how." Where breast feeding is widely practiced, the effort should be to preserve the practice while not calling undue attention to the techniques. In a traditional society with an accepting, matter-of-fact attitude toward the ability to nurse, lessons that raise questions could be confusing and cause anxieties that could be counterproductive.

THE DRAMATIC decline in breast feeding in the low-income countries, especially in rapidly growing urban areas, means a staggering loss in one of the primary determinants of nutritional status. The cost is substantial, both in high mortality and morbidity rates and in outright economic loss. Moreover, fertility rates are also affected, since breast feeding probably has prevented more conceptions than all other forms of contraception.

The silent loss of such a major resource is cause for concern. Steps can be taken and the size and implications of the problem should be examined and techniques be carefully designed to deal with it. For the vulnerable infant and young child, an effective public effort to counter the current trend may be of greater significance than any other form of nutrition intervention.

## CHAPTER EIGHT

# The New Foods

The prospect of meeting the nutrition needs of the young with appropriate food at the appropriate age is enhanced by new technologies that have dramatically reduced the cost and effort of providing good nutrition. Although no panacea, these technologies are of major significance. Despite all the talk about the scale of the malnutrition problem, attempts to combat it have been modest, chiefly because of the absence of a powerful low-cost method for short-cutting the slow and passive reliance on income growth.

The widespread acceptance of malaria programs is an illuminating case in point. Although thoroughgoing analyses of the economic benefits of reducing malaria were lacking, and planners guided by a surplus-labor theory were skeptical there could be benefits, a massive program was accepted for worldwide implementation. This acceptance may have been due partly to the effective advocates and to the international steam they generated. But it also reflected the fact that advocates of malaria prevention had a powerful technology that appeared to offer good prospects for substantial if not total elimination of a problem that affected large numbers of people at a very modest per capita cost and in a short time. Malnutrition today affects vastly more people than malaria ever did. But malnutrition is not carried by a vector that obligingly parks on the wall; compared to it, malaria presented a relatively simple technical problem. Now, however, the nutrition picture may change.

Hope today lies in foods that a decade ago would have been dismissed as fanciful. Perhaps more important, new food concepts have evolved that may lead to substantial advances. Man can now sprinkle synthetic micronutrients while milling flour; the child fed a few slices of bread baked from that flour has the vitamin, mineral, and protein equivalent of a diet studded with fruits, vegetables, and milk. Or man can produce a whole range of palatable new foods, bolstered by nutritious oilseed products that until a few years ago were considered unsuitable for human consumption.

The value of such feats is clear when nutritional need is contrasted with consumption in low-income countries. Earlier reference was made, for instance, to large numbers of children with serious vitamin A deficiencies, which lead to impaired growth, increased susceptibility to infection, and visual handicaps that can be as severe as total blindness. To meet its vitamin A requirements through traditional means, India would require 200 percent more fruit and nearly 300 percent more vegetables,[1] with all of the increases going to the nutritionally needy. But for less than 2 cents per person a year in raw material costs, nonconventional forms of vitamin A can be added to existing food staples.

The new nutrition technologies can be divided into two broad categories: those concerned with the enhancement of the nutritive value of existing foods by fortification and those concerned with the formulation of new foods. (Genetic seed improvement might also be categorized as a new nutrition technology.) Key to the success of both approaches are new low-cost nutritious ingredients, a large number of which have been developed in recent years.

## Fortification

Where foods can be centrally processed, one of the most attractive means for better nutrition is fortification—bolstering the nutritive value of processed foods already prominent in the diet.* The principle of fortification challenges the long-standing belief that the consumer must consciously desire and be involved in nutritional change. "Health is not something you can do to people, they have to do it to themselves"[2] is a common theme in nutrition forums. Scientific knowledge for better nutrition "cannot . . . be used where it is needed unless the people themselves want to use it, know how to do so, and are prepared to accept the changes necessary for its effective use";[3] this, the prevailing attitude of the professional community of a decade ago, is maintained in some quarters today.

---

* One purpose is to restore vitamins, minerals, and protein lost during processing: the milling of cereals, for example, removes the germ and bran, and with them most of the vitamins and minerals and the better part of the protein. Another is to increase the level of nutrients beyond those in the raw product and to inject other nutrients. The restoration of lost nutrients is generally termed "enrichment." Carrying the process further, or adding still other nutrients, is called "fortification." For purposes of simplicity, the term "fortification" will be used to apply to both.

*Early Efforts*

The use of existing foods as carriers for additional nutrition is not new, but mass exploitation of the idea to benefit nutritionally needy countries is. In the mid-1930s a substantial segment of the U.S. population was deficient in iron, thiamine, niacin, and riboflavin, and diseases clearly caused by nutritional deficiency—anemia, beriberi, pellagra, and ariboflavinosis —were prevalent. Those scientists and public health officials searching for remedies first considered widespread use of vitamin pills but recognized the difficulty of getting them to those who needed them most. The group next considered public programs designed to increase the consumption of non-processed grain. But this, too, was discarded because of lack of success in earlier efforts and the slowness of nutrition education. Large-scale distribution of special foods to the needy was also considered, but was not regarded as economically feasible. The group finally concluded "the way to get the needed nutrients back into the diet was to add them back to the flour and to get them into the one food most common on most tables— namely, bread. . . . It was a simple matter to determine how much of the thiamine, niacin, riboflavin and iron should be added to the bread so that five or six slices a day per person would bring . . . these nutrients up to the human requirement and thereby prevent the deficiency diseases which were so widespread."[4]

The fortification would not alter the bread's acceptability to the consumer, nor would the cost cause the baker to increase the price of his product or seriously disturb his profit.[5] The formal proposal, in 1940, to fortify processed wheat stirred congressional and public debate. Several of the arguments raised are echoed today in other parts of the world: people should use only natural foods; synthetic fortification will create an imbalance of nutrients; the National Institutes of Health is a tool of the drug industry looking for business; the value of fortification cannot be proved.

It was not until World War II, when public attention turned to the need for a strong citizenry, that a National Mandatory Enrichment Policy finally was issued. The order was rescinded at the conclusion of the war, but nearly 92 percent of all commercial white bread and nearly all retailed flour in the United States continues to be enriched. Thirty-four states require it by law.

Many of the deficiencies that were on the rise in the United States in the late 1930s have virtually disappeared. Of the vitamin deficiency diseases then measured in the hundreds of thousands of cases, it is now difficult to find a case for study. The number of deaths due to pellagra in 1966 was 1.1 percent of the figure for 1941. Of course, a great deal else was happening during the same period, and much of the nutritional improvement might have taken place anyway as a result of the buoyant economy. The isolation of the fortification variable is reflected, however, in studies of chronic alcoholics, whose bread-and-gravy diets went unchanged during the period of national economic growth. Much beriberi and pellagra were found among the alcoholics in 1941. A study of the same group in 1946, after nutrients were added to the bread, found no trace of these diseases.[6]

An even more dramatic claim for fortification results from experience in Newfoundland, where infant mortality was high, tuberculosis increasing, and diet deficiencies prevalent. A 1944 law required all margarine to be fortified with vitamin A and all white flour with niacin, iron, thiamine, riboflavin, and calcium. After four years a remarkable improvement was noted, and by 1953, infant mortality rates had dropped 63 percent, and stillbirths 59 percent; tuberculosis was reduced 81 percent, and the once common beriberi had disappeared.[7]

In the Philippine province of Bataan, severe beriberi was common in 1947. By late 1950, with the introduction of thiamine-enriched rice, the disease had declined 89 percent among 63,000 people studied, and no beriberi mortality was reported.[8] In immediately adjoining areas, where rice was left in its normal processed state, the incidence of beriberi increased during the same period. Despite the success of the experiment, a nationwide rice fortification program was never implemented in the Philippines. The experiment, however, encouraged Taiwan to institute a large-scale project for its armed forces that resulted in a dramatic decline in thiamine deficiency.

In Great Britain, measures instituted during and after World War II, when more than 50 percent of the British food supply was cut off, included fortification with calcium and a higher extraction rate that reduced nutrient losses in the milling of wheat. The national health at the end of the crisis was generally regarded as better than before the emergency began. In 1921 three-fourths of the children in New York City showed signs of rickets. Now, due in great part to the widespread vitamin D fortification of milk, infantile rickets in the United States is extremely rare.* The iodization of salt is an outstanding example of effective fortification. In the heart

---

* A similarly wide success has been the dramatic reduction in the rate of dental caries—reduced by as much as 65 percent—following water fluoridation in communities in the United States and Canada.[9]

of the endemic goiter belt of India, the prevalence of goiter among those consuming fortified salt declined from 38 percent of the population to 15 percent in five years, and down to 3 percent in ten years.[10] There was a total absence of goiter and related cretinism and deaf-mutism among children born during the period. Among those who used unfortified salt, the incidence of goiter rose. These striking results were matched in Guatemala, where endemic goiter dropped from 39 percent in 1952 to 15 percent in 1962 to 5 percent of the population in 1965. In neighboring Central American countries, where salt went unfortified, the goiter rates did not decrease during the same period.[11]

### The Limitations

Fortification is not without its limitations. Only those people who rely on marketed processed foods benefit. The fortification of milled cereals, for example, will not help people in a rural subsistence economy who grow and grind their own. In Bangladesh, fewer than 20 percent of rice eaters purchase their rice in a commercial market. Moreover, a viable fortification project depends on large-scale central processing. In rural areas where inhabitants buy locally grown and processed grain, special equipment and controls would be required in thousands of small rice and wheat milling units.

Fortification also implies broad coverage, reaching those who do not need the help as well as those who do. Thus, to reach preschool-aged youngsters of low-income families, nutrients may have to be given to people of all ages and all income groups (some of whom will benefit) who consume the same product. This may be an uneconomical means of providing nutrients to the target group. Inevitably fortification raises the cost of the final product, though usually only by a fraction. If the cost is passed on to the consumer, he may reduce his purchases of other foods or the quantities of the fortified product he buys. Unless fortification is mandatory or the cost is absorbed by the government or the manufacturer, cheaper unfortified brands of the processed food will be available. The consumer who needs the fortifiers most is least likely to pay the premium.

The costs of fortification are recurring, unlike those of nutrition education which is designed to change a habit and should at some stage become unnecessary for a specified group, or of genetic seed improvement which also would have an end in sight. Moreover, public sentiment occasionally puts restraints on fortification efforts; the fear that fortification "adulterates" food is epitomized in the campaign to prevent fluoridation of water in the United States. Fear of unknown hazards of the nutrients, and especially suspected dangers of uncontrolled levels of intake, heighten public concern.*

### The Advantages

Despite its limitations, fortification is an attractive mechanism to provide better nutrition. It does not require changes in eating, cooking, or purchasing habits. Ideally, added nutrients do not affect the traditional character of the food: it looks, feels, tastes, and smells exactly like the unfortified product. Generally, fortification is not a costly way—often it is the least costly—to provide nutrients to the needy, and even the "nutrient wastage" incurred in the broadside delivery to the nonneedy does not alter this fact. Few, if any, special marketing measures are required for fortified products—no special packaging, promotion, or merchandising, no separate distribution apparatus.

The benefits of fortification appear in a much shorter time than those of projects to formulate new foods, to improve seeds genetically, or to promote education in nutrition. A large-scale fortification activity can be mounted and put into operation in a matter of months; it involves few decision makers and few administrators. A new supplementary child feeding program, by contrast, may require a host of approvals and involvements at the federal, state, and local levels in its development as well as an army of field operatives to run the feeding activity.

Although fortification may fail to benefit rural areas where centrally processed cereal foods are not marketed, swelling populations in urban areas are easily reached. They often are nutritionally critical groups, for processed foods increasingly displace fresh foods in urban diets. (It may be feasible to reach rural populations with some fortified foods, such as salt, tea, or sugar. For example, 90 percent of all sugar in El Salvador passes through one refinery.) One benefit of fortification is that it seldom reduces the total food supply; synthetics or oilseed residues seldom used

---

* The public fear of food additives—preservatives, emulsifiers, mold inhibitors, binders, bleachers, and other nonnutrient agents designed to improve texture, flavor, appearance, and storage—should not be allowed to slip over to fortification. Fortifiers should be identified not as additives but as "requirements" for processed foods to meet established minimum nutrition levels.[12]

for human consumption are the most frequent additives. Even if consumed in larger-than-intended quantities, fortifiers rarely pose a health hazard.*

Where target groups can be reached with processed foods, fortification is among the simplest of the options available for improving nutrition— entailing less cost, less time, less administration, and fewer clearances than other measures, and no special distribution apparatus. Since much depends on local circumstances, a number of questions should be addressed in determining the feasibility of any given project: Is the food carrier consumed by a sizable portion of the target population? Is the carrier processed centrally in units large enough in size and few enough in number to permit controlled fortification? Can the carrier be fortified without affecting the taste, odor, or appearance, and therefore the acceptability, of the food? Will the fortified product permit further processing or cooking (and storing under local conditions) without major losses of the added nutrients? Is the processed food consumed in relatively constant amounts so that fortification levels can be calculated accurately? Can the food carrier be fortified without significant alteration of its cost to the consumer?

## The Costs

The costs of vitamin and mineral supplements in processed foods is extraordinarily small (see Table 10). Fortification with vitamins A and D adds 0.04 cent to the cost of a quart of milk, and fortification of processed cereal grain with standard vitamins and minerals averages 0.02 to 0.03 cent per pound. The iron compound necessary to fortify salt costs 4 to 6 cents per capita per year, the iodate one-sixth of a cent. If only one in five consumers of the fortified food is in need, the total cost per beneficiary still is generally low. At these prices, vitamin and mineral fortification should be undertaken when central processing presents the opportunity.

---

* In the few nutrient instances where intake in substantial excess of that planned may create a problem, the risk of side effects in a fraction of the population must, as with other public health measures, be weighed against the consequences of failure to take the step.[13] Concern has been raised, for instance, about the possibility of parents feeding dangerously large quantities of salt to their young because they know the salt is iodized (or "medicated") or, as has been proposed, fortified with iron. There are no known examples in which this has happened, whether because parents do not react this way or a child's palate will not tolerate excessive quantities of salt. Hypothetically the danger exists and should be treated with care—but it must be compared to the dangers if the fortification did not take place.

TABLE 10. *Cost and Source of Selected Vitamins and Minerals*

| Nutrient | Source | Cost per year to supply 5-year-old's total need, dollars[a] |
|---|---|---|
| Vitamin A | Cod liver oil | 3.08 |
| | Raw carrots | 0.48 |
| | Butter | 28.14 |
| | Synthetic fortifier | 0.02 |
| | Mass dose | 0.02 |
| Vitamin D | Cod liver oil | 4.94 |
| | Fish | 32.17[b] |
| | Synthetic fortifier | 0.01 |
| Thiamine (B₁) | Shelled peanuts | 24.17 |
| | Dried beans | 8.67 |
| | Whole wheat flour | 26.73 |
| | Synthetic fortifier | 0.01 |
| Riboflavin (B₂) | Nonfat dry milk | 30.54 |
| | Eggs | 18.40 |
| | Whole wheat flour | 99.28 |
| | Synthetic fortifier | 0.01 |
| Niacin | Chicken | 34.55 |
| | Whole wheat flour | 43.44 |
| | Dried beans | 33.02 |
| | Synthetic fortifier | 0.02 |
| Calcium | Fresh milk | 30.78 |
| | Dried beans | 22.28 |
| | Spinach | 29.74 |
| | Micronutrient fortifier[c] | 0.08 |
| Iron | Liver | 16.85 |
| | Dried beans | 10.53 |
| | Spinach | 11.21 |
| | Micronutrient fortifier[d] | 0.13 |

Sources: Benjamin T. Burton (ed.), *Heinz Handbook of Nutrition* (2nd ed., McGraw-Hill, 1965); John W. Gage, *The Cost of Fortifying Foods with Vitamins* (Hoffman LaRoche, 1970); "25 Million Children May Go Blind," Express News Service (India), July 6, 1968; World Health Organization, *Requirements of Ascorbic Acid, Vitamin D, Vitamin B₁₂, Folate and Iron*, Technical Report No. 452 (WHO, 1970).
   a. Ingredient cost only; does not include cost of carrier.
   b. Varies with type of fish.
   c. Calcium phosphate
   d. Ferrous sulfate.

Protein supplementation is more costly than vitamin and mineral additions but is still considerably less expensive than conventional protein sources. The cost of fortifying wheat with soy flour is a tenth the cost of providing the equivalent protein in the form of milk. Costs depend on the nature of the protein fortifier and on the deficiencies of the product and diet to be fortified.

Mass use of a nutrient drives its cost down dramatically (see Figure 2). Synthetic vitamin A, which in 1951 cost 15 cents per million international units, has gone down to under 5 cents as production has increased. Riboflavin costs have dropped from $100 to $30 per kilo as annual output has grown from 20 to 400 tons. Ascorbic acid has declined from $23 to $4 per kilo since vitamin C usage has increased from 500 to over 4,000 tons per month. Lysine costs have dropped from $30 a kilo in 1956 to $2 in 1971. The cost to enrich 100 pounds of flour with vitamins and minerals in 1941 was 17 cents; in 1967 it was 2 cents.

In analyzing fortification possibilities, the first question commonly is how much the nutrients add to the cost of the product. If adding iron to wheat flour increases the cost by a fraction of 1 percent, which could probably be absorbed by the manufacturer, the instinctive reaction is to con-

FIGURE 2. *Decline in Costs of Selected Synthetic Nutrients, 1940–70*

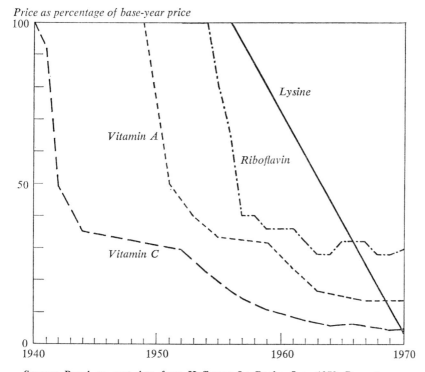

*Price as percentage of base-year price*

Source: Based on cost data from Hoffmann–La Roche, Inc., 1972. Percentages are figured from the following base-year prices: for vitamin C, $71 per kilogram in 1940; for vitamin A, 30 cents per million international units in 1949; for riboflavin, $100 per kilogram in 1952; for lysine, $30 per kilogram in 1956.

sider it a worthwhile investment. If fortifying salt with iron would add 10 percent to the price, the initial tendency may be to dismiss the move as economically infeasible. It is the absolute costs of the alternate means of achieving a nutrition goal that should be compared, however. The cost of fortifying salt seems high because, unlike most processed products, salt initially costs very little. In terms of cost per day, even a 10 percent increase in the cost of salt (perhaps to be covered by subsidy) may be a less expensive way of reducing iron-deficiency anemias than a more modest increase in the cost of a higher priced product. If, as is often the case, the salt is the only way to reach rural people,[14] the addition of iron to refined wheat flour is of little value to that group.

*Who pays.* When fortification costs are minute, they become buried in the processing cost. The modest charges for vitamins and minerals added to flour, for instance, are usually borne by the baking industry. When protein is added, however, cost becomes a factor, and the question is who pays. If the consumer is to bear the cost, should the government make fortification mandatory? If so, will the consumer, because of the higher price, buy a smaller quantity of the fortified food or less of another basic food? What are the nutritional tradeoffs?

If fortification is not mandatory, will the consumer freely choose to purchase the higher priced product? Those who most need nutritional help probably will not. The nutritionally needy, often unlettered, consumer is least likely to understand the virtues of the fortification—especially since, by design, the added nutrients are undetectable—and least likely to afford the additional costs. Moreover, fortified staples that look identical to unfortified but are differently priced could be misrepresented. The only safeguard would be to provide the fortified product in packaged form, which would raise its cost still further.

The obvious alternative to the consumer's paying the increased price is outright subsidization by the government or by external aid agencies (they would be unlikely, however, to support such projects on a continuing basis). The decision to underwrite a fortification project should be based on a comparison of the subsidies and costs with other ways of reaching the same objective.

A means of limiting the burden on the consumer has been proposed in India. The government would require fortification of *atta,* a mesh of wheat used in making the *chappati,* the staple of the north Indian diet. Through its price controls, the government would encourage the miller to spread the fortifying costs to consumers of all processed wheat products; upper income groups, who consume mostly refined wheat flours, would carry much of the expense while fortification of the *atta* would cost the beneficiaries less than they would otherwise pay.

### Carriers and Potential

A carrier can be selected either by identifying centrally processed foods eaten by the target population and determining what nutrients these foods can carry, or by beginning with the necessary nutrients and finding suitable carriers. The most common carriers currently are wheat flour, bread, milk, water, salt, margarine, cooking oils, rice, pasta, breakfast cereals, confections, and processed corn products.

Thus far, however, fortification efforts have been concentrated in the industrialized countries. The exceptions include rice in Thailand and the Dominican Republic; small quantities of tea in Pakistan; margarine in Brazil, Costa Rica, Chile, and Turkey; and wheat products and cooking oil in India. The opportunities to help reduce or even eradicate nutritional deficiencies in low-income countries are vast. There is room for much more imaginative use of the fortification vehicle and more persistence in seeing efforts through to implementation. If, for example, a country's entire salt or sugar supply were fortified with iron or vitamin A, the national incidence of nutritional anemia or blindness might be substantially reduced.

Achievement of the full potential of fortification technology, however, will require a more systematic review of the opportunities than has so far been made, and a more sustained, solution-oriented effort to exploit them —the sort of effort that has succeeded in other areas of food technology. Many of the innovations in soy usage, for example, resulted from a comprehensive search by the industry for new product uses. But no such business constituency is interested in finding an iron compound suitable for, say, salt fortification. This may, in fact, be the primary reason for the small number of fortification projects and the faltering progress of those that exist. Initiative must, in such circumstances, come from government.

In sum, under appropriate circumstances, fortification is one of the most attractive alternatives available to the government official responsible for nutrition betterment. He can now for very small expense obtain significant nutritional results. For those needy whom it can reach, this approach probably has greater leverage on human suffering, at a lower cost, than any other option. Even in the rare cases in which fortification is more expensive than alternative techniques, it is likely to be the quickest method of reaching large numbers of people. While longer range work continues on such other options as upgrading the nutritive value of seed varieties, fortification can, at a minimum, serve as a good interim measure. As India's former food secretary who instituted much of the work in nutrition there concluded, fortification "may be our brightest hope at least in the short run for quickly reaching a large number of people with better nutrition at little cost."[15]

Besides its obvious value of improving nutrition inexpensively, fortification has other interesting developmental implications. It is a concealed form of income supplementation—for specific purposes. It achieves this without need of a massive organizational or administrative apparatus such as health services, welfare activities, or child feeding programs require.

When conditions for fortification are appropriate, governments should require it.

## Formulated Foods

In the early 1960s widespread interest was aroused in the international nutrition community about the development of low-cost nutritious foods from nonconventional sources. Partly the excitement was caused by increased recognition of the importance of malnutrition, but uncertainty about continuing supply from existing nutrition sources played an important role. For more than a decade, U.S. milk contributions had been the mainstay of overseas institutional feeding programs of voluntary and international relief agencies. In many countries, planning was based on the expectation that the flow of milk donations would continue. The milk, however, was available primarily because of U.S. price support policies, not in response to foreign nutrition needs. The overseas feeding programs were the fortunate by-product of a domestic surplus-disposal problem. Suddenly, in 1964, there was jolting realization that U.S. milk surpluses would amount to only one-half, perhaps as little as one-fourth, those of the previous year and the prospects beyond were as dim. Recognizing that there was a bottom to the bottle, and that for some time the poor countries could not themselves provide the milk (even if they did, this would be an expensive means of meeting the need), food aid program administrators sought help from both industry and the scientific community.

The main objective was to develop a low-cost substitute for milk. To avoid dependency on others' surpluses, emphasis was put on the use of ingredients that were or could be produced in the country of need. Those involved in the deliberations and the ensuing product-development work concentrated their search on low-cost nonconventional protein. From the outset they sought to develop a blended food—a mixture of processed cereal and nutritious and widely available oilseed. They were heavily influenced by the success in the 1950s of Nevin Scrimshaw and his colleagues in Guatemala at the Institute of Nutrition for Central America and Panama (INCAP) who had developed an acceptable mixture of corn and cottonseed flour that could be produced locally at a cost substantially less than that of milk. The scientists had demonstrated not only that such foods were good nutritionally, but that children ill with the worst kinds of nutritional disorders could be restored to health by a diet of such food. The principle—long used successfully for animal rations—is simple: combine traditional cereal grains that are deficient in one or more of the amino acids that make up the protein with foods that are rich in them. The principle had been instinctively followed for centuries. In south Asia, pulses (*dal*) commonly are eaten with the wheat-based *chapatti;* in the Middle East, ground chickpea (*hummos*) or sesame paste (*tahini*) with round wheat breads (*pita*); in Latin America, *frijoles* with *tortillas*; among poor blacks in the United States, hominy grits with black-eyed peas; all of the combinations increase both the quantity and quality of protein. (A favorite cereal-oilseed mix in the United States is the peanut-butter sandwich.)

The format for producing a premixed food was established in the production of INCAP's Incaparina and the earlier development of a South African product called Pronutro. But their distribution was limited. A project of a much larger order of magnitude was required. Two formulated foods were developed in the United States, CSM (corn-soy-milk) and WSB (wheat-soy blend); by 1971, nearly 2 billion pounds of the two products had been produced for international distribution. Similar foods, some commercial, some sponsored by governments or international agencies, were produced in Colombia, Brazil, Algeria, Lebanon, Tunisia, Ethiopia, and India. Of the sixty-two projects initiated by 1971, nearly half were in Latin America.[16] The largest, in India, produced Bal Ahar (Hindi for "child's food"). In 1970 it constituted two-thirds of all the special foods produced in low-income countries; 100 million pounds were programmed in 1973, and future production was projected upward.

The new blended cereals have several virtues. They are substantially lower in cost than most conventional forms of animal protein, vitamins, and minerals. They can be tailored to meet the specific nutritional needs

of a target group in a target area, providing calories in the process. They
can be designed and distributed primarily as children's foods (the rest of
the family sometimes uses milk intended for a child, but they are less likely
to eat a food specifically formulated for toddlers). Unlike most conventional protein sources, they require no cold storage. The two major constraints are the cost of blended cereals—lower than that of animal protein,
but higher than that of cereal staples (much of that due to packaging and
distribution)—and the unfamiliarity of the product.

### Product Range

Blended cereals are the most popular but only one of a range of new
foods. These important innovations designed to satisfy dietary needs might
be divided into: facsimile foods, such as simulated meats or milk; variations of existing foods, such as soft drinks; and new eating concepts, such
as a nutrition pill to add to the family cooking pot.

*Facsimile foods.* Imitation food is intended to be as nearly like the taste
and appearance of a food already part of the diet as possible. Margarine,
made with such nonmilk fats as cottonseed, soybean, and safflower oils, is
the best known and most successful example of the transformation of low-
cost vegetable materials into an imitation product. For many years the
Seventh-Day Adventists, a vegetarian religious group, have used simulated
meats; they developed artificial chicken and ham, vegetable hot dogs, and
imitation hamburgers. Now, a sophisticated technology employing techniques and equipment similar to those of the synthetic-fiber industry produces what is known as textured protein; protein oilseed isolate is spun
into fiber that is fabricated into meat analogs designed to extend or substitute for basic meat dishes. Less expensive extruded meat analogs, sized,
colored, and flavored to simulate diced meat, are marketed in Japan,
Europe, and the United States, but their cost at present limits their applicability for low-income countries. Toned milks, filled milks, and imitation
milks—all designed to resemble regular milk—also fall in the facsimile
category.*

* Milk toning is the addition of water and nonfat dry milk to milks otherwise
high in butterfat. Much of India's milk comes from buffalo and has a butterfat content twice that of cow's milk; milk toning has been used effectively there since the
late 1940s to stretch the milk supply. Filled milks are those in which the butterfat of
cow's milk has been replaced by vegetable fats added to a skim-milk base. In imitation (or wholly nondairy) milks, now being marketed in several parts of the world,

*Variation of existing products.* Food "variations" make no pretense of imitating current products, but do take advantage of consumer preferences. For example, a number of companies have produced protein beverages that are bottled and marketed to take advantage of the demand for soft drinks. A caramel-flavored beverage is sold in Brazil, a fruit-flavored one in Surinam, a banana-flavored one in Guyana, and a chocolate-flavored one in Iran. Vitasoy is the most dramatic commercial success of the protein products; marketed as a chilled drink for warm weather and a warm drink during cool weather (like tea or chocolate elsewhere), its 80 million bottles a year account for 25 percent of Hong Kong's soft-drink market. In the same category are variations of snack foods, frozen bars, cookies, candies, and, most prominently, children's gruels. Incaparina, for example, was patterned after *atole,* a corn-based beverage commonly used in Central America.

*New eating concepts.* The "new eating concept" is in many ways the most difficult change to make, since it requires a complete alteration in purchasing and eating patterns. An example of this in the United States is Instant Breakfast, which is designed to offer a quick and convenient way to consume a nutritionally balanced meal, or its forerunner Metrecal which incorporates essential nutritional needs in a dietetic beverage. Abroad, extensive efforts—not noteworthy for their success—have been made over the years to market Multi-Purpose Food, a powdered product that, sprinkled on cooked foods, enhances their nutritive value. In the same family is the Nutricube, a small cube full of nutrients, which is supposed to be dropped into the family cooking pot.

For the most part, formulated foods are of good nutritional value; many, especially the blended foods and textured proteins, can be tailored to meet the deficiencies of a target group. They have the advantage of adding to the food supply since they use materials not generally part of the human diet. Many of the new foods do not require refrigeration and so can be shipped and stored more easily than fish, dairy products, and other traditional protein foods. Except for those in the "new eating concept" category, most of the new foods require no change of eating habits.

---

both the milk and the butterfat are replaced by vegetable protein and vegetable fat, usually from soybeans but sometimes from groundnut or coconut. The new dairy products are not without problems, most of them concerned with palatability. But differences in taste and texture are not always displeasing to the consumer. A distinct advantage of the vegetable-based milks may be their digestibility by those groups with low tolerance for cow's milk.[17]

*The Costs*

Costs vary widely. Although most of the facsimile foods cost less than the products they imitate—rehydrated extruded meat analogs are 10–21 cents per pound; textured soy in India would be one-fourth to one-sixth the cost of meat (spun fibers cost about 25 percent less than meats)[18]— they are nonetheless expensive for the nutritionally needy. Milk substitutes are the exception; with mass production they may be half the price of regular milk. The variations on existing products are more costly than the foods they replace but are generally substantially cheaper than the traditional means of providing the same levels of nutrients. A kilo of processed cereal blend, for example, may cost two to four times more than ground corn but a small fraction of the price per kilo of the same nutrition in conventional form. In Colombia a peso can buy four times as much protein value in the form of Incaparina as in milk and five times more than in eggs.[19] Costs of products in the new eating concepts category depend on the food—prices range from 10 cents to 65 cents a pound, with 25 cents a common figure; prices of the equivalent protein range from about 30 cents to over $2.50.

*Criteria*

Certain criteria should be applied in the development of formulated foods, whether for public institutional feeding or for commercial ventures.[20] The product should be of good nutritional quality. It should be designed to reach nutritionally vulnerable groups. It must be culturally acceptable. It should fit into an existing eating pattern so that a nutritionally significant quantity will be consumed. It must be regarded as something of value, sufficiently attractive that the consumer will buy it in preference to alternatives. It must be less expensive than traditional forms of nutrition; if it is to be a commercial product, its price must be within the reach of the needy. It must store without refrigeration and be designed to minimize infestation. It should, if possible, be composed of ingredients that are locally available, or could be produced locally. It must be free from toxicity and other hazards.

Several formulated foods have met these criteria and are already being used or are ready for large-scale distribution. Others still have obstacles— some technical, some economic—to overcome. Yet the remarkable advances in new products indicate that remaining problems are surmountable.

## The Ingredients

Whether speaking of fortified or formulated foods, whether of distribution through the commercial market or government institutional feeding programs, the success of the "new foods" depends on the "new ingredients"—that panoply of food components unknown a decade ago or, if known, seldom thought of as capable of being consumed by humans. Attention here is concentrated on protein ingredients, partly because the technology for adding vitamins and minerals to existing foods is already well established, is cheap, and poses no particular problems, and partly because protein-calorie malnutrition has attracted the interest and concern of the international nutrition community, especially the United Nations.* The deficiency of protein, it should be recognized, is only one of several nutrition problems facing low-income countries,† and in some countries may not be the major one.

### The Oilseeds

The family of foods that has received the most attention as fortifiers or ingredients of the formulated foods are the oilseeds; in a 1971 survey, for

---

* In 1955 the World Health Organization (WHO) established a Protein Advisory Group to study the nutritional and safety aspects of protein in foods. In 1960 the Food and Agriculture Organization (FAO) and the UN Children's Fund (UNICEF) added their sponsorship, broadening the group's mandate to look at technological, marketing, and economic aspects of nutrition, particularly supplementary feeding of infants and other high-risk groups. Since 1971 the sponsorship has included the World Bank.

† Whether there is a protein shortage is a matter of some controversy in the nutrition community. One school holds that if people only ate more of the traditional diet, protein problems would be solved automatically. In many circumstances, especially those affecting adults and older children, this is no doubt true. There are, however, important exceptions: (1) when roots or tubers form the staple of the diet, as in large parts of Africa, South America, and south India; (2) when the concern is the small child who, being provided with ample quantities of nutritionally adequate food, simply may not be able to eat enough of it to satisfy his protein need (feeding children four or five times a day, which has been suggested as a way of overcoming this difficulty, is not practical); (3) when a child's protein needs are increased because of losses resulting from poor absorption brought on by the kind of acute infection that is common among poor children; and (4) when family food habits do not provide the child the traditional diet (as, for example, when pulses are withheld). Moreover, neither diets nor ratios of foods in diets are what they traditionally were in some areas, as in India and Pakistan where the cereal-pulse ratio has increased dramatically.

instance, 93 percent of the new foods reviewed used an oilseed as the protein base.[21] In general the oilseeds are both low in cost and high in nutritive value. Their most striking characteristic, however, is abundance. Approximately 110 million tons are harvested annually, mostly in countries of nutritional need. The 1970 oilseed production contained on the order of 55 million tons of protein—enough to meet, several times over, the total protein requirements of the world. With token exceptions, however, oilseed protein is not consumed by those in need. In fact, many of the protein-deficient countries are large exporters of oilseed meals. India is the world's largest exporter of groundnut and sesame, and ranks only after the United States as an exporter of all oilseed meals.*

As its name implies, the oilseed is grown mostly for its oil, which is used primarily for cooking. The oil is separated from the seed either by traditional screw pressing or, more recently, by solvent extraction. The residue "oilseed cake" (also called presscake or meal) can be refined and used as the protein ingredient for human-grade foods. The meal of major oilseeds, which is about 50 percent protein, is used most often, however, as animal feed or fertilizer. Ironically, in some countries this by-product of vegetable oil poses a disposal problem.

Because the meal is a by-product, it is an economically attractive protein source. The price of the typical oilseed is 7 cents a pound, of the residue cake 4 cents. From this, an oilseed protein flour can be produced for 12 cents a pound; by comparison, nonfat dry milk costs at least twice as much, and other forms of animal protein upwards of eight times as much. The quality of oilseed protein is not as high as that of animal protein but is considerably higher than that of cererals alone. Although certain of the oilseeds are deficient in one or more of the essential amino acids, they are generally high in those that cereals lack; hence the virtue of mixing the two. A combination of cereal with oilseed may be better than the oilseed alone.

In short, the oilseeds are the world's least expensive and most available source of protein. The principal difficulties in exploiting them for human consumption are color, toxic factors, digestibility, and palatability.

*Soybean.* The soybean, versatile, low-cost, and easy to produce, constitutes 43 percent of the harvest of the world's seven major oilseeds. Two-thirds of its production, however, is concentrated in the United States,

* The exports cannot be viewed solely as a nutritional loss because they provide an important source of hard currency—for Nigeria, 15 percent of its export earnings—that could contribute to nutritional betterment.

where in two decades (1949–69) soybean acreage more than quadrupled —from 10 million to 43 million acres. After corn, soybean is the second-largest U.S. crop, valued at $2.5 billion per year. It has become the largest American export crop, at $1.4 billion per year.

Except in mainland China (in all likelihood the second-largest soybean producer) and several other countries in the Far East, soybeans are not a traditional crop in low-income countries.*

Although most of the world has only in recent decades thought of soy as a protein supplement, it has been consumed in the Far East for millennia; an estimated 8 million tons of cooked or fermented soybean products are eaten each year. One of the major categories of soy products used in the East are those obtained from aqueous extract, the most popular form being soy milk. This, in turn, can be made into *tofu,* a curd consumed by Japanese at the average rate of over 20 pounds a year, comparable to the U.S. consumption of hot dogs. The *tofu* can be processed still further into a cheese food called *sufu.* Another major category of soy products are fermented foods, the most popular of which are *shoyu* (soy sauce), *natto* (a side dish of fermented soybeans), *miso* (a paste product used as a seasoning or base for soups), and *tempeh* (a fungal culture roasted or fried in patties). Two of every three Indonesians consume *tempeh* daily, getting a substantial part of their nutrients from this product which contains anywhere from 15 to 25 percent protein.

Like all oilseeds, most of the world's soy is crushed for oil (which makes up 19 percent of the bean). The meal by-product furnished nearly two-thirds of all oilseed meal processed for animals in 1970. Recently it has been developed for human use in the form of soy flour, soy concentrate, and soy isolate. The three forms differ in sophistication of technology (and thus usefulness), in price (from 6 cents to 38 cents a pound), and in protein level (from 50 percent to 90 percent). They are used in infant foods, beverages, cereals, breads, confections, and simulated dairy and textured meat-type products. They supply the protein base for Vitasoy, the Indian baby food Bal Amul, the later formulations of Incaparina, and Pronutro. In Brazil, efforts are under way to fortify cassava with soy, and in several countries new composite wheat flours, that use up to 16 percent soy, are being tested.

Soybeans are the least expensive of the major oilseeds in terms of price

---

* In recent years, however, soybeans have been successfully grown in India and Brazil; in the latter they have increased more than eightfold—to over 5 million tons —in six years.

per pound of utilizable protein and are also the most nutritious. Unlike cottonseed and groundnut, they have, when cooked, no toxic or antinutrition factors. Moreover, they fit nicely into traditional cropping patterns, enriching the soil rather than, like sunflower, draining nutrients from it. Because of these advantages, soy has become the standard for price and quality against which the other protein ingredients are measured.

Soybeans do have drawbacks. As noted, they generally are not grown in the developing countries where protein is most needed. Except in the Far East, the habit of eating soybean products has not been developed, unlike some other oilseeds such as sesame and groundnut. The bitter, beany taste of soy is sufficiently unpleasant to many people outside the Far East that it must be masked.

*Cottonseed.* Cottonseed production is second only to that of soybeans among world oilseeds; because most tropical and subtropical countries produce cotton, its oilseed is widely available in areas of protein need. Whereas other oilseeds are grown primarily for their oil, cottonseed oil is a by-product of cotton-lint production. Thus, the protein derivative is yet a further step removed from the original purpose of the crop. The Indian subcontinent, the United States, the USSR, and mainland China together produce three-quarters of the world's annual total of 22 million tons, one-fifth of which could be edible protein.

Use of cottonseed in edible foods is the result of early ecological concerns. Less than a century ago it was regularly discarded, usually dumped into rivers. When it was recognized that this posed a health hazard to those depending on the rivers as a water source, as well as a danger to fish, interest was stimulated in finding uses for it.* Until recently it was salvaged principally for use as animal feed and fertilizer.

The major problem cottonseed presents for human consumption is a toxic pigment it contains known as gossypol. When the gossypol is reduced to acceptable levels for food, it still gives off an undesirable, yellowish-green color and also lowers the nutritive value of the product. Two ingenious methods have been devised to remove the gossypol. In India a "liquid cyclone" mechanically extracts the pigment, and in Italy a solvent is used to penetrate and destroy the potency of the gossypol glands. A genetic breakthrough has provided a glandless variety of cottonseed that

---

* For similar ecological reasons, development of another protein source, whey protein concentrate, is under way. In the past the whey not used as animal feed was discarded, a practice now prohibited in some countries.

eliminates the problem of extracting the gossypol. Altering the seed, however, has produced an undesirable change in the fiber of the cotton, where the financial value of the crop lies. In addition, the glandless varieties are more vulnerable to insects and probably will require more use of insecticides, a significant economic consideration.

Only modest quantities of cottonseed have been processed and incorporated into human-grade products, the greatest use being as the protein base in early formulations of Incaparina. In the United States cottonseed has been used since the 1930s in a flour known as Proflo to improve baking characteristics. Cottonseed flour costs from 12 cents to 30 cents per pound. Slightly more than half its weight—upwards of two-thirds in the gossypol-free varieties—is protein.

*Groundnut.* The groundnut (so named because, unlike other oilseeds, it grows underground) is also known as the peanut, monkeynut, goober, or earthnut. It grows abundantly in hot climates, where malnutrition is most prominent. India produced 6 million tons in 1970, substantially more than one-third of the world's total (it required 18 million acres, an area twice the size of Switzerland). The second largest producer was China with 2.7 million tons, followed by the United States, Nigeria, and Brazil. Two-thirds of all groundnuts in the world are crushed for their oil, which is sufficiently attractive to have become the most popular cooking oil among the French. The presscake is most often thought of as an animal feed or as a fertilizer, which imposes a major impediment to its greater use as a human food. In the last decade, cases of aflatoxin contamination have caused additional concern about the use of groundnuts. The toxic fungus, on groundnuts from Brazil, caused the sudden death in the early 1960s of 100,000 English turkeys and large numbers of ducklings and pheasants. Shortly after, the same fate befell large numbers of ducks in Kenya that had eaten locally grown groundnut. Subsequently, aflatoxin was found in 15 percent of the peanuts sold for human consumption in Uganda. Experiments on rats indicate aflatoxin in groundnuts may be carcinogenic, yet in mice it apparently has no effect; no ill effects have been demonstrated in man.[22]

Aflatoxin in groundnuts probably results from harvesting practices. In certain agricultural areas, farmers dampen the ground to make it easier to pull the plant from the soil. As the nuts sit in the dampness, a mold that is sometimes toxic eventually forms. Indian technologists have devised a technically sound but logistically complex system for drying the nuts mechanically. In several projects in India, bad nuts are removed by hand. Broad-scale elimination of aflatoxin, however, will probably require changes in harvesting, handling, and storage.

Except for the problems of imagery and of aflatoxin, the groundnut compares favorably with other oilseeds. Its nutritive value is not as high as that of other oilseeds, but the flavor and color of groundnuts incorporated in a product are of less concern than those of most of the other oilseeds; in some areas, the nutty odor and taste are commonly accepted.

Unlike most of the other oilseeds, the groundnut is already a popular consumption item in certain regions. In Africa, groundnut-based sauces and stews are common, and in the Far East groundnuts sometimes are included in the cooking. Generally, however, only a small fraction of total production is used as human food. The prime exception is the United States, where three-quarters of the peanuts produced (1 billion pounds a year, or 5 pounds a person) are eaten, mostly in the form of peanut butter or salted peanuts. In India, on the other hand, less than 1 pound per capita per year is consumed.

Since interest has developed in using oilseeds as a protein base for other foods, forms of finely ground groundnut have been incorporated in wheat products, confections, milk substitutes, children's foods, and some formulations of the additive concentrate known as Multi-Purpose Food.

*Sesame.* Sesame is perhaps the most ancient of all oilseed foods. It has been consumed in the Middle East for millennia, is mentioned in early south Asian Sanskrit, and is important in ancient Hindu ceremony still practiced today. Because of its desirable flavor, a larger proportion of the sesame produced is consumed directly as food than any other oilseed. In the Middle East it is popular in such dishes as the white paste *tahini,* and *halavah,* a sweet popular in the Arab world. In Africa, sesame seeds are used in soups and porridge; in India with sweet meats; in parts of Latin America mixed with corn in bread; and in Europe and the United States in baked goods. The seeds are pressed for an excellent oil, noted for its resistance to rancidity, which is the preferred cooking oil in Japan. The residue of seeds from which the oil has been removed is a high-quality animal food. Sesame production is dominated by India, which produces 30 percent of the world's crop. Substantial quantities are grown in mainland China, and lesser amounts in Latin America and Africa.

Sesame is nutritionally one of the best oilseeds and is free of toxins. Perhaps the reason such a desirable oilseed constitutes only 2 percent of the world's oilseed production is that its pod, when ripe, opens so easily the seed are often lost (whence the "open sesame" of *Ali Baba and the Forty Thieves*). Attempts to develop varieties of tighter pods have led to lower yields, smaller pods, and lower quality seeds. Because of the fragility of the pod, oil processors often do not take the trouble to remove the undesirable hull and the cuticle, and their residue product is thus fibrous, bitter, and of a dark color. Simple, inexpensive forms of processing are being used in the United States and parts of Latin America. Until their use becomes widespread and harvesting becomes more economical, sesame is likely to remain a minor member, in terms of quantity, of the oilseed family.

*Coconut.* Coconut flour is a potential protein ingredient for weaning foods, especially in the Philippines, Indonesia, south India, Ceylon, Malaysia, the South Pacific islands, and other areas where the coconut is abundant. The Philippines' 185 million trees annually produce nearly a third of the world's 17 billion nuts. The coconut is the country's largest foreign exchange earner, yearly bringing in $150 million or a quarter of all income from exports. More than a third of all Filipinos are said to depend on the industry for a livelihood.*[23]

The dried kernel of the nut, known as copra, consists of 20 percent protein. Although physically different from the other oilseeds, the cocount is, like them, grown today primarily for its oil, and the defatted presscake is used as animal feed.

In some societies coconut is popular as a human food, but only a small portion of production is used in this way (since most coconuts grow wild, data are not precise). In comparison with soybean, cottonseed, and groundnut, coconut has had limited development as a protein for incorporation in human-grade weaning foods. However, coconut flour is commercially produced for use in Malaysia, Thailand, and the Philippines. In some areas, home-produced coconut milks and coconut creams are popular.

Apparently, the flavor of coconut is universally accepted. The nut has a high fiber content, however, which leads to difficulties in processing digestible foods, and because current processes for animal feed are highly unsanitary, the copra can be toxic. Even though it has a low protein content, the coconut is high in protein quality; its amino acid composition is better than that of other oilseeds.

---

* The coconut has served many purposes in areas where it is produced. In Sanskrit, the word for coconut palm means "the tree that furnishes the necessities of life" —food, milk, fiber, oil, fuel, and wine.

Coconut often is grown in regions where other oilseeds are not. Nevertheless, relatively few coconut-protein products have been developed. This may be due to the assumption that they would be costly. The average yield is one ton of copra for a hundred trees, or twenty pounds per tree—an inferior yield in comparison with other oilseeds. One hectare of land produces enough protein for only two people; soybeans grown on the same amount of land can provide enough protein for forty.[24] Moreover, it takes fourteen years of cultivation before the coconut tree begins to bear fruit.

*Sunflower.* The sunflower seed has rapidly assumed prominence, now ranking second only to soy in world vegetable-oil production. From 1961 to 1968, world sunflower seed exports quadrupled, increasing by an average of 40 percent a year. This dramatic climb is principally due to an improved variety of seed that increases both yield per acre and the amount of oil extracted—nearly double that of a decade ago. The cost of sunflower, at 3 cents a pound, is the lowest of the oilseeds.

Although one of the advantages of the sunflower is that it can be grown in conditions of near-drought, relatively little has been produced in the hot, dry low-income countries. Nearly two-thirds of the 9 million tons grown annually is produced in the Soviet Union, and much of the remainder in Eastern Europe and Argentina. The sunflower, too, is grown primarily for oil and its by-product, which is used as high-quality animal feed. Only recently has serious thought been given to use of the meal in human foods, the first product being a baby food produced in Chile. Initial work suggests that processed seed also can effectively be used in cereals, baked products, beverages, and meat analogs. It has a bland and acceptable flavor and apparently does not produce the flatulence or other gastrointestinal problems that accompany certain other of the oilseeds. Nor have any toxic substances been identified. Its major drawback is an undesirable darkening of products in which it is used; the development of an industrial dehulling process to eliminate the problem has been reported from the Soviet Union.

*Rapeseed.* Like the sunflower, rapeseed production has expanded rapidly and is now fifth in importance among the oilseeds. Production doubled from 3.8 million tons in 1961 to 7.6 million tons a decade later; major producers are India, China, and Europe. Rapeseed is cultivated primarily for table greens, animal forage, and oil. In eastern India the oil is preferred over all others for the preparation of curries.

Given the substantial production, surprisingly little has been done to explore the possibilities of deriving edible meal from rapeseed. As a potential food source it appears to be high in nutritive value, but its brownish color will require attention, as will problems of digestibility and toxicity. A detoxified rapeseed is considered feasible; its protein content of 55 percent may make it an attractive source of edible protein for human food formulation.

Other oilseeds that may prove valuable ingredients of human food are mustard seed and safflower seed. Thus far, only modest attention has been directed to these.[25]

### Grain Protein Concentrates

In the milling of grains, much of the protein value is lost. After processing, 100 pounds of wheat generally is reduced to 60 to 75 pounds of flour. The remainder, known as mill feed, is a nutritionally rich portion of the wheat that is customarily used for animal feed. Mill feeds have been bypassed as human food because of their high fiber content, which affects their digestibility and baking characteristics. In the mid-1960s a simple method of milling portions of the mill feeds was devised to produce a wheat protein concentrate (WPC) with little fiber and a high quality protein.

A 70:30 mixture of wheat flour and protein concentrate has many advantages over regular flour. It contains 25–50 percent more protein than regular wheat flour. The amount of lysine, the amino acid most deficient in wheat flour, is bolstered in the mixture. The wheat fractions that are added to the flour cost 5 cents per pound, 20–30 percent less than the cost of flour; hence 70 pounds of wheat flour mixed with 30 pounds of protein fractions cost less than 100 pounds of regular flour. Using the concentrate as an additive stretches the availability of flour by 30 percent without raising land usage. Moreover, few equipment changes are required for the process.

The concentrate still presents some problems of acidity and, at high levels of consumption, digestibility. When used in heavy proportions, the wheat concentrate produces breads similar in both color and taste to whole wheat bread, which is not acceptable to some audiences. The product's stability, and thus its effect on baking quality, are still uncertain.

To date, wheat fractions have mostly been used to fortify wheat flours and to extend bakery products. They are a prime ingredient of WSB (wheat-soy blend), a prominent commodity distributed in the U.S. Food for Peace program. Along with sesame flour, they have been used as the protein base in Frescavida, a powdered beverage tested in El Salvador, and in the preparation of a high-nutrition cookie in the United States.

Wheat protein concentrate deserves more attention than it has received, however. The 5 million tons of mill feed that the United States annually produces is converted into approximately 100,000 tons of animal protein when used as feed; it could be converted into five to ten times that much protein if consumed directly by humans in the form of a wheat protein concentrate.

In developing countries that grind much of their wheat as whole wheat, few fractions are available to add to the flour. It may be economically sound for these countries to import wheat fractions for incorporation in their locally milled products. Addition of the concentrate can add substantially to the nutritive value of whole wheat flour[26] as well as more highly milled products.

Rice, like wheat, loses many of its nutritious constituents in the processing. The bran removed during milling has a high vitamin content and is 12–13 percent protein. Making a rice concentrate with the bran, however, poses greater complications than making a concentrate of wheat. Rice bran has a high fiber content and includes oil that must be extracted before the protein can be used. Further, rice is seldom ground into flour to which a concentrate could be added. Nor do rice-eating societies usually have an alternative ground cereal staple that could be fortified with rice fractions.

### Single Cell Protein

Single cell protein—or SCP—is in the words of the UN Protein Advisory Group "potentially a major new protein source."[27] The name SCP itself leads to a certain amount of confusion, perhaps by design; it is probably preferable to such less-ambiguous alternatives as "petroleum protein" or "microbial protein." Single cell protein is actually a generic term for protein flour derived from any of a series of unicellular microorganisms— yeast, bacteria, fungi—that can be grown on a variety of abundant and inexpensive culture mediums, such as oil waste, natural gas, molasses, paper-mill waste, sewage, sweet potatoes, starch, and so on. Also part of the SCP family—but sufficiently different to be singled out for special treatment—are algae.

Microorganisms have been used for food production for centuries. In the making of soy sauce, sauerkraut, vinegar, yogurt, beer, yeast for oven baked products, and certain cheeses, the organisms are part of the food process itself. Only in the past decade has serious attention been directed to putting the single cell organisms to work to produce mass quantities of protein.

The supply of raw materials that can produce single cell protein is virtually unlimited, and they are cheap, most of them being industrial or agricultural waste products. The waste from world oil production alone, for example, could provide enough tons of protein annually to meet existing needs some seven times. Thus, in a world of increasing food demand and potential long-range food and feed scarcity, SCP offers promise of an abundant additive protein supply.

Because the organisms are continuously at work, single cell protein can be produced in very short periods. Whereas a 1,000-pound steer produces 1 pound of protein in twenty-four hours, and 1,000 pounds of soy produce 92 pounds, it is possible for 1,000 pounds of single cell organisms to produce 1,000 pounds. In other words, cattle double their mass in one to two months, chickens in two to four weeks, grass and some plants in one to two weeks, but SCP in less than two hours.[28] The production speed of SCP also offers unique advantages in genetic experimentation—it produces a complete generation of products every three to five days.

Single cell protein makes few demands on skilled labor. In India it takes a million people to produce 1.2 million tons of fish a year, but Assam petroleum could supply the same amount of protein with the work of 100 men.[29]

Since SCP is grown in a reactor or fermenter, it is independent of the vagaries of the weather and it makes no special demands on farm land. It requires so little space that half a square mile could produce 10 percent of the world's protein supply.[30] And SCP raises few waste-disposal problems because nearly all its constituents are used.

Despite its many assets, the future of SCP for human consumption is not clear. A low-cost SCP product will require a substantial production facility and market. A 50,000–100,000 ton plant is necessary for economic production, since the unit costs are 40 percent greater in a 10,000 ton plant than in a 100,000 ton plant. Even at that volume, SCP, although cheaper than milk, may not be competitive with oilseeds. Costs are estimated to range from 14 cents to 40 cents a pound. In some processes, technical problems remain to be solved in the recovery of the protein.

Raw materials for producing single cell protein may come from petroleum waste, from which the paraffins or waxy components of the crude oil are used; natural gas (predominantly methane); alcohols (particularly methanol and ethanol); and carbohydrate wastes such as sugars, starches, waste materials from food processing operations (citrus, molasses, lactose from whey, materials from potato-processing plants), and cellulose (wood pulp, waste paper). Natural gas can support only bacteria, but the others can be used for propagation of either bacteria or yeast. Fungi also can probably be grown on these substrates. Substantial quantities of pure water are necessary to grow the organisms, as well as minerals and power. The costs of these factors must be weighed against local, or perhaps regional, demand to determine whether production can be economical.

*Algae.* Algae are a special brand of single cell protein. Their production depends on a large body of water and a great deal of sun. Much of the living material in the ocean feeds on algae; the estimated quantity available is more than 100 tons yearly for each person in the world.[31] Jules Verne, about a century ago, suggested using algae for human food, but only since 1963 has the notion been seriously investigated. In that year, 80,000 Africans were discovered to be consuming daily an average of 250 grams of a food called *dihe*, dried cakes made from the blue algae of Lake Chad. The material, which is 70 percent protein on a dry basis, is skimmed from the lake, placed in small holes in the hot sand to dry, then baked and sold in cake form for a token price. The resulting product is used as a meat substitute or mixed as a thick sauce with millet balls and is the major source of protein in the diet. Further investigation of algae's use turned up a not dissimilar product. Montezuma's chronicler, Bernal Díaz, in a 1519 account, reports witnessing at a public market "fish mongers and others who sold little loaves which they made from some sort of slime taken from the lagoon, having a flavor like cheese."*[32] Substantial quantities of algae, some harvested, some cultivated, are consumed by the Japanese, but they are used for flavoring rather than as a protein food.

*Uses of SCP.* At the outset, SCP will be used to meet the increasing demand for animal-feed ingredients, perhaps to replace the 6 million tons of fishmeal and soy imported yearly by Europe. Thus the supply of animal protein for some—although usually not the neediest—portions of the society will increase; eventually SCP may increase the availability for direct human use of other protein sources now used for animal feed by replacing them.

The Soviet Union is already involved in large-scale SCP feed produc-

---

* In 1972 a one-ton-a-day plant to produce algae for human food was opened in Mexico, not far from where algae was collected 450 years ago.

tion and British Petroleum is operating a 20,000-ton-a-year pilot plant for feed in France. Work also is under way in Taiwan, Japan, Czechoslovakia, India, and China. Several petroleum companies are devoting attention to SCP, some in cooperation with large food firms (Standard Oil, for example, with Nestlé) to develop a human-grade product.

Thus far, single cell protein for human consumption has been used mainly as a flavoring material or as torula yeast for vitamin B. (Yeast was proposed by the League of Nations in the late 1930s as a means of meeting the needs of the malnourished. In World War II the Germans used it as a food supplement.) Torula yeast is included in some formulations of Incaparina and Pronutro and in the United States in commercial baby foods, processed cereal products, pasta sauces, spreads, soups, and confections. Addition of SCP improves the nutritive value of the foods without detriment to texture or taste.

Of the various microorganisms that can be grown, bacteria and yeast grow most quickly and are most efficient in conversion of nitrogen or carbon into protein. They also have a higher protein and amino acid content. The major advantage of fungi and algae is that they can be recovered more simply and less expensively than bacteria and yeast.

Single cell protein plainly has promise as a protein source, especially because of its long-range availability. The major technological breakthroughs in its utilization have been made; the requirements now are for small gains in several areas. Several hundred thousand tons of SCP will probably be produced as animal feed by the late 1970s. Large-scale production of a purer product for human use is still some years away. Solution of the safety and nutritional problems is within reach, but the economic questions remain large.

### Fish Protein Concentrate

Fish is one of the best forms of protein and potentially one of the cheapest, but except in coastal areas it is difficult and expensive to get to consumers. Because of their perishability, many fish are wasted or used as fertilizer. Fish protein concentrate—commonly called FPC—is designed to overcome the perishability problem and to make fish previously not used for human consumption an edible product at a low cost. Almost all the oil and water is removed from the fish, and the resulting protein concentrate is processed into a dry flour that requires no refrigeration.

Fish meal has long been an ingredient in poultry and pig rations; at least a third of the fish caught are used in this way. After soy, fish meal is the most important of the internationally traded meals; the volume of 5 million tons in 1968 nearly doubled the 1960–64 average. In Peru, which produces 40 percent of the world's total, fish meal is the major foreign-exchange earner, constituting three-fifths of all exports (production grew from 12,000 tons in 1953 to more than 2 million in 1968). Other protein deficit countries, such as Chile and Morocco, also ship out the bulk of their fish meal.

Fish protein concentrate is much more refined than fish meal. Whereas the meal is made from almost any fish caught and is processed under crude, unsanitary conditions, FPC is made from selected varieties and is processed by solvent extraction. In its most sophisticated and costly form, FPC is a dry, light colored, tasteless, odorless powder containing at least 80 percent protein of excellent nutritional characteristics. Adding 5–10 percent FPC to cereal boosts the nutritional composition to a level comparable to that of animal protein. A 5 percent addition of FPC to white wheat flour more than doubles the utilizable protein in a diet using wheat as the sole source of protein. Nine-tenths of a pound of rice combined with one-tenth of a pound of FPC provides the protein equivalent of nine eggs.[33]

FPC has been incorporated in breads and infant foods in South Africa, corn products in Guatemala, hard bread in Sweden, baby foods in Ethiopia and Chile, pasta in Chile, biscuits in Brazil, flavored-beverage tablets in Pakistan, and a variety of wheat products in Peru. It has been tested in sauces, candies, *chapattis,* curries, soups, and gruels. Small amounts of high quality FPC are not detected in processed foods, but large amounts or imperfectly processed FPC prove objectionable in either taste, odor, or color.

More serious than these difficulties is the cost of FPC as a fortifying additive. Both a modern fishing industry and expensive and elaborate processing facilities are required—an economically reasonable project would require a 5,000-ton-a-year FPC plant, costing $4 million. Beyond that capital outlay, FPC costs 16 cents a pound to process plus 1 cent per pound for raw materials.* The total cost of FPC is about 22 cents a pound, more than twice the cost of most oilseed flours.

---

* In projects in Sweden and the Soviet Union, processing takes place aboard floating factories—in the case of Sweden, a reconverted whaling factoryship—attended by groups of trawlers (eleven and thirty, respectively).

The pendulum has swung from the early enthusiasm that promoted FPC as a kind of nutritional messiah. In the late 1960s, interest had reached such a pitch in the United States—sustained by several sea-state legislators whose constituencies would benefit directly from FPC production—that the Vice President of the United States participated in a high-level policy committee on FPC. The product was oversold, for technical problems had not been worked out when large-scale production was initiated. Most of the FPC produced under the first major U.S. government contract did not meet government specifications, and the manufacturer went bankrupt.

Besides problems of cost and technology, FPC faces difficulties of public acceptance. The lengthy public debate over the safety and aesthetics of FPC—as well as the initial stand of the U.S. Food and Drug Administration which had the effect of legalizing shipment abroad while prohibiting domestic sales—marked FPC as a second-class food. The product's acceptance is further limited by religious and social restrictions on meat products in some areas that would prevent use of the concentrate as a widescale fortifier of cereal staples, its most economic usage.

Where does all this lead? Although the nutritive value of FPC is excellent, its complex technology and high capital investment and processing costs seem to limit its potential impact. The UN Protein Advisory Group's working committee on FPC concluded it could not be recommended to developing countries because it "would not generally be competitive with other supplements."[34] Thus the future of fish protein concentrate hinges on either a less costly production technique or a less sophisticated and hence less costly product. To date, much of the technical effort has been directed to eliminating the fish taste and odor, but this has been achieved only by high-cost production. In areas like Indonesia and West Africa, where the fish flavor and smell are acceptable, a less sophisticated product may be marketable at half the cost of the bland one now being sought.*

In sum, either additional technological advances must occur or the goal must be lowered and the product directed to a more limited public that likes fish. Otherwise, it is unlikely that fish protein concentrate will have much impact on the nutrition problem in the near future.

---

* In some circumstances an overall nutrition contribution might be made by feeding an FPC milk-like product to calves (its cost is half that of cow's milk). In Chile 180,000 calves a year are slaughtered (and the potential protein lost) because milk is in such short supply that Chile cannot afford to have cow's milk fed to the young animal instead of being available for human consumption.

*Leaf Protein Concentrate*

Since the early days of World War II, when a German food blockade was feared by the British, efforts have been under way to identify suitable forms of grass and green leaves that might be incorporated in the human diet. The leader in this work—N. W. Pirie, an Englishman whose zeal is unmatched by that of any other proponent of a specific nutrition intervention—has sought to take advantage of the efficiency of photosynthesis for converting nitrogen into protein. His technique is to crush ordinary leaves, pressing out the juice, which is then coagulated by hot water—much as the white of an egg is poached. The resulting protein is a dark green solid with a strong flavor akin to that of tea or hay and a texture not dissimilar to that of cheese.

The original notion was that leaf protein concentrate (LPC) could be produced from the waste leaves of sugar beets, sugar cane, and water hyacinth. When protein yields proved low, special forage crops such as alfalfa were proposed as sources of LPC. Although there are wide differences in the nutritive values of various leaves, estimates of 60 to 70 percent crude protein in the concentrate are not uncommon.[35] The protein has good biological value and high vitamin A content.

Assuming the technical problems of objectionable color and taste can be overcome, the major need is for an economical refining and production process.[36] Leaves must be available at the proper stage of maturity in large quantities. Their bulk creates logistics problems that make costs of LPC production higher than those of any of the nonconventional alternatives. The Protein Advisory Group figured that the crude product from alfalfa would cost from 10 cents to 20 cents per pound and that marketing costs and profit could increase the total 50–100 percent. A more sophisticated product acceptable in human-grade foods would cost two to three times as much, perhaps 35 cents to 50 cents a pound for the concentrate or 65 cents a pound for protein. Those figures are based on the economics of a unit capable of annual production of 25 million pounds. The notion of small-scale village production units advanced by LPC advocates has been judged impractical.[37]

The leaf protein concentrate experiment, like that of fish protein concentrate, points up the need for nutritionists to be concerned with economics and acceptability in the evaluation of new foods as well as with biological value. The notion of taking advantage of the efficiency of photosynthesis is an attractive one. After all, leaves constitute the largest potential supply of protein, and already—in the form of grasses, alfalfa, and other forage plants—serve as the basis of animal protein. However, leaf protein concentrate still awaits a major technological breakthrough before it can be considered practical.

### Synthetic Nutrients

Synthetic nutrients offer one of the more promising methods of manipulating foods to obtain better nutritional value. Vitamins have long been manufactured in chemically pure form for low cost—at least ten vitamins are produced by chemical synthesis*—and, where employed extensively, probably have had marked national nutritional effects. It is now suggested that the protein value of foods can be improved through the addition of synthetic amino acids, which can be produced either by chemical synthesis or by fermentation.

The economic benefit of adding lysine and methionine to improve the protein quality of chicken and pig feed has long been known to feed companies. The recent dramatic decline in prices of synthetic amino acids now makes their widescale use economically attractive for human feeding as well.† Substantial quantities of Japanese flour are fortified with lysine, and bread baked from this flour is fed to 9 million Japanese students in school feeding programs. Pounded rice, bean noodles, and rice cakes are frequently laced with lysine, as are instant noodles, a popular Japanese food. In the United States, lysine has been included in breakfast cereals and breads, and one major food firm has market-tested a lysine-fortified flour.

Lysine has been added to Guatemala's Incaparina to boost the protein

* Synthetic food supplements include vitamins A, C, E, K, thiamine, riboflavin, niacin, pyridoxine, folacin, choline, and pantothenate.

† The price of methionine and lysine is approximately $1 a pound. Threonine costs approximately $7 a pound, tryptophan $20 a pound; with quantity production, the prices will be reduced to $3 and $5. A plant that could provide lysine economically would require production in the millions of pounds and an estimated capital cost of $6 million. The question is not only the investment but also the outlet for such quantity. Few countries would have use for the minimum production required. This suggests possible need for regional production units for certain of the fortifiers.[38]

value of the cottonseed, and the amino acid has fortified tens of millions of loaves of India's Modern Bread as well. It has also been used in emergencies: in 5,500 tons of German-donated wheat flour shipped to Bihar in 1966–67, and in bulgur wheat sent to Biafra in the late 1960s. Shortly before the change of governments in 1968, Peru issued a decree (never implemented) that lysine be included in all processed imported wheat; since nearly all wheat was imported and processed in five mills, the conditions for fortification were nearly perfect.

Synthetic amino acids offer a number of advantages. They improve the quality of the protein in cereals, all of which are deficient in one or more amino acids. The utilizable protein in wheat, when it is the sole source of protein in the diet, increases 66 percent with the addition of lysine; corn-meal, 70 percent with lysine and tryptophan; and rice, 78 percent with lysine and threonine.[39] Sorghum and millet, common foods of the poor, are helped considerably by lysine, but the fact that only small quantities of these two foods are centrally processed limits opportunities for fortification. In controlled studies of animal and human growth, amino acids added to simple cereal diets have stimulated statistically significant increases in growth.[40]

Amino acids are among the least expensive options for improving protein quality. Only modest technical change is required to add amino acids in the milling process, and for urban areas this may become the simplest form of protein fortification. Because small quantities are required, the costs of storage and transportation are lower than those of most alternative forms of protein fortification. The amino acids are colorless and generally odorless and they do not alter the texture, taste, or color of the product they fortify. Unlike oilseeds, they can also be used to fortify whole grain.*

The average per capita cost of vitamin, mineral, and lysine fortification of a wheat diet is 0.6 cent a day, or $2.37 a year (compared to $2.75 for fortification with soy); of wheat flour with lesser amounts of lysine, 81 cents; and of whole wheat, 36 cents.[41] Fortifying a diet consisting of 70 percent cereals with lysine would increase the average food budget about 4–6 percent.

Yet, not all nutrition advocates are enthusiastic about the addition of

---

* Artificial kernels encapsulating vitamins, minerals, and amino acids can be added to rice or whole wheat, or the grain itself can be impregnated or sprayed with a concentrated solution of the amino acid.

amino acids as a remedy for protein deficiencies. The potential hazard of an amino acid imbalance was at one time a matter of concern. Now the main issue is the uncertainty of impact: because diets differ so greatly in size and composition and by age and income groups and season of the year or day of the week, can the precise needs of any single group be isolated and met? Large field studies under way in Thailand (rice), Tunisia (wheat), and Guatemala (corn) may provide a better idea of the applicability of amino acids under real conditions.

Perhaps in areas where protein deficiencies clearly exist, and the diets of target groups as a whole are deficient in one or two amino acids, their addition to appropriate carriers would be a sensible, effective instrument. This becomes more and more likely as synthetic amino acid costs decrease and as nutrition problems intensify in "reachable" urban areas. Amino acids are no panacea, however, and their indiscriminate use is unlikely to represent efficient resource allocation.

IN RECENT YEARS, scientists have developed a remarkable array of low-cost, nutritious food ingredients to be used in formulating new foods and fortifying old. Technologies are at different levels of advancement and different levels of promise. Not all of the proposed ingredients will be successfully produced and used, and some do not merit further investment as possible nutrition supplements. But a number of new ingredients already are at hand, and encouraging beginnings have been made on others which are now more than laboratory curiosities. Moreover, the early work has established principles and approaches to nutrition problems that can be carried beyond present product considerations.

Of the specific ingredients, the oilseeds are the most attractive. And of the oilseeds, soy perhaps has the greatest potential. Its major limitation currently is the lack of significant production, unlike other oilseeds, in many of the countries of nutritional need. This, however, has started to change. Meanwhile, most of the other major oilseeds have great capacity for nutrition contribution.

Single cell protein and fish protein concentrate must come closer to matching the price and quality standards of the oilseeds if they are to be reasonable; no such feat is on the horizon. Until a better product is achieved, single cell and ground fish products will be used primarily as animal feed. Leaf protein concentrate is even further back in the pack. Wheat protein concentrate has bright potential and deserves much more attention than it has received. The use of synthetic amino acids requires sharper focus than it has received, but under appropriate circumstances may merit considerable exploitation.

In sum, one can look with confidence to any of several of the new ingredients as a promising base for programmed solutions to major nutrition ills. Whether these ingredients can be incorporated into diets of the nutritionally needy remains a perplexing issue, however. Two vehicles have been attempted: the commercial marketplace and public institutional feeding programs. Both pose problems; yet, properly oriented, both have significant potential.

## CHAPTER NINE

# Problems and Promise of Private Industry

If the new food technologies are to have a nutritional impact, it is necessary that the newly created products somehow reach the hands of the malnourished. To meet this need, nutrition authorities have directed much attention to the potential contribution of private industry. The problem requires both technical and marketing ingenuity and these, after all, are the very qualities that have made possible the food industry's extraordinary impact on eating habits of the richer countries.

Enthusiasm favoring the involvement of private industry has been based on several general assumptions:

• The food industry has the technical know-how to develop and produce acceptable, nutritious foods at a price the needy will be able to afford.

• Once the foods are available, they will reach significant numbers of the needy.

• Having been reached by these foods, the needy will benefit from better nutrition levels.

Implied in each of the above are that:

• The ventures will be profitable.

• Developing countries will welcome investment in projects for low-cost, nutritious foods.

In actual practice these assumptions have proved to be overoptimistic. Though more than a hundred projects to feed the malnourished have been initiated, and scores of new products developed with the aid of the food industry, no great significance should be read into the flurry of corporate nutrition activity. First, under current conditions, the number of needy people who will benefit from this activity is extremely limited. Second, current business efforts are likely to be counterproductive when the impression of widespread corporate action breeds a false sense of security among government officials responsible for a nation's nutritional well-being. Third, business corporations are not established for purposes of benevolence; they can undertake socially responsible ventures of significant magnitude only if the ventures will be profitable; prospects for profitability are not promising unless the existing pattern of corporate involvement in nutrition and government's part in that involvement change.

## Industry's Engagement

In the middle 1960s, a slowly developing public concern about malnutrition (that had been evident for several years in the headquarters of United Nations agencies) began to emerge in official Washington. Almost intuitively, certain government officials turned to industry because of its legendary success in developing, producing, promoting, and distributing foods. In the United States an estimated 98 percent of all food was passing through equipment of the food processing industry. The average annual consumption of baby foods by children under three years in the United States had gone up from less than 11 pounds in 1940 to 80 pounds in 1965. Similar growth, on a different scale, was taking place in food industries elsewhere. In India the production of baby milk foods rose from 3,600 to 15,600 tons in eight years, and the food industry as a whole—although still of modest size and impact—increased tenfold between 1952 and 1966. In Taiwan, processed foods constituted a quarter of the total value of the country's manufactured products and 40 percent of its total exports. From instant *tortilla* mixes in Latin America to instant *julabi* mixes in India, the impact of food industry initiatives was increasingly being felt in the less affluent countries.

The sheer size of some of the multinational food corporations suggested them as natural allies in a nutrition effort. A comparison of their gross annual sales with the gross national products of the developing countries reflects something about their respective economic sizes. General Foods ranks ahead of Ecuador, Coca-Cola ahead of Kenya; Nestlé matches Uganda and Tunisia combined; and Kraftco's sales were triple the gross national product of either Bolivia or Paraguay in 1970. Fifty-two developing countries have gross national products smaller than the annual sales of Swift and Company.[1]

Besides government officials' confidence in industry and awareness of fledgling nutrition efforts under way (for example, development of the cereal blend, Incaparina), there were specific reasons supporting the belief that business could launch an effective campaign for low-cost, nutritious foods. The successful establishment of the low-calorie processed foods industry was an attractive precedent.[2] Commercial technology had evolved to meet a recognized need, which in turn dramatically affected American eating habits. In 1960, 13 percent of American families consumed low-calorie soft drinks; five years later the figure was 67 percent. Much the same was true of products with reduced cholesterol content and tooth-decay inhibitors as well as special foods for low-salt and diabetic diets.

Another promising sign was the development and production of blended animal feed. Through sophisticated use of oilseeds and synthetic amino acids, food companies had formulated nutritious, low-cost meals for animals, often superior in nutritional balance and value to foods consumed by man. Oilseeds were also being used to provide man with less expensive and, in some instances, preferred substitutes for traditional animal products. For example, Americans in the late 1960s consumed more than twice as much margarine as butter, a reversal of the consumption pattern in the early 1950s; approximately 80 percent of their whipped cream toppings were derived from vegetable sources; and vegetable-based coffee whiteners (consumed yearly at a pound per capita), filled milks, substitute ice creams, and other such ersatz dairy products had become commonplace on the dinner table.

Still another cause for official interest in business involvement was the successful corporate role in the broader field of agricultural development. The green revolution—itself of nutritional value—was the result, at least in part, of private ingenuity and investment in the production and marketing of fertilizers, pesticides, and other aids to modern agriculture.

The mix of ingredients vital to all of the successful activities consists of research and development expertise, marketing skills, management ability, and investment capability. It was natural for government officials, and often for the scientific community, to look to business for help.

Flattered and actively courted, industry in the United States responded to the inducements, though not without reluctance. While business leaders saw 5,000 new food products introduced annually in the United States, they also saw 4,500 failures removed from the supermarkets within a year. They recognized that, given their unfamiliarity with the additional impediments of working in a developing country, the odds would be even less attractive than this one-in-ten survival rate at home. They voiced concern about the limitation of food distribution channels, the difficulty of altering food habits, and the risks involved in selling to low-income families—generally regarded as an unprofitable segment of the market.

Moreover, while the achievements of the food companies were undeniable, the ability of governments and international agencies to channel anew the talents that had led to those achievements was less certain. What the U.S. government had in mind was full industry involvement in product development, commercial distribution, and marketing, with standard government help, leading to productive and profitable activity. But business leaders, recognizing the risks in a largely uncharted field, were less adventurous. They had envisioned selling food to governments and international agencies for distribution in institutional child feeding programs.

Although some companies lost interest, most food industry leaders eventually accepted the nutrition challenge, convinced that solutions to malnutrition problems hinged in large part on private enterprise. As the vice president of an international food firm put it: "Food companies will go overseas in unprecedented numbers and they will go to previously undreamed of places. Business will respond to the challenge because there is increasing recognition that we cannot maintain freedom and free enterprise in a few wealthy countries surrounded by misery."

By late 1966, most of the major international food companies had initiated laboratory research on low-cost protein foods.* Soon market testing was initiated for new varieties of baby cereals, soft drinks, imitation milks, candies, snacks, soups, and noodles, and by 1968 a dozen of these new products were on the market.

### The Motivations

What were the specific reasons underlying corporate decisions to "respond to the challenge"? A number of food and pharmaceutical companies operating in India indicated they became involved in the nutrition effort for a variety of reasons:†

---

* When progress was slow, the U.S. government prodded American corporations (and later, foreign) with attractive grants of up to $60,000 for exploratory work in countries of potential commercial operations.

† This section is based on responses to a questionnaire and interviews with executives of twelve foreign and twelve Indian food and pharmaceutical companies. They were conducted with the understanding that the respondents would not be identified; thus no source is given for many of the quotations in this chapter.

*Relations with the host government.* A visible concern for the well-being of the local populace, dramatized through a nutrition project, would be useful to foreign companies in future dealings with the government on matters concerning licensing, production expansion, capital repatriation, remittance of profits, taxation, and so forth. Domestic firms, which had their own problems with licensing and taxation, similarly recognized the value of being identified with such a social issue.

*Foreign companies' relations with their home governments.* Favorable response to a request (for example, from Washington) for nutrition involvement abroad might be useful in broadening corporate relationships with the home government and with specific government personnel.

*Relations with the public.* The use of a nutrition project for promoting both company "soul" and product quality to the general public and, more specifically, to family food purchasers (as well as doctors and other professionals who influence food-buying habits) might improve sales of the company's entire line.

*Product profit.* The prospect of a new product or product line with major sales and profit potential from a vast, untouched market was obviously alluring; in some instances, part of the attraction was the projected use of excess plant capacity.

*Competition.* Even without a clear view of a potential profit in sight, some companies embarked on protein activities so that they would not be left behind in what might materialize as a major market. One official said, "We don't dare not to be in it."

*Social good.* Concern for the human condition and a sense of public service responsibility to help the starving and ill-fed were frequently expressed motives for corporate involvement in nutrition.

All of the foreign companies and many of the local ones reported that corporate image was the most important general factor influencing their decision to become involved. There was also a strong thread of social responsibility, which is difficult to measure but, contrary to common skepticism, appeared genuine in many instances.

The profitability of new products was seldom the sole reason for entering the nutrition market, and in some cases it was not the dominant one. It is obvious, however, that all but the "social good" motives relate to profitability in the broader corporate sense. The problem is that where image is a prime motive, corporate contributions to national nutrition are likely to be token.

Moreover, when product profit is the prime motive, most of the consumers of a nutritious product will not be those poor people for whom nutrition programs are intended. More than half of the companies stated that their new products were aimed at the middle and upper income levels. As an executive of a British subsidiary in India says: "It is a sad fact that most nutritional food products marketed by commercial firms are aimed at the segment of society least in need of them."

### The Realities

Although industry appears to be uniquely equipped to deal with the malnutrition problem, entrepreneurs in processed nutritious foods have encountered serious, often unanticipated, difficulties. The problems have inhibited and, in some cases, have aborted commercial ventures; they also cast a cloud on some of the assumptions posed at the outset of this chapter.

*Product costs.* One of the original assumptions was that the food industry could offer nutritious products at a price the needy could afford. With vitamins and minerals available at negligible costs and an increasing variety of protein raw materials available at reasonable costs, it was thought that products could be developed to sell at a low price. But for all the ingenuity that has gone into the development of new products, technologists have not yet been able to come up with a food that can be priced low enough to reach and help the masses of people who most need it.

• Industrial processing inevitably elevates a product's cost beyond that of its staple base: the retail price of Incaparina in Guatemala is nearly four times as high as the cornmeal it replaces; moreover, it costs 20 cents a pound, while the average Guatemalan earns only 88 cents a day. Packaging costs frequently are a problem, especially in poor societies where only small quantities of a product can be retailed at a time: One executive of a British firm in Bombay reported: "For our range of food products, the expense of packaging alone adds, on an average, between three and five rupees a kilogram to their cost. Thus, if we could obtain the ingredients for nothing, market and distribute them for nothing, and made no profit, they would still be too expensive for the multitude who need them most."

• Procurement of raw material is uncertain and therefore costly: According to an Indian business executive, "raw materials are not available because there is little demand; there is little demand because high prices do not allow an expansion of the market."

• Tariffs pose another problem: One large U.S. company in the Philippines had to change the protein base of its product because the tariff on imported soy flour rendered it too costly. When the organization considered building a plant in Manila to serve other parts of southeast Asia, it discovered that other countries would impose tariffs of 35 percent to 50 percent on any products entering their markets. One executive complained: "By the time we have paid duties on raw material and duties on finished goods, I am sure you can appreciate that we no longer have a low-cost, high-protein food product. All of this work, involving research investments of millions of dollars, has been carried out; and I know of no major food company which has not finished its work on several products. But being able to make them and market them, in view of the above problems, are two entirely different matters."[3]

• Technological obstacles cannot be overcome: In India, one international company devoted triple the time planned to meet desired standards for cottonseed flour, and even then the product lacked the anticipated sophistication. Peruvita, a privately produced protein-rich cereal food extensively promoted in Peru, failed in part because of its "wet dog" odor and flavor, imperfect formulation, and short shelf life. A soft drink company had problems with a difficult-to-describe "after feel" in the throat. And in Brazil, CPC International's enrichment of Maizina made the product more attractive not only to customers but also to insects. At times the new products fail to live up to the nutrient levels claimed for them. When the desires of the consumer and the nutritionist do not coincide, nutrition inevitably receives lower priority. Nutritionists have often in return scoffed at the nutrition contribution of certain of the new foods, especially the protein-based soft drinks; their disfavor makes the promotional support of the medical professions and financial subsidies from government difficult to solicit.

The effort to commercialize Incaparina in Panama exemplifies the kind of unexpected difficulties that raise product costs. The El Salvador–Honduras war cut off shipments of cottonseed flour, curtailing production for six weeks. Defective polyethylene-lined bags produced in Panama caused substantial product loss. An imported packaging machine failed to operate. And early production batches of the food went rancid in the humid shops, leading to major consumer dissatisfaction.[4]

*Reaching the market.* By late 1968, many businessmen, government officials, and academics were voicing their conviction that the sizable international demand for more protein-rich foods would ensure an ample market for a great many companies.[5] Not that there ever was an illusion that the market was simply there for the asking, but many people now admit that they expected greater consumer response than has occurred. And there are no apparent signs of a sizable increase in demand in the near future. Those who require the new foods have no money to buy them, and most of those who have the money do not need them. A middle group, which may have both the money and the need, is small in most developing countries.

In many places, there is no tradition of a weaning food, and in some, there is no established custom of purchasing processed food. Moreover, the buying pattern for new foods is too inconsistent for a new product to have a nutritional impact. Even Incaparina, with its impressive penetration into all levels of Guatemalan society, has not been consumed in nutritionally significant quantities.*[6] (It has been estimated that for a new product to be nutritionally useful to a child, sufficient stimulus must be provided to encourage a hundred separate purchases a year.)[7]

Inadequate commercial channels are another problem. Although there is increasing penetration into the countryside, most business is urban-oriented. The number of nutritionally needy living in urban areas in the developing countries is very large, yet the largest fraction of the needy often live far from normal means of transportation and commercial delivery points. For people in the hinterland a commercial market is often only a small stall with a low inventory—a few packets that will be sold before the reorder.

*Raising the nutrition level.* The attractive product that lures a new purchaser usually displaces another food in his diet. Many consumers in low-income countries spend 65 percent to 80 percent of their income on food and can afford no more. Some companies promoting new foods overlook the consequences to the purchasers. In New Delhi the four largest daily newspapers from 1968 to 1970 tripled the space devoted to food advertising; nutrition-related themes dominated the advertisements. Such advertising is often aimed at convincing parents that only certain high-priced nutritious products will keep their children well and alert. As a result, low-income purchasers are sometimes seduced into spending a disproportionate amount of their income on canned baby foods and similar items at the expense of more needed staples.

In West Bengal, some families were found to be "leaning on patent baby foods which they purchased at exorbitant rates, sometimes in the black market, although they could purchase cow's milk locally at much

---

* Monthly sales in 1972 were the equivalent of one glass of milk per person.

lower cost. They thought these baby foods had extraordinary food value and were far superior to cow's milk for the health of infants."[8]

In some parts of the world, companies have taken blatant advantage of nutrition consciousness. In the Caribbean, nurses are employed to obtain names of new mothers from hospitals; then—often competitively—they race to the women's homes to give free samples and related advertising. The products are "convenient, attractive and almost totally inappropriate for less developed regions. . . . The food industry in developing countries," one expert reports, "has been a disaster . . . a minus influence."[9]

*Corporate profit.* Although many corporations have initiated nutrition projects for other than profit motives, they have generally expected that the projects would be profitable. Few companies, however, have been satisfied with their financial return; and the prospects are not encouraging. General Foods' chairman puts industry's nutrition dilemma this way: "There is no question that these people (those toward the bottom of the socioeconomic totem pole) are in dire need of more and better nutritious food. At the same time, it is virtually impossible for a private business establishment to develop, distribute, and sell enough of the kinds of foods these people need and still break even, much less look for any profit motive."[10]

Some international companies have been unrealistic about the possibilities of applying their skills in unfamiliar cultures. Sophisticated production, marketing, and advertising techniques sometimes have been of less value than expected, in part because of low education levels and the absence of comprehensive distribution and communication channels. The kinds of market information normally available to a large company about to begin a commercial venture are simply not available in a developing country. Skilled manpower is in short supply. There are also shortages of equipment, parts, raw materials, and, according to one executive, "intangibles like standards and concepts of product integrity."

Commercial distributors have sometimes met unexpected competition from institutional feeding programs that use donated foods. The commercial sale of Multi-Purpose Food to the Madras government collapsed, reportedly, because free food suddenly became available under a voluntary agency's child feeding program. The developers of Incaparina have long complained about the "counterproductive effect" of U.S.-donated CSM distribution. And companies complain of unfair competition from government-run enterprises that are not trying to maximize profits.

*Host country interest.* A number of food companies have found the climate for their investments less warm than they expected. For foreign firms, much of the cold shoulder comes from local companies concerned with the intruding and better financed competition. In one country, for instance, local and foreign companies had agreed, at least in theory, that the simultaneous introduction of many nutritious products would help educate the public, yield experience from which all companies could benefit, and bring help from the local government (an industry might get favored treatment; a single company probably would not). In the face of actual competition, however, local companies often made substantial efforts to prevent other products from being marketed.

More importantly, the expected welcome mat and general support from local governments sometimes have been difficult to find. When a commercial food project—local or foreign—is approved, the sanction sometimes is conditioned by a string of requirements considered inhibiting by businessmen. In Brazil, for instance, a weaning food containing protein attracts a 22 percent to 25 percent tax. And in India the government sometimes requires the inclusion of an export component before a project proposal will be approved. Also in India, official policy has strongly supported the notion that research and development be carried out by government-sponsored food technological institutes rather than by private enterprise.

One corporate concern that goes beyond the food industry is the frequent requirement that equipment be locally produced. A major commercial fish project collapsed after three years of negotiations because the government demanded that half of the trawlers be purchased from local dealers. Since the amount of foreign exchange involved was not great, the negotiating officer of the international company suggested that there was a confusion of objectives. "Is the objective to catch more fish to improve nutrition," he asked, "or to subsidize the local boat building industry?"

Another common requirement—again one that is not limited to the food industry—is that foreign companies collaborate with local investors. One problem with these arrangements is that multinational food corporations, bent on long-range expansion of sales, generally prefer to reinvest profits—a notion not always attractive to the local businessman accustomed to quick dividends.

In some countries these problems—technology, equipment, collaboration—become issues upon the application for a license to permit local commercial food production. The objectives of licensing may have little to do with nutrition. They often are aimed at geographic dispersion of industry within the country; assistance to small business, which sometimes means restricting growth of larger firms and thus inhibiting research and expansion by those firms most likely to succeed; and limiting foreign exchange costs through official preference for indigenous companies (especially when locally developed processes are available or potentially available). India, for instance, welcomes foreign investment "only if the know-how for the product is not indigenously available."[11]

Whether the result of ideological design or bureaucratic sluggishness, sanctions for commercial food production sometimes take extended periods—often years—to obtain. Approval for Cerealina by the government of Brazil took eighteen months. In Mexico, products of two international firms were held up awaiting government approval of advertising copy. Licensing decisions in India involve a multitude of committees and public officials at all ranks. One $200,000 project, in which an American firm was collaborating, was rejected after two-and-a-half years of deliberations that directly involved the prime minister, the deputy prime minister, and the chief minister of Gujarat. Licensing problems are not restricted to foreign firms; one all-Indian company in Bombay devoted two years and many trips to Delhi to obtaining its license to produce protein foods. In a South American country that professes a national nutrition policy, it commonly takes years to register a new food product name. (One multinational firm circumvented the problem by adopting the word "Duryea" for its processed food milled from high-lysine corn; the name was selected not because it related in any way to nutrition or even to food, but because the title had long been registered and used by the company—on starch boxes; Mr. Duryea was the Frenchman who invented wet milling for starch.)

*Mutual distrust.* In some countries, distrust between the local government and the food industry raises problems, at times reflecting a failure of communication and understanding. Public officials question the motives of businessmen, and the attitude is often reciprocated. Even when government goes to the food industry for help and offers potential business (such as the production of food for distribution in institutional feeding programs), the relationship is fraught with difficulties.

Food executives complain that local governments fail to establish well-defined goals. In some countries a cardboard package containing a protein-rich food attracts bugs, but a package designed to resist bugs attracts excise duties. A food policy may be invoked but not adequately filtered down through the bureaucracy. In one Asian country, policy makers publicly advocated priority for protein foods, but no document proclaiming this ever reached the proper ministerial bodies. Consequently, in the same month that an international soft drink company received approval to produce a diet drink, it was turned down in its request to market a protein beverage.

The difficulties are not limited to less developed countries; international businessmen often find working with the bureaucracy of their home country or the United Nations agencies frustrating. Time delays, duplication of effort, and unnecessary paperwork are complaints sometimes heard from those seeking help in their food projects.

## Governmental Interventions

Because most of the technical and marketing expertise in food is lodged in the private sector, industry is uniquely equipped to help overcome malnutrition. For a variety of reasons, many related to economics, ventures in the processing of nutritious food for the very needy have had little nutritional significance. Nor is it likely that business can, under current procedures, make a major contribution in the future.* If business is to play a large role, substantial change is required in conditions that have thus far inhibited the contribution.

The cornerstone of such change is financial support from government to a consumer food industry, the very notion of which is anathema in some national capitals. Yet the issue is not governmental support but nutrition. It would be precipitous for governments to dismiss out of hand what may be the best existing instrument for reaching masses of people. The conditions that would make it possible for industry to contribute to nutrition objectives should be carefully examined. Then the implied public costs of meeting those conditions—through financial supports, guarantees, technical assistance—should be computed. Whether governmental assistance to industry is an effective and financially attractive means of achieving a particular objective can then be judged against alternative actions.

### Conventional Marketing

To date, corporate involvement in food projects has been primarily in development of a nutritious product and sale of the product through nor-

* This conclusion recognizes changes are now afoot: for example, costs of fortifying nutrients are declining, a body of commercial experience is being compiled on which to base new projects, and governments have an increasing appreciation of need for answers to nutrition problems.

mal commercial channels. To make that participation nutritionally helpful to those in need and financially attractive to industry, government can offer many kinds of support: (1) Create tax policies favoring firms producing low-cost, nutritious foods that meet specified standards (Peru offers a ten-year income tax relief to companies producing foods with at least 30 percent protein); where there is consumer tax on food, tax exemption can be given for special nutritious products. (2) Allow duty-free imports of equipment (a special attraction, since most equipment is multipurpose and will not be used exclusively for the nutrition project). (3) Provide land, warehouses, government-owned plants, or other physical facilities at little or no rent. (4) Offer special, low-interest loans. (5) Underwrite the costs of product development and market studies. (6) Guarantee the capital investment in nutrition projects. (7) Guarantee sales to assure a plant size adequate for economically viable production (in India's Bal Amul project, the government purchased excess production in the early stages for use in institutional feeding programs, in a way that promoted commercialization). (8) Guarantee the availability of raw materials, perhaps at the price the government must pay for them. (9) Sponsor research in packaging that would be useful to the industry as a whole. (10) Provide radio and other mass media facilities to promote products. (11) Offer preferential transportation and storage rates. (12) Encourage use of government institutes for laboratory and clinical testing of commercial products. (13) Create marketing departments in government technical institutes to improve their usefulness to industry. (14) Provide training facilities to develop skills needed by industry. (15) Eliminate or reduce restrictive requirements—on licensing, for instance—and streamline procedures that must be maintained. (16) Solicit assistance for firms—capital, material, technical—from foreign governments and international and voluntary agencies.

Should the government conclude that some of these indirect supports make sense vis-à-vis the alternatives to achieving better nutrition, it must create a climate friendly to the entrepreneurial mind. Further, its objective must be clearly understood and stated—for instance, as better nutrition for children, rather than protection of local public technological institutes or subsidization of a fishing boat building industry. Policies will flow from the objective, and specific activities from those policies. Government should take an active role in encouraging projects. If governments act only on requests, the limited number of government licenses will not always go to the most experienced or well equipped food firms. Companies best suited to do the job should be identified and their participation should be aggressively solicited.


### Unconventional Opportunities

The traditional view of industry's role in nutrition is a limited one. Opportunities exist that go considerably beyond standard notions of product commercialization, opportunities that avoid most of the impediments discussed earlier. Here are some examples that draw heavily on India's experimentation with nontraditional business-government interactions in the nutrition field:

The *atta* project, designed to produce more nutritious *chapattis,* is a significant illustration of private sector–public sector collaboration; the government contracts with private companies for the purchase of fortifying ingredients as well as the processing and marketing of the final product.

Food companies can work with governments to produce processed foods for distribution in public institutional feeding programs. In production of Bal Ahar the Indian government contracts with private companies for the processed oilseed flour, the premix of vitamins and minerals, and the mixing of the complete product. Similarly, through U.S. corporate eyes the one significant financial success in the nutrition field is CSM. The U.S. government annually contracts with the private sector for over $30 million (375 million pounds) of this high-protein cereal blend for free distribution abroad.

Corporate distribution facilities can be used to market low-cost foods produced under government programs. India's family planning program provides an example of how this would work for the food industry. A consortium of large private companies uses its wide distribution network to sell condoms at a government-subsidized price (three for 2 cents) that is 85 percent below the actual cost. Analysis had indicated that this was the least expensive method for meeting a family planning objective. In India, corporate distribution networks, although not as comprehensive as in Europe, are a significant resource; Hindustan Lever's products, for instance, are sold in 300,000 shops, and commercially packaged tea in 1.4 million shops. Coca-Cola reaches some of the most remote populated areas of low-income countries.

Skills of private industry can be marshaled to devise education programs that create greater nutrition awareness. Both an individual commercial product promotion and an institutional advertising campaign, carried out by an association of commercial firms, have been effective educators in India.

Industrial research capabilities and facilities can be made available for government programs. The *atta* fortification project was facilitated by the use of equipment designed by Roche, a Bombay pharmaceutical house. The company also resolved a government dilemma concerning the value of undertaking research on lysine, which India did not produce and could not afford to import. Roche went ahead and developed lysine in its laboratories to demonstrate that, if lysine proved to be a worthwhile addition to the Indian diet, it could be produced locally.

Private industry can help with segments of projects, government and industry each performing part of a process in a way that taps the comparative advantage of each. Or government can contract with a company or consortium of companies to do the complete job in meeting a predetermined nutrition objective. This may include designing a product to meet certain specifications; devising a system of distribution—commercial or institutional—that will reach the needy; and developing appropriate educational materials to accompany the distribution.

Managerial and marketing talents of industry can be made available in a variety of ways, including basic planning of national nutrition strategies and programs. Also, private and public sectors can collaborate to lower the prices of such conventional protein foods as fish, dairy products, and land-based crops of nutritional significance. Corporate experience can be helpful in designing and carrying out projects for more effective processing, storage, transport, and distribution. This implies the possibility of more business participation in basic agricultural practices (for example, in the rapid commercialization of seed varieties with higher nutritive value).

Industry can contribute to better nutrition by more selective marketing of nonnutritious—and antinutritious—foods. To be sure, selective restriction of the mass media message is difficult, but more sensitivity should be applied in the use of local promotional techniques. Firms that persist in employing marketing practices that clearly run counter to the government's nutrition objectives (for example, the aggressive promotions designed to influence early cessation of breast feeding) should be subject to official regulatory action. Governments should consider requiring a minimum nutrition level in foods that are known to be widely consumed or that are in the process of supplanting other foods to the detriment of the national diet. For example, consideration should be given to requiring inclusion of nutrient supplements in all soft drinks[12] as a condition for licensing and public distribution. (The notion of government intervention to prevent food adulteration is accepted.) These suggested steps are an extension of the principle of food regulation in the public interest.*

All of these less conventional government-business interactions require that industry respond to national need, provide the services it uniquely has available, and in some instances provide skilled personnel to assist the government. Most large companies already recognize the importance of including government's needs and policies in their marketing equation. However, if industry's capabilities are to be exploited in special noncommercial ways, government must take the lead. Private enterprise cannot create policy. It can encourage and help create a favorable public climate and may even embarrass a government into action, but it cannot lay down the rules. Nor can it operate in a policy vacuum. Should a government decide that involvement of the private sector is worth the costs, the success or failure of participation by private companies will depend on government receptivity, government policies, and government actions.

NUTRITION authorities have devoted substantial time and program energies to involving private industry in producing new nutritious foods. Although food companies have in many cases responded enthusiastically, there is little to show in the way of nutrition improvement. Nor are prospects bright for reaching a significant portion of the needy with proprietary foods marketed in the conventional manner (even taking into account the lengthy gestation period sometimes required for new food projects to emerge successfully). Problems are many, but the major impediment is the inability to reconcile the demand for corporate profit with a product low enough in cost to reach the needy in large numbers.

Although the food industry has the potential to make a major contribution, it probably cannot do so unless it is subsidized. Without government incentives, industry is unlikely to create nutritious products that have a

---

* Clearly, those commercial actions and antinutritious products that are harmful to society should be subjected to regulation. Whether government should regulate those nonnutritious products that do no good—but do no direct harm—is a vexing issue. (The harm is indirect; every soft drink purchased by a poor person probably displaces something nutritionally more useful in the diet of someone in the family.) The costs—administrative costs of regulation as well as costs to consumer sovereignty—should be weighed against the costs of other options government has available to achieve the same nutritional ends.

significant demand among the poor and at the same time yield profit. The rich resources of the food industry do not come free. Governments must provide the proper climate and offer incentives to obtain the commercial involvement needed to make a major nutritional impact. Opportunities for government help clearly exist. The pertinent question is not whether government support to industry is palatable, but whether the cost and relative significance of conventional private sector involvement compares favorably with alternative ways of achieving the same nutrition objective.

Perhaps more important than industry's conventional food marketing role are certain unconventional opportunities for industry-government cooperation. Corporate distribution networks, advertising expertise, research, and technological skills all can be applied to national nutrition goals. In all of this, the onus is on government to provide the objectives, policies, programs, and favorable climate that will be critical factors in encouraging or discouraging a contribution from the private sector.

## CHAPTER TEN

# Feeding Children through Public Programs

Of all the conscious efforts in low-income countries to get nutritious foods to the needy, by far the largest are the institutional child feeding programs, which provide meals through schools, health centers, and other organized facilities. They are the most expensive of nutrition programs, costing approximately three-quarters of a billion dollars a year (two-thirds in the form of foreign food aid), and they account for upwards of 95 percent of all budgets in economically developing countries directed to child nutrition. They are the most widespread of nutrition programs, reaching about 125 million children in about 100 countries.[1] And although highly agreeable in their public face, they are the most controversial of programs among nutrition's cognoscenti.

## The Advocates' View

Advocates contend that institutional programs help to keep masses of children alive and healthy through an extensive network of facilities already in place. Such programs alleviate the problems of selection, preparation, and distribution of food in the home and avoid many obstacles that might otherwise prevent the foods prescribed from reaching the mouths intended.

Champions of child feeding programs also suggest that they lead to a better education system and to all this implies for national development. Not only does school attendance improve, but the students are more attentive and receptive to learning. Preschool-aged children who are included in the program reflect the benefits once they reach school. Properly presented, the program is also an opportunity for nutrition education.

Finally, the supporters of institutionalized child feeding assert that the program offers several social and political benefits. For example, feeding programs have been credited with improving food habits. They also are said to make community and government aware of nutritional needs and to stimulate interest in meeting them. They provide government an opportunity to fulfill its social responsibility to the people, and in the process, to accept foreign aid that is not as vulnerable to domestic political attack as other kinds of assistance.

## The Adversaries' View

Quite a different view is taken by a school of internationally recognized nutritionists who claim that conventional child feeding programs have been nutritionally counterproductive: even though the food comes free, the costs of administration, storage, transport, and so on, are too great a financial burden for local governments to bear; the funds could have greater nutritional impact if spent in other ways. Furthermore, foreign assistance for feeding programs discourages local manufacture of low-cost foods. "Give away techniques," in the view of the Food and Nutrition Board of the National Academy of Sciences, "... will not solve either their problems or ours."[2]

Critics of the programs also question whether they benefit children in the appropriate age and economic groups. Generally, less than 10 percent of the youngsters are in the more vulnerable preschool-age group; and seldom are large numbers of the neediest youngsters in the population reached. Moreover, critics warn that where the younger group is reached, the food giveaway may induce bad nutrition, especially if it serves as an incentive for early weaning as free milk appears to have done in Chile.[3]

Opponents also point to the heavy workload imposed on health clinics and schools in the weighing and distribution of food, filling out of reports, and, in many instances, food preparation, to the detriment of basic health treatment and education. Some critics are concerned about both the black market in donated foods and their use in religious proselyting. They allege that the free food transfer is by no means as politically and socially acceptable as its advocates would have it seem.

Finally, the detractors claim that such programs relieve local governments of their responsibility to confront the needs of their people and to shape national priorities to meet them—in short, that child feeding programs tend to create psychological, nutritional, and political dependence.

As can be seen, the arguments of the two camps are not always joined. Moreover, both advocates and adversaries on occasion rely more on emotion than on hard data. The pros and cons of child feeding programs need to be closely examined if costs and benefits are to determine what nutrition activities should be carried out.

## Development of Feeding Programs

Institutional feeding programs can be traced back at least as far as the mid-nineteenth century, when the Paris National Guard established a fund to provide school lunches for needy children.[4] Victor Hugo, who is mentioned as the first patron of this program, continued to advocate the concept even after his exile to Germany, where in 1865 he financed out-of-pocket hot meals at a local school. Child feeding projects gained such momentum in Germany that by the end of the century the Social Democrats introduced into the Reichstag a bill authorizing school feeding in every German city. After substantial debate, the proposal was defeated, not because of the expense or of doubt about the program's value, but for fear that the program's popularity would induce a further flow of families from farms to cities. In the early twentieth century, military concerns accelerated child feeding programs in both Germany and England when substantial numbers of recruits were rejected as physically unfit.

Most of the early feeding activities were privately financed. For example, school feeding was initiated in Japan in 1889 by a Buddhist priest with food furnished as alms; it was not until 1932, amidst economic depression, that a nationally funded program was launched. The Netherlands in 1900, in the first national legal recognition of a government's responsibility, authorized local governments to make meals available at school for youngsters unable "through lack of food to attend regularly." Within three years the Danes had legalized similar programs and the Swiss had made them compulsory.

Not all countries were receptive to institutionalized public feeding. Belgium objected to the concept on grounds that it intruded on the role of parents. Finland permitted school lunch programs but, to avoid any sense of dependence, stipulated that they must be accompanied by school gardens.

Few large feeding programs were reported from the colonized countries before their independence. An exception was India where programs were conducted in Madras as long ago as 1925, but it was not until the late 1950s that statewide programs became a major factor in the Indian education system. In Brazil also there were early programs, but mass distribution began only in the early 1960s.

Although early programs differed from one another, they were generally on a small scale, sponsored by private charitable groups, directed specifically to the poorer children, and often concerned only with milk distribution. As programs evolved, governments began to take over their sponsorship, dispensing a broader range of foods and embracing children of all economic levels.

### International Involvement

As they had during and after the First World War, several of the more affluent countries expanded their programs to help feed the needy abroad in the distress brought on by the Second. Their efforts were channeled through the United Nations Relief and Works Agency (UNRWA), the United Nations Children's Fund (UNICEF), and the World Food Program of the Food and Agriculture Organization (FAO). Chief among the countries that offered bilateral aid was the United States, whose foreign food grant programs reach about 65 million children a year. From 1954 to 1971, $5.6 billion worth of U.S. food was donated abroad through U.S. programs.*

The U.S. overseas programs in the early postwar years appear to have served as a convenient focus for several quite different objectives. First, they responded to a clear need that the United States had the power to alleviate. The popular press and congressional hearings of the day reflected genuine concern for the destitute abroad, which by itself probably would have been sufficient to motivate large feeding programs. The format of the program had the further advantage of providing a channel through which

* These food grants are separate from concessional sales (including sale for local currencies and IOU-type credit arrangements for hard currency), which constitute 80 percent of U.S. foreign food aid. About one-third of all U.S. aid, or $25 billion since the end of World War II, has been in some form of food program. This accounts for 3 to 4 percent of total U.S. farm output.[5]

the general public could help directly. The U.S. government gives food to the voluntary agencies (of which CARE, Catholic Relief Services, and Church World Service are now the largest) and with private contributions, the voluntary agencies then administer, distribute, and promote the foods.* The U.S. government also gives food to international agencies (UNRWA, UNICEF, and the World Food Program) and provides food directly to governments through grants or concessional loans.

In the fifties the feeding programs provided one answer to the mounting U.S. problem of surplus foods brought on by rising farm productivity and U.S. agricultural support policies. The heavily political subsidies bestowed not inconsiderable benefits on portions of the farm community.† Furthermore, as feeding programs and donated foods became more sophisticated, U.S. food processing firms also benefited, and the voices of their strong lobbies apparently did not go unheard in Washington. Frank Ellis, for ten years a top operating official of the Food for Peace program of the Agency for International Development, credits the success of the child feeding activity to a combination of motives—altruism, politics, and profits.‡

The postwar overseas food aid programs were marked by their simplicity of intent and crudeness of operation. They were also characterized in recipient countries by flourishing black markets which were of sufficient magnitude in some cases to become an established part of the local culture. The clasped hands symbol that appears on all U.S. donated foods allegedly became one of the best-known food trademarks in the world. John Kenneth Galbraith, U.S. ambassador to India, describes early food distribution through religious agencies as "a kind of heavenly gate to an enormous black market." In Calcutta, milk descends "through a hierarchy of distributors and each level sells half, more or less, and passes half on to the next grafter for the next division. Not much remains for the ultimate poor after this geometry."[9] In India the black market and the difficulties resulting from sizzling government audit reports reached such proportions

---

* CARE, whose administrative costs usually are borne by the host government, reported that in 1970 it converted each dollar contributed by its 1.5 million regular donors into $8.42 worth of aid.[6]

† The yearly cost to the U.S. budget for this program has ranged from $3 billion to $5 billion. Because of the federal price support measures, the consumer pays some $4.5 billion more for farm products.[7]

‡ Ellis's persistence was responsible for much of the program upgrading outlined in the following pages. A 1965 Interdepartmental Nutrition Task Force was asked to look into roles for the United States in international nutrition. The heavily Ellis-influenced recommendations—generally regarded as pie-in-the-sky when they first appeared in the Task Force Report—have now mostly been realized.[8]

that one frustrated international agency closed down its large food distribution program.

In most countries, problems of food diversion have been reduced to a "manageable" scale. The field director of one voluntary agency reports it operates with losses roughly equal to the shoplifting costs built into American retail prices. Donated foods are now rarely found in the bazaars where black marketing once flourished.

Major reasons for the improved field management were the more stringent requirements imposed by donor countries and the tighter controls of recipient governments themselves. The Dominican Republic, for example, instituted severe criminal penalties for misuse of food aid. Also, the distributing agencies, which depended heavily on volunteer program distributors who seldom had any training, began recruiting professional administrators, often with business backgrounds.

Matters also improved with a change in the program concept. The early programs distributed food to families in bulk quantities. Consequently, there were many diversions between the distribution center and the family pot. Today, most of the food is prepared and served at the institutional site, and most of the feeding is directed to the youngsters. In Brazil, 11 million students are fed through a sophisticated national network encompassing over 96,000 primary schools. In India, 92 percent of the 17 million beneficiaries of organized feeding projects in 1970 were children,* nearly all reached through institutional feeding programs.

The nature of the foods themselves also changed. Where milk and milled cereal staples (especially wheat flour and cornmeal) were once the major foods in aid programs, items less acceptable to the black market have taken their place.† Among them are bulgur wheat, a parboiled and cracked form of whole wheat, and cereal and oilseed blends such as CSM (corn-soy-milk) and WSB (wheat-soy blend). Recipient countries have begun to blend donated foods with local ingredients, processing them through local industrial facilities. The most striking example is India's Bal Ahar.[10]

Traditional foods are being improved through fortification—milk with

---

* The remainder were mainly adults participating in food-for-work projects and their families.

† Today's foods are not as marketable because they are unfamiliar, and at times disliked. This is not always by design. One of the early batches of Bal Ahar in India by mistake contained 10 percent salt. The substitution of this food for milk powder in feeding programs instantly solved the black market problem.

vitamins A and D, processed cereals with a variety of vitamins and minerals. In 1970 the first shipment of lysine-fortified bulgur wheat was sent to Nigeria and in 1971 three soy-fortified products—cornmeal, bulgur, and rolled oats—became available.

### New Considerations

Although officials have devoted time and resources to assessing and upgrading the nutritional and administrative sophistication of feeding programs, less systematic assessment has been made of their basic value. Measures of success usually have been based on numbers of children reached, effectiveness of the distribution system, commodity costs, and nutritive value of the foods provided, rather than on which of the children were reached, the effect of these programs on the nutritional status and growth of these children, the resulting changes in the education system, or the return on the investment as compared with other forms of nutrition expenditures.

Feeding the destitute in the wake of war, famine, or other disasters, in which imported foods often mean the difference between survival and mass death, is hardly open to criticism. It is another matter to apply the same rationale to a much broader program under quite different circumstances. While both are propelled by the same humane motive, there are major conceptual and administrative distinctions between emergency and non-emergency feeding programs. Whereas disaster conditions permit little choice, one might legitimately ask whether the current mode of providing nutrition to youngsters is the most effective way of being helpful in more normal times.

This question takes on added importance with the uncertainty of the future of foreign food aid. In the past, recipient governments often bore considerably less than half the total cost of institutional feeding programs, thanks to the heavy supply of donated foodstuffs. Henceforth they may have to pay for a larger share of the food. As of 1972, these foods are no longer readily available—at least from the United States, which formerly provided two-thirds of all donated foods. U.S. surpluses of some of the foods long popular in the feeding programs are diminishing, partly as a result of the 1972 wheat deal with Russia, and a general budgetary tightening is in evidence. Moreover, the slight additional costs long presumed to be entailed in giving food to those in need turn out on closer scrutiny to be not so modest after all, especially when taking into account the costs of processing and of nonsurplus foods sometimes provided in the programs. As reasons for farmers' subsidies are reviewed, it becomes apparent that it is less expensive (although not always preferable) to pay farmers not to grow the food than to accumulate surpluses to be sent abroad for donation programs. Justifications for grant foods are now more stringently policed, and the easy, almost automatic, program approvals are a thing of the past.

## Costs and Benefits

What then is the return developing countries can expect to receive on a nutritional investment in institutional child feeding? The answer depends in part on whether foods are donated from abroad or provided by the country itself, the latter being an increasingly feasible assumption. The effectiveness of the program in meeting nutritional objectives is of course an important part of the evaluation.

Even when foods are donated, local nonfood costs can run more than one-third the costs of the foods. The host country must pay handling charges from the time of arrival at the port of entry; rail, truck, and other transport costs within the country; administrative costs to meet wages and overhead for program officials, cooks, warehousemen, auditors, and others; and operating expenses for facilities, fuel, cooking utensils, and in some cases eating utensils. In addition, most countries receiving U.S. help are now required to pay half of the ocean freight on their food shipments, a not insubstantial amount. For locally processed products like India's Bal Ahar, the recipient government also pays for some of the ingredients and the processing and packaging costs. In Liberia the national government pays one-third and the local community pays an additional 10 percent of the total cost, the latter including food. In Colombia the national and local governments contribute 19 percent of a $2.3 million program, and the Turks pick up 58 percent of the total costs of programs in their country (see Table 11).

An untallied but considerable cost of feeding programs is the time required for preparation and serving of the food, especially when it involves diversion from another activity. Every hour a school master (or student) or a health center employee devotes to cooking could be one less hour given to education or health services. Another indirect cost that some critics cite is the inhibiting effect of donated products like CSM on com-

TABLE 11. *Cost of Institutional Feeding Programs in Selected Countries*

| Country | Participating children | Total cost, dollars[a] | Cost per child per year, dollars[b] | Percentage contributed by U.S. sources[c] | Percentage contributed by recipient[d] |
|---|---|---|---|---|---|
| Turkey | 2,240,000 | 20,829,477 | 9.30 | *42* | *58* |
| Liberia | 45,000 | 590,263 | 13.12 | *56* | *44* |
| Costa Rica | 362,000[e] | 1,565,496 | 4.32 | *19* | *81* |
| Colombia | 158,807[f] | 2,331,375 | 14.67 | *81* | *19* |
| Brazil | 11,014,961 | 41,680,793 | 3.78 | *31* | *65*[g] |

Sources: Data compiled from statistics of CARE and from Government of Brazil, National School Lunch Campaign (CNAE). Data are for fiscal year 1969 for Turkey and Liberia; for fiscal year 1971 for Costa Rica, Colombia, and Brazil.

a. Excludes construction costs of nutrition centers.

b. Based on 180 days in Turkey and Colombia, 160 in Liberia, 140 in Costa Rica, 118 in Brazil.

c. Costs of PL 480 commodities (Commodity Credit Corporation value), ocean freight, and some CARE expenses.

d. Includes contributions by national and provincial and local governments.

e. Includes 12,000 children in mother/child health centers (operating 365 days).

f. Includes 25,525 children in mother/child health centers (operating 365 days).

g. World Food Program of the UN Food and Agriculture Organization contributes 4 percent.

mercialization of Incaparina in Guatemala. The benefit that the affected product or venture might have had must be weighed against the value of the feeding program. What would happen had there been no program and what might be anticipated if the program came to a sudden stop? As their advocates contend, donated foods can pave the way for commercial ventures by exposing potential customers to new products and new food concepts. The classic example is General MacArthur's introduction of milk and bread into school lunches in postwar Japan. After a generation of children had been regularly exposed to these foods, both became standard Japanese fare.* The commercially marketed Bal Amul might never have been introduced had it not been for ongoing institutional efforts to introduce the product and the concept of blended foods to potential customers.

## The Beneficiaries

Once its costs have become clear, the next step in judging the value of a program is to establish whether it reaches the age and economic groups

* Partly as a result of this change, Japan today is the leading purchaser of U.S. farm exports. Japanese food imports from the United States totaled $1.1 billion in 1970, the largest amount of food ever transferred between two countries.

for which it was intended. In nearly all countries with institutional feeding activities the major recipient is the schoolchild, with a sprinkling of preschool-aged children also benefiting. Given the nutritional priorities of the very young, such an allocation of limited resources is questionable. But students, unlike younger children, are easily accessible through the built-in distributional mechanism the school provides. The food programs, like the early programs to inoculate children against tuberculosis, are aimed at those most easily reached rather than the most vulnerable.

*The very young.* Those younger children who receive institutional help usually get it through nursery centers, maternal and child health clinics, and mothercraft and child rehabilitation centers; but these are too few, and often such feeding programs as they operate are irregular. In India, assuming totally effective food programs, all such outlets could reach only 6 percent of the total population under school age. Plainly, new vehicles must be found to help massive numbers.

Taking one approach, India has achieved some success in using the school itself as the feeding site for preschoolers. This program, begun during the famine emergency of 1966–67, has continued as the most effective means of reaching large numbers in this age group. Its advantages are obvious: the presence of the schools and the existence of feeding activities and their utensils, storage facilities, and already hot fires. The major drawback is the commotion the younger children create at the school, which could be alleviated by using the school facilities when classes are not in session.

Another means of using the school mechanism for preschoolers, one that has been tested in India and Bangladesh, removes this problem: schoolchildren take food home to their younger siblings. Under this approach, however, the food is less certain to reach the destination. Furthermore, youngsters who have no older brothers and sisters in school would not benefit; but they are not as prone to nutrition problems as children in large families. This approach involves the parents and thus could have the added benefit of inducing parents to modify family eating patterns.

School feeding may also benefit younger children indirectly. A child who receives food at school may get less at home, while his younger brother or sister gets a larger share of the food that comes into the household. Through this kind of substitution, the value of a school feeding program for the school-aged child comes into question, but it may be an effective way of reaching the preschool-aged youngster in many households. This effect has yet to be adequately measured.

*The poor.* Do the programs reach the neediest economic group? Just as it is harder to reach a child the younger he is, so is it harder to do so the poorer he is. In many places the neediest youngsters often are unable or incapable of going to school at all, or last only briefly if they do begin. The Education Ministry of Zambia has raised the question of how many new schools can be built with the money being invested in feeding programs for children who already have the opportunity to go to school. Furthermore, schools in poor, remote villages are the least likely to have feeding programs; and for that matter, the poorest communities—and states and nations—are the least likely to have programs. Often they lack the awareness that such opportunities exist, let alone the initiative and funds to launch an activity. Bihar, the state hardest hit by the famine in India in 1966–67, was the poorest state and also the only large one that had no child feeding program. In most countries the size and location of the programs are planned not only on the basis of need but also on the availability of administrative skills and other resources necessary to carry out the program. Because in general the wealthier the state or the nation the greater these resources, those needing the most help often are unable to receive it.

That it may be ten times as difficult and costly to reach children to whom no convenient channel exists as to reach others who would not be as needy but may also benefit from the food should not of itself serve as a deterrent. The more relevant issue is the relative value to the nation of reaching only a tenth as many youngsters.

### Nutritional Impact

Hunger in the classrom generally is believed to lead to lethargy, apathy, and inability to pay attention.[11] There are few hard data, however, on which to base judgments about the usefulness of feeding programs in combating these problems. This probably reflects both the long-standing assumption that institutional feeding activities are valuable and the inordinate difficulties in carefully measuring their impact.

Such evidence as exists is not definitive. Japanese nutritionists suggest that school lunches played no small part in the significant increase in the physical size of the "under thirty" Japanese generation. The typical Japanese fourth grader no longer fits in the chair his parents occupied a generation ago; twice since the end of the war, desks in Japanese schools have been moved out for larger ones, and architects are now designing doorways for homes and offices six inches higher than before.[12] Several studies in south India have reported a well-balanced diet supplement provided at school resulted in statistically significant increases in weight and height, in school attendance, and in classroom performance.[13] In the old Orange Free State, absenteeism fell from 9.5 percent to 6.9 percent in the three years following introduction of a feeding program.[14] Suspension of a lunch program in Puerto Rico led to a marked reduction in attendance, while attendance at the Bantu Schools in South Africa varied in relation to the food supplied.[15]

On the other hand, in the Philippines and El Salvador protein supplements provided over extended periods brought no significant change in health status.[16] Although the Philippine program later was modified to correct the caloric deficit thought to be responsible for the lack of change, at the end of the second phase the nutritional condition of the students still had not improved significantly. The general conclusion was that the evaluators' lack of control over food consumption in the home and elsewhere—unmeasured by the evaluations—masked any improvement that might have been measurable. The Philippine study exemplifies the dilemma faced by the serious evaluator in attempting a rigorous examination of an institutional feeding program. After three and a half years and substantial expenditures of money, time, and scientific talent, an Orissa (India) study[17] could offer only vague conclusions concerning nutritional impact.

The one unambiguous finding of the Orissa study was the absence of any significant physical differences between students who participated in school feeding programs and students who did not in a random sample of 24,000 schools. However, a careful correlation of physical measurements and number of feeding days showed that a well administered and consistent program produced positive nutritional results.* The failure of the feeding programs may lie not in the concept but in their implementation—insufficient or poor food, or inadequate administration.[18]

*Improving Feeding Programs*

The effort to get optimum value from a feeding program may call for increasing or upgrading the foodstuffs used. Or an already adequate sup-

---

* The study also demonstrated that attendance went up 10 percent with a feeding program; food in school was a supplement rather than a substitute for food at home; and programs that had children sit and eat together had the significant social effect of breaking down caste tradition.

ply may be made to produce a reasonable payoff if some neglected peripheral problem is solved.

*Food quantity.* The nutritional impact of feeding programs often is limited because the child gets only a glass of milk or some comparable token supplement or, if the meals are larger, gets them irregularly. A government that is unable to increase its feeding budget might increase the quantity of food in its program by encouraging participating communities to provide portions of the ration. Already in Turkey, 60 percent of the food used in the program is of local origin; in Costa Rica, 52 percent. Under some circumstances, encouragement of school gardens may provide additional foods for school meals and teach children the rudiments of horticulture as well. When government supports serve to increase a country's agricultural production, a portion can be set aside for use in institutional feeding programs as a kind of tithing on new resources. Or the commodity mix of a program could be altered to offer greater quantity for the same cost. For instance, funds spent on milk for children with significant caloric deficiencies could be spent more effectively on a grain-based supplement. At times, more food may be obtained by simply asking for it; the attendant nonfood costs will rise, of course. (Feeding programs generally develop somewhat haphazardly, when a foreign agency offers a program to a host government—the program seeks its audience, rather than the reverse. Governments seldom examine alternative sources of donated foods. Some "shopping" may be in order.) Often, program costs could be reduced—or supplies increased at the budgeted cost—if foods were shipped in bulk by the donor nation and added to the general food supply, thus circumventing a complex distribution apparatus. Central governments could give the proceeds from the sale of this food to school systems and other bodies to procure foods from the local market.

*Food quality.* In many instances the value of the feeding program could be enhanced by improving the quality of the food served. Some of the means for increasing quantity would also have the effect of improving quality through the introduction of foods of higher nutritive value. Specific steps to improve quality can include upgrading foods through fortification —or by further boosting of normally fortified foods. For example, a program that provides only a part of a child's annual vitamin A and iron needs could easily provide a year's supply on school days. Because vitamin A can be stored, it might even be given in concentrated doses once or twice a year. Iron is less easily stored but can bridge days out of school. Because most of the foods to be fortified are donated, the small cost of increasing levels of fortification would probably be readily absorbed by the donor government.

Quality might also be raised through higher protein content in the cereal grains that are supplied. This means a change in purchasing specifications by the original buyer of the grain. The protein content in wheat, for instance, may vary from less than 10 percent to over 15 percent; it is usually near the lower percentage because of its effect on the baking property of the wheat, an irrelevant consideration in the way wheat is used in most feeding programs. To ensure acceptability, a conscious attempt is now made to provide foods that closely resemble those already eaten in a community. Nutritionally this may be the wrong tack. Often a better nutritional contribution can be made if the traditional diet is supplemented by foods not commonly available. Timing of meals could also improve results. In some instances a school breakfast may be more useful than a midday meal, at least in terms of classroom attentiveness. Efforts to improve children's diets through distribution of the most popularly known nutrient concentrate—the vitamin pill—have been notably unsuccessful.

*Regularity of supply.* The on-again, off-again nature of institutional meals in many countries is often the result of dock strikes (both in donor and in recipient countries), port congestion, unreliable internal transport, political procrastination, and poor planning. Local or regional inventories should be adequate to cover unanticipated stoppages and slowdowns. And donor commitments should be long term. Congress ties U.S. agreements to food availability, an unknown from year to year. While in most years, quantities have been sufficient to meet requests, certain programs have been curtailed in lean years. The uncertainty of supply makes receiving countries reluctant to invest scarce resources in the equipment and other facilities needed for a successful program.

*Food utilization.* Foods sometimes do not make the expected nutritional contribution because of poor consumer understanding of how they should be used. In Chile, only 48 percent of the expectant and nursing mothers given free milk at health centers were found to be using it as expected; the rest were diluting it or giving it to other members of the family. In south India, such women often took milk home for the men of the family. Nigerian mothers failed to recognize powdered milk for what it was, thinking it a medicine; the amount of water they added to it (and thus the strength of the milk they drank) varied considerably. Inadequate

understanding that begins at the distribution center could lead to nutritional injury; four-fifths of the milk used in a Latin American feeding program, for instance, contained harmful bacteria.[19]

All this points to the need for more extensive and more effective education efforts. It also suggests closer attention should be paid to the cultural appropriateness of the foods supplied and to improving field testing
of the programmed commodities. One voluntary agency's shipments to the
tribal areas of Madhya Pradesh included cans of string beans. The destitute tribals had never before seen tin cans and, of course, had no can
openers. Their only implements were bows and arrows and axes, and it
was the latter they used.

*Packaging.* Perhaps the single most severe limitation on the nutritional
value of feeding programs is imposed by inadequate packaging. Loss due
to tears and breaks is considerable. So is loss due to rancidity and infestation. A child in Andhra Pradesh, asked about the difference between food
at school and food at home, responded, "Food at school has bugs in it."
More than half the bags of shipped U.S. food inspected in one survey had
rips or punctures large enough to admit beetles—and one pregnant beetle
can multiply a million and a half times in the six months it generally takes
for the journey from mill to mouth.[20] Once the bag reaches port, it is
handled anywhere from twelve to thirty times, often with unauthorized
hooks (making lifting easier) by dock workers unable to read the warnings, which are seldom printed in their language. Moreover, the bag will
have to withstand "a range of temperature and humidity well beyond that
projected for domestic products. In addition, it will be stored for several
months—and, in some cases, for a year or more—under substandard conditions with inadequate protection against insects and rodents."[21]

*Field management.* Thin management and inadequate controls are not
uncommon to institutional feeding programs. Reports in the files of audit
offices around the world point to weak administration, which results in
waste and diversion of food. Although some distribution agencies have
made solid improvements by hiring professional managers, others have
not. An extensive study of the administration of the Indian program found
that in the same locale management effectiveness varies widely.[22] Programs are especially weak when their sponsoring agencies lack field staffs;
for instance, personnel in UN agencies that have no field program super-
visory staff become little more than signers of food transfer documents.
With the current interest in multilateral food activities, the need for a

strong managerial hand in the international agencies' programs is especially significant.

*Preparation and distribution.* One cost of feeding programs is the time they take from other activities. The overburdening of the teacher or health worker that they always threaten led in Bihar to a brief teacher strike. The problem can be alleviated by simplifying the reports that consume extensive time and effort at each step from schoolmaster to international headquarters. A standardized reporting form could satisfy the needs of all the agencies and governments involved. In addition, efforts can be undertaken to lessen the load involved in food preparation. One approach is to distribute ready-to-eat commodities. Another is to centralize food preparation along the lines of the south India model. A typical central kitchen there prepares food for fifty schools and 4,000 youngsters, saving one or two hours a day for the teacher or health worker; providing better storage (hence less rancidity, infestation, and theft) than in schoolhouse or health center; requiring less fuel; and offering greater certainty of daily feeding. (After lack of food, wet fuel wood and absence of the cook are the most common reasons meals are not served.) Even larger assembly-line cooking facilities have long been used in Mexico and Peru. In communities where school lunches are not available, local food vendors can be selected and licensed to carry out the feeding program, as was done in Nigeria. Since the local vendor's food is often the only food available during the school day, institutional influence on what he serves and his standards of sanitation has obvious merit.

*Nutrition education.* Better nutrition through educational efforts could be partly accomplished through feeding programs. Little has been made of the opportunity to use the frequent contacts with children in the programs to work toward longer range improvement in nutrition. Effective student involvement in school gardens and food preparation could give the feeding program lasting value. In Israel the practical knowledge that upper elementary grade children gained through planning and preparing school meals was thought of sufficient value both intrinsically and as a means of changing home food habits to offset the time lost from more traditional courses.[23]

*Health measures.* Many of the nutrients provided in feeding programs are lost because of the poor health condition of the beneficiaries.[24] Gastrointestinal disease, particularly important because it is so common and may interfere directly with the absorption and utilization of food, can be curtailed. Systematic immunization programs against common diseases may in some instances be effective, and deworming sometimes may be helpful. Although the cost of the medication may force a cut in the number of children benefiting from a feeding program, the overall nutritional value of the program may rise.

*Related nutrition programs.* Feeding programs frequently are carried out in isolation from other community and national efforts to improve nutrition. They seem at times to obstruct other efforts—perhaps inhibiting the marketing of locally processed foods—or to ignore opportunities to complement health, family planning, or education services. Coordination with related ongoing efforts, or even mutual assistance, should be an objective of feeding programs.

## The Politics of Feeding Programs

Child feeding programs are politically attractive, for they are direct, highly visible, and generally well received. Salvador Allende, Fidel Castro, and Indira Gandhi, responding directly to the most obvious nutritional needs of their people, have campaigned on promises of milk programs and other institutional feeding for their nations' children. Governments can lean heavily on foreign aid for feeding programs, in ways that are less sensitive and less politically volatile than in other fields. Interestingly, the stigma against concessional purchases, which politicians in some countries have publicly committed themselves to end, does not seem to apply to donated foods aimed to benefit children.

Although child feeding programs are clearly political assets, they are by no means without drawbacks. Food recipients sometimes resent being put in what they regard as a welfare role; the degree of their resentment varies by culture, but is often significant, especially when the mother or child must admit need to qualify for the food aid. A feeding program in Uganda drew strong criticism: "The result of this well-meaning philanthropic venture is tragic. Gift foods should be handled as therapeutic agents but, like all drugs, are potentially dangerous, especially where there is the risk of dependency."[25] In India, villagers complained about a midday meal program: "Why should our children eat the yellow corn or maize *uppma* and drink powder milk when we produce the best rice and possess the highest milk-yielding buffaloes in the village?"[26] Occasionally, ulterior motives are suspected. Even the least sophisticated notice when food is used for political purposes or religious proselytization—for example, when a religious agency in Chile uses its food program vehicles for electioneering and to shepherd people to the polls. Misunderstandings also arise. In a Gujarati village near Baroda, participation in the lunch program dropped 30 percent as parents perceived the main purpose of the program to be to "fatten the boys and later recruit them for the army."[27] In a part of East Africa, milk distribution increased enmity toward government officials because it violated local taboos.[28] Any form of dissatisfaction with the food or the administration of the program (irregularity of feeding, paperwork burden, and so on) may rub off on the government.

Although from the donor's point of view the feeding programs may represent the best of humanitarian instincts, the projected image is not all glitter. A *Times of India* columnist saw such programs as a means of satisfying "vanity, of carrying the White Man's Burden, of practicing typical Christian virtues, of refusing to accept or conform to the country's law, customs, local traditions, behavior, responses, and attitudes."[29]

The U.S. program is hampered by a congressional obsession with recognition of the donation—generally attained with patronizing labeling—and the requirement that the donor be identified on containers, vehicles, reporting forms, and anything else connected with the program.* Plainly, the practice of national self-aggrandizement by donor countries is misdirected. According to a leading African health and nutrition official, the donors are insensitive to the antagonisms they raise.[31]

MOST of today's widespread child feeding programs began largely as relief efforts motivated by compassion, political attraction, and the need of affluent countries—primarily the United States—to dispose of surpluses. The programs have expanded dramatically, reaching and probably bene-

---

* Few food labels in the world are as well known as the clasped hands of the U.S. Food for Peace program. But the handshake is an unknown form of greeting to many or does not carry the same meaning as in the West (touching the hands of others is in some places regarded as unhygienic). Moreover, until the recent change in the symbol, the fact that the hands pictured were both white was another puzzle. The common reaction in Africa and Asia to two white hands shaking one another did not always fulfill the standards of gratitude expected by some in the donor country. "The typical food aid recipient . . . does not grasp the concept of vast political units on the other side of the world. Even *less* could he understand or identify with the faceless 'people' of such an entity. Some children who have learned that their daily school milk comes 'from America' have told us that America is the name of a cow. This makes a great deal more sense to them than a 'friendly' nation half-way around the world, or the people thereof."[30]

fiting hundreds of millions of children. How much benefit and to what children is less clear.

A plain need exists for critical examination of the programs' current impact as well as potential impact if they were upgraded. Program costs and the added cost of widening the programs should be compared with the costs of other means of meeting nutritional goals.

The costs of a feeding program should be figured both with and without foreign food grants. An institutional feeding program that makes sense while food grants are available may no longer be a wise investment if the government has to bear a larger share of the costs. Or, the return may be sufficiently attractive that food needs for child feeding programs should be included in projections of national requirements for food.

Donor countries ought to question how important food aid is compared with other forms of foreign assistance. If surplus stocks are not available, is it worthwhile for them to grow extra food to service food programs? The feasibility of eventually transferring program responsibility should also come into question. Both U.S. and UN programs schedule takeover by the host country in their plans—perhaps knowing such a transfer is impossible. In some instances it may not be in the best interests of a host country to divert funds from other programs to sponsor a large feeding program when aid is no longer available. Moreover, the transfer principle overly narrows nutrition objectives; it focuses the recipient's commitment on feeding programs, without regard for investments in fortification, seed improvement, nutrition education, and so on.

Like the host country, the donor country or agent must have a clear objective. Is the purpose of its program limited to getting the local government to shoulder innovative programs—the ambition that animates much foreign assistance—or is it to feed significant numbers of malnourished children? The U.S. AID mission to India in 1968 chose the latter option, concluding that the creation of a self-sufficient institution capable of making a continuing contribution to the country's development was not the central concern. To allow institution building to dominate would, it was believed, be an inversion of priorities and a serious mistake.[32]

Greater clarity of objectives and improved programming of the feeding projects are needed. Institutional feeding programs clearly offer opportunities to meet nutrition objectives. But these opportunities commonly are missed, largely because those administering the programs become concerned mainly with food distribution rather than the broader need of which the distribution is part. Consciously or unconsciously, and despite the controversy they may have raised, institutional feeding programs have helped to better nutrition, and in certain instances may be the only sure method of providing needed nutrients to particular target groups. Some of the programs probably could have been more effective if conducted differently and addressed to different audiences, and some of the resources they consumed might have been more profitably used in other ways. Major attention should now be given to an empirical examination of the programs. It should be recognized that there are several reasons for child feeding programs and to view them solely for nutrition considerations would be overlooking other benefits, including broader contributions to a child's well-being.

Since the institutional feeding program is the largest conscious nutrition activity under way and nothing of comparable size waits in the wings, existing programs should not be held up in the name of a comprehensive study. Nor should a replacement program designed to achieve a nutrition objective in some better way be allowed to supplant the current feeding program before it has been implemented and is operating on at least a comparable scale.

## CHAPTER ELEVEN

# Lessons from the Indian Experiment

Much of the most interesting nutrition thinking and experimentation is going on in India, where substantial steps have been taken to build a national nutrition policy, to launch a national program, and to establish projects—both operational and experimental. A special section of the country's Five Year Plan is devoted to the subject. This is not to suggest India's nutrition problems have been solved or are even well on the way to solution. But an encouraging and probably irreversible beginning has been made.

Despite the limitations of projecting experiences from a single country onto a larger international screen, a review of the reasons behind some of India's policies and projects and the broader lessons that emerge from them may be of help to other countries concerned with nutrition needs.

## Genesis of an Involvement

Nutrition as a profession is no stranger to India. For the past half century, India's laboratory and clinical work has ranked with the finest in Asia. As in most nations, however, the linkages between the scientific community and the government and political policy makers have been few. Laboratory findings have often remained in the laboratory. Until recently, the policy maker saw malnutrition as a welfare problem and addressed it accordingly.

It took the Bihar famine of 1966–67 to dramatize the magnitude and implications of malnutrition. Ninety million people in eastern India were trapped in the worst drought since the country became independent. Pictures of both bloated and wasted, malnourished bellies appeared regularly in the world press, accompanied by predictions of a vast natural disaster involving millions of starvation deaths.

Fortunately, the forecasts proved to be wrong. The Indian government mobilized a massive relief program and, aided by substantial quantities of food from the international community, was able to hold the line until the next monsoon. The experience (described in Appendix A) made a deep impression on the Indian officials who participated in the relief effort.

During the same period, government officials began to be concerned by findings reaching India that suggested a link between malnutrition and mental development. They already knew that malnutrition was the major cause of childhood deaths. They were also aware that poor food affected bodily growth and thus physical performance. However, for the first time they began to see a connection between nutritional deprivation and the sluggishness commonly observed among the extremely poor. When the head of the national nutrition research laboratory reported that 80 percent of India's children suffered from "malnutritional dwarfism,"[1] some Indian political leaders publicly expressed fear that India might be raising a generation of substandard citizens.[2]

One response to the famine crisis was an accelerated effort by the government to raise grain production. Successful introduction of new, high-yielding seed varieties, combined with widespread use of fertilizer and modern agricultural methods, led to rapid increases in production. In the two years following the famine, acreage planted in high-yielding varieties increased fivefold. Fertilizer consumption more than doubled and, perhaps of greater significance, so did local production of fertilizer. In one year the total number of tractors increased from 51,000 to 81,000, and half of the new tractors were locally produced; foodgrain production reached 95 million tons compared to 72 million tons in the famine year and a previous high of 88 million tons. By 1971, India was producing 106 million tons of cereal grains,* and in the process had built a buffer stock.

Although all of this was of obvious benefit to the well-being of the population, it was an insufficient answer to India's nutrition dilemma. There was no assurance that the additional food or the income generated by the crop increases would be broadly distributed. In fact, to some it seemed likely that if the agricultural revolution continued along its path

---

* Even with bad weather and a war, the crop estimate for 1972 was approximately 100 million tons.

of the late 1960s, the already difficult income distribution problem and its related tensions would be further aggravated.[3]


## Program Approaches

To the Indian policy makers and administrators who turned their attention to nutrition it was apparent that many highly nutritious foods—natural and processed—were beyond the reach of all but the very affluent. This was especially true of foods for very young children.


### Fortification Innovations

Experience had demonstrated the difficulty of altering established and preferred food habits. If diets could be improved inexpensively without requiring conscious decisions by consumers to buy, cook, or eat differently, the likelihood that they would be successful was greater. Consequently, early in the new effort, attention focused on using established food as carriers of additional nutrients. The first large venture into fortification of cereal foods came with the introduction of Modern Bread in January 1968. During the drought years of the mid-1960s, the Food Ministry had made a concerted effort to increase bread consumption since wheat, unlike rice, was available in large quantities from abroad. With help from Australia and Canada the government established nine Modern Bread plants, capable of producing 100 million loaves of bread a year, in the major cities of India. To each loaf was added the synthetic form of the amino acid lysine, to increase the bread's protein value, plus vitamins and minerals tailored to India's major nutritional maladies.

Early skepticism that only the urban wealthy were bread eaters and would benefit proved to be wrong. In Bombay, 40.6 percent of those with family incomes under $26 per month in 1969 were daily bread consumers. In Calcutta, 29 percent of two-to-four-year-olds ate bread. Also, bread increasingly reached into nonurban areas. In 1970, 40 percent of all bakery products were consumed in rural areas, only half the amount consumed being baked there. (Three-quarters of India's large bread producers reported that 10–30 percent of their sales were rural.) Although bread is not yet a major item in the general Indian diet, commercial bread production is expanding rapidly—by 250 percent in the 1960s (45 percent from 1968 to 1970), and at a projected annual compound growth rate of 13.2 percent from 1970 to 1975.[4]

The influence of Modern Bread on increased production is difficult to measure, but it is interesting that most of the major bread producers emulated Modern by introducing fortification into their products and by stressing better nutrition in their advertising. More important than bread sales, however, was Modern Bread's success in dramatizing the possibilities of fortification. In 1969 Secretary of Food A. L. Dias announced that India had adopted a policy of fortification,[5] soon reflected in a large-scale project designed to fortify a traditional Indian food, *atta,* the ground wheat product popularly used to make the dietary staple, *chapatti.*[6] Premilled *atta,* the least expensive form, is often bought by those in the lowest economic group. Beginning in 1970, premilled *atta* sold in Bombay and Calcutta incorporated sizable doses of vitamins and minerals, and protein in the form of groundnut flour.

Although it reaches the bottom of the income ladder, fortified *atta* benefits mainly the urban population. Nearly 80 percent of Indians live in rural areas, where it is logistically impossible to undertake a wheat fortification program because most of the wheat eating portion of the country's 565,000 villages have their own village grinding equipment. As a result, a search was made to identify low-cost, centrally processed foods that already reached all elements of the population.

The most attractive item meeting these criteria was salt, already used in some areas as a carrier of iodine to combat goiter. Salt is universally used—those not part of the monetized economy barter for it. And salt production is relatively centralized—the annual Indian production of 4.8 million tons is limited to fewer than two hundred salt works (roughly half of it in twenty-four large works, most of which are located in Gujarat). Distribution of salt can be at least partially controlled by the central salt department and by the regulatory mechanisms of the state governments. Nutritionally, salt is an attractive carrier because it is used consistently throughout the year, an important consideration given the seasonal variation of the rural Indian's diet. Most important, salt is consumed in relatively constant quantities by all Indians, urban and rural, vegetarian and nonvegetarian, rich and poor. Those in need of the greatest nutritional help, in fact, may be the heaviest consumers—it is often the only flavoring agent they can afford.

The vast majority of Indian women and small children suffer from nutritional anemia. Salt with iron added could reduce this condition significantly at a cost of about $4 million a year, or a 10 percent increase over current costs. Calcium can be added to salt without increasing the cost.[7] Iron and calcium fortified salt have been successfully tested in the laboratory and clinic, and incorporation of other nutrients is being examined.

Research also has begun on the fortification of tea. Contrary to common belief that tea was almost solely an adult drink, surveys completed in 1970 and 1972 showed that in some states tea was given regularly to 78 percent of the "under five" population. And unlike nearly all other food products, it was consumed in quantity by rich and poor in both rural and urban areas (in Calcutta, for example, 93 percent of both the highest and lowest income groups surveyed take tea regularly).[8] In Gujarat, 87 percent of villagers gave tea to their children, including 84 percent of the lowest income group (family incomes of under $13 per month). A study covering all of India found that 54 percent of tea drinking families gave tea to their children.[9] Moreover, per capita tea consumption is increasing dramatically, averaging a 6 percent increase annually from 1956 to 1968.

Interest in tea fortification stemmed partly from the discouraging findings of an investigation into the possibility of fortifying rice. Because the vast majority of Indian rice eaters cooked their rice in large quantities of water, which was then discarded,[10] any fortifying elements would probably disappear also. In the case of tea, it was the residue itself that was consumed. Professional tea tasters in Calcutta and London tested Indian fortified tea without detecting a difference in the character of the product.[11] Investigation of the value of fortified tea[12]—particularly as a carrier of vitamin A—is in the early stages.

Another unsuspected fortification vehicle was discovered from a survey undertaken in Calcutta to identify child feeding practices. Low-income families, it was learned, commonly used *sago,* a low-nutrient product made from small globules of tapioca, as a weaning food (children under twelve months of age averaged 1.2 servings a day). Moreover, 80 percent of all *sago* was produced in one town in Tamil Nadu, simplifying control. Thus, *sago* was an excellent prospect for carrying nutrients to a target group.[13] The same survey pointed as well to a popped rice known as *muri* that is consumed by substantial numbers of low-income Bengali children.

The above fortification examples are not put forth as panaceas or as projects necessarily worth emulating elsewhere, but rather as conceptual approaches that may have broader applicability.

*Initiative of the Private Sector*

A second feature of the Indian experiment was the role of private enterprise. In contrast with most other developing countries, India has sizable and sophisticated food processing and pharmaceutical industries. Yet it was only after the Bihar famine, in mid-1967, that a group of business leaders met to evaluate industry's responsibility and commercial opportunities in meeting the country's nutrition needs.[14] The group has grown to a thirty-two-firm (and three government institutes) organization—known as the Protein Foods Association of India—designed to do collectively what few single firms can afford to do alone.

One of its prime objectives is to make reliable market data available to manufacturers. Thus a series of regional food habits surveys was its first large project. Little was known of what people ate (by income, cultural group, and community size), why and how it was prepared, and how it was distributed within the family. The western regional study pinpointed several foods popular with the lowest economic classes that might be improved through fortification or genetic development of seeds (for example, while most of the attention devoted to upgrading the protein level of cereals had focused on wheat and rice, the survey indicated that the people who need help most eat sorghum and millet). Similarly, specific widely consumed condiments emerged as potential carriers of better nutrition to the lower classes.

To create greater public awareness of the nutrition problem and keener receptivity to new foods being developed by individual firms, the industry group launched an institutional advertising campaign. It involved all mass media—including a film released to 3,500 cinema houses throughout the country.[15]

The aim of these activities was to accelerate the introduction of a series of nutritious foods onto the market. By 1972, twenty-seven new beneficial products were under development, being market tested, or being sold. Many of the projects, however, had run into problems. They forced consideration of new marketing mechanisms, including involvement in products made possible by government-financed feeding programs.

The government's response to the interest and initiatives of industry was positive, if belated. Throughout 1969 a joint government-industry committee conducted hearings into problems of the food processing companies with an eye toward meeting industry needs for food standards, more flexible licensing procedures, and possible incentives.[16]

*Redirecting Child Feeding Programs*

A third element of India's nutrition effort was the school and preschool child feeding program. Sizable numbers of children were reached for the first time during the Bihar famine, and the visible effect of the feeding on the youngsters was dramatic. In the late 1960s nearly 17 million Indian children received a regular meal under the program. The meals often included Bal Ahar, the low-cost, locally produced blend of donated American wheat and inexpensive Indian oilseed protein. After a stumbling start, production had increased to 55 million pounds in 1972, and prospects for still further widespread use of the cereal blend appeared favorable.

Institutional feeding programs were believed to have an effect on learning ability and classroom performance. The child with an empty stomach, it was sensed, was neither alert nor receptive. Nor was he physically or mentally equipped for the rigors of formal education. (The extensive evaluation of institutional child feeding programs known as the Orissa study was undertaken from 1967 to 1970 to learn more precisely what the effects were.[17]) At one point the president of the ruling Congress party raised the issue of nutrition and educational performance with a group of officials who had a major role in India's economic policy. After learning from them that some $300 million a year was spent for primary education, the Congress president asked whether it would not be better to spend a portion of these funds to equip the child nutritionally to cope with the school experience. The implications of this exchange reflect the evolution of nutrition as a public policy issue in India.

*New Concepts in Nutrition Education*

The Indian experiment also attacked the problem of nutrition education. Better use of the existing family food budget via better consumer understanding had long been recognized as important to nutritional improvement. Nowhere, however, had experience in bringing this about been encouraging. Both the effectiveness and economics of the traditional extension approach to nutrition education were open to question.

The preferred approach in India isolated the problem as not so much one of nutrition as of communication. Mass media and commercial advertising agencies were brought into education campaigns. They made a conscious effort to avoid the earnest "four food groups" clichés of the standard nutrition posters and to introduce instead appeals playing on universal values. The initial advertising for Modern Bread, which featured health and the addition of lysine, was withdrawn in favor of what turned out to be a highly successful campaign built around other appeals; after consumer interest was awakened, the nutrition theme was reintroduced, with some success. *Vanaspati,* a vitamin fortified oilseed-based fat used in place of the more costly, traditional *ghee,* saw greatly increased sales with the shift from a straight nutritional to a "mothers who care" campaign.

The emotional play on universally expressed human needs, such as survival and the minimization of suffering—including suffering due to loss of child—proved to be an effective way of reaching consumers. Another valuable aid in designing campaigns was recognition of basic societal influences. A mass media advertisement, for instance, was based on the popular Tamil proverb "Does your child eat with his mouth closed what you feed him with your eyes shut?" A film in the same campaign, leaning on the Indian penchant for astrology, was titled "Your Child's Plate Is His Horoscope." The dominant saffron-orange color used for promotional materials and product packages for Bal Amul and Modern Bread reflects demonstrated Indian preference for the color, perhaps due to the positive identification of the color with the saffron robes of the *sadhus* (holy men).

Adventure comic books with a nutrition message were distributed to millions of children who never before had been exposed to this medium. Market research techniques were employed to learn what people eat, why they eat it, and what they regard as good for them. Studies showed a higher understanding of how food affects health than expected—but often a misunderstanding of the benefits of specific foods.[18]

Special efforts were made to reach people where they regularly congregate. The government produced ten movie shorts on nutrition to reach the millions of ardent Indian film goers, and instruction for dietary improvement was transmitted by All-India Radio through both community and private receivers.

### Analytical Approach to Solving Nutrition Problems

Perhaps for the international nutrition community the most significant innovation in the Indian program was the employment of development planning techniques to solve nutrition problems. The first attempt to evaluate alternate cost solutions was a comprehensive nutrition plan presented by the Ministry of Health in 1968.[19] Although it was not so sophisticated as some analysts would desire, the plan successfully initiated the use of analytical techniques to determine a policy for meeting nutrition needs. A much broader systems approach was started in 1970 in the southernmost state of Tamil Nadu (for a description, see Appendix D).

Other activities also were being pursued, with varying degrees of success. Indian scientists pushed ahead with research to develop higher protein seed varieties. The government undertook a $140 million program designed to improve the quality and quantity of urban milk supplies. Cottonseed, historically used for animal feed, was processed experimentally for human consumption. Cultivation of soy beans, high in protein but virtually unknown in India until the mid-1960s, was introduced, with per acre yields rivaling those of experimental stations in the United States.* A milk substitute to be used with tea—the way most Indian milk is consumed—was successfully developed from oilseeds. As in several other countries, research was initiated on fish protein concentrate and on single cell protein.

By 1972, plans were well under way to implement a massive integrated child welfare program featuring nutrition feeding of small children and pregnant and nursing women, education of the mothers, special prophylactic measures against nutritional anemia and blindness, immunization, preschool education, and health care.

Attempting to pull together the multiplicity of activities was an interministerial committee at cabinet secretary level, chaired by the Planning Commission. This group in 1969 helped develop the nutrition chapter of India's Fourth Five Year Plan.[20] Eighty million dollars was budgeted for a nutrition program in the plan; several times that amount was being considered for the Fifth Plan.

## Lessons Learned

From this experience, certain principles of nutrition programming and planning have developed that deserve highlighting.†

1. Most significant is the scale of thinking about nutrition. The neces-

---

* The decision was the result of extended debate in government councils. Some officials felt the energies and resources necessary to introduce soy should be used to perfect the groundnut, an oilseed already in abundance in India but of limited usefulness for human consumption because of aflatoxin. But soybean enthusiasts had convincing arguments of higher yield, export potential, and nutritive value. Little attention, however, was directed to the matter of transforming the soybeans into edible material. Fearing that the lack of facilities for processing the 1971 crop might be a disincentive to future soy production, the government provided a price support for soy to maintain and encourage farmer interest.

† More specific program and project conclusions are presented in Chapter 12.

sity of working within the confines of overstrained health ministry budgets has kept nutrition experts in many countries from facing up to the magnitude of both the challenge and the opportunity and thus from taking the kind of quantum jump planned in India. There are officials in New Delhi working on the premise that a massive attack on malnutrition could nearly eradicate certain nutritional diseases. This is a scale of thinking perhaps never before envisioned for nutrition.

2. Recognition that programs do not develop according to a predetermined master plan has brought flexibility to nutrition operations. Although ultimate objectives must be clear, opportunities—often unexpected—must be seized and parlayed as they arise. For example, early nutrition efforts in India were sidetracked because of the Bihar famine, but the widespread public concern aroused by the famine gave the impetus that otherwise might have been missing for development of a child's food.

3. An important bureaucratic principle emerged from the Indian experiment: If the existing framework doesn't work, don't work within the existing framework. Too often, as at the start in India, attempts are made to fit a new far-reaching program into established institutions. But frequently the mode of operation of traditional ministries and research institutions is not conducive to new concepts and experimentation. To escape the bureaucratic quicksand, the Indian officials instead of tailoring their needs to existing institutions developed new organizational arrangements. In the process, a number of existing organizations (though not always their field services) were infected with a nutritional commitment that led to productive contributions to new programs.*

4. A common question in the development business is whether a new concept or program can best be introduced at the base working level of the bureaucracy, with the aim of projecting a technically well-supported project upward in the hierarchy, or started at the very top, so that its effects can trickle down. In the limited experience in India, neither answer was correct. Both routes were tried. The technical forces, although often highly qualified professionally, did not carry sufficient influence to move the bureaucracy. The ministerial level, although attracted to the political value of a nutrition concept, was often so preoccupied it could give nutrition no more than fleeting attention. What worked for India was the effort of a small, informal, unorganized constellation of enlightened busi-

---

* In addition to the Food and Agriculture, Health, Education, Industries, and Information ministries, the Ministry of External Affairs was involved and in 1968 initiated an action-oriented nutrition resolution in the UN General Assembly.

nessmen and scientists, a devoted newspaper editor, and—most important —senior civil servants. These interested men never met as a group, and in some cases were not personally acquainted with one another. They were conscious, however, of their mutually reinforcing roles; their interactions were responsible for the critical steps leading to a formal national policy and heavily budgeted program.

5. The Indian nutrition effort forced attention to a sophisticated application of new technology, both scientific and managerial. In developing societies, transfer of complex modern technology that might bring leap-frog advances is often talked about and rarely applied. The need to find substitutes for foods that richer nations already consider inexpensive— and to find ways to bypass stubborn traditional food habits—has forced India to begin applying the new nutrition technology.

Much of its nutritional progress may be attributed to India's willingness to explore and experiment beyond conventional boundaries—notwithstanding the doubts, often the consternation, and always the lack of unanimity of scientists and bureaucrats, both Indian and international. Had Indian government programmers heeded the well-intentioned critics of such concepts as bread fortification, salt fortification, and the formation of an industrywide action group, the nutrition momentum might never have developed.

6. One result of the new style of programming was recognition of the need for a more systematic look at ways to improve a child's nutritional well-being. Over the years many solutions have been advocated. A set solution is easy to sell; it is specific; its costs can be detailed; its effects are presumably measurable. This, however, may be looking through the wrong end of the telescope. Rather than starting by examining specific food or fortification possibilities, India began to examine what a child eats, how it gets to him, and where in the delivery system intervention is feasible and most helpful. A slight twist of the market mechanism may mean more to the nutrition of a child than all the new foods that could be devised and produced. A shift in production incentives, retail price policies, or ration shop procedures could well be a major part of the answer. Indian nutrition planning began to take such factors into consideration.

In carrying out its intent, India undertook several significant planning and evaluation projects. They were not allowed, however, to hold up existing nutrition activities—or to hinder new ones based on current best judgments.

7. The success or failure of nutrition projects, it was quickly recognized, often hinged on factors that seemingly had nothing to do with nutrition. Thus the practical considerations weighed in the nutrition program included the political attractiveness of a project, its visibility, the length of time required to see results, the potential reaction of commodity interest groups, prospects for imitation, long-range effects, managerial competence, clearance requirements, administrative constraints, and so on.

Modern Bread was selected as the first fortification venture in India partly because it was easy, quick, inexpensive, and visible and required the involvement of relatively few people. Plainly, there were more important ways to improve Indian nutrition—one of them to grow more pulses. But this implies changes in land use and, as such, risks controversy. It was quickly apparent that many officials would be involved—formally and informally—in any decision to change agricultural objectives. And it was evident that nonnutrition considerations—both relevant and reasonable—would weigh heavily on their attitudes. By contrast, a new policy to fortify Modern Bread meant concurrence of Modern Bakeries' chairman (who was also the secretary of food) and its managing director. Those attempting to improve nutrition in India opted for reality. There was no illusion that fortification of bread would solve India's nutrition problems, but they chose to do the doable, holding the longer view that the project could, if effective, contribute to something more significant. In short, there is an important psychological dimension to development, and there is nothing more effective in creating momentum than a successful start. This may mean expending energies initially on projects selected for high visibility, short gestation times, and a high probability of success. A project shaped by these criteria may produce less direct payoff than longer term alternatives, but it may be the best means of attaining the ultimate nutrition goal.

8. At a certain stage, nutrition problems move away from the domain of technology toward the domain of administration. Patient research and experimentation by the scientific community obviously are critical. However, the programming of operational elements, often overlooked in the past, proved to be an essential component of India's program. The biggest difficulties, once the research has been completed, no longer are technical or clinical problems; they are budgeting and managerial, logistical, and marketing problems. Solving them requires different talents, different temperaments, different skills—often a combination of skills that straddle the traditional disciplines.

9. One administrative feature almost always included in India's program activities was operational evaluation. An experiment, by definition, will include failures. Too often in the development business, however, no objective measurement is made of how programs are working; or an academic evaluation is made that is not helpful in programming and decision making. The research element that was part of nearly all the Indian nutrition activities forced attention to the life styles and needs of specific age, income, and geographic segments of the population. As a result, officials began abandoning the misleading averages and aggregates that commonly had been used.

10. The Indian nutrition experience reflects a fruitful style of technical cooperation, one that offers an illustration of a direct problem-solving approach, with all the broadness of operational scope this implies. Indian specialists, and their foreign counterparts, pursued problems that cut across the classic functional sectors—and across departmental organization charts—of development programming.

The India experience demonstrated that academic and research institutions of industrially advanced countries can make a contribution to meeting nutrition objectives. This contribution, however, has been limited by the tendency to espouse formulas from afar for remolding traditional societies. The usefulness of foreign research efforts will be enhanced to the extent that institutions adapt to the realities of local operational problems and programs. Solutions that appear theoretically sound from a distant laboratory often turn out to be infeasible in the context of the highly personal, highly traditional, and socially motivated eating habits of a low-income society.

## Nutrition and Politics

The Indian experience pointed up the attractiveness of nutrition as a political issue. Although politicians recognized that no single factor could meet the minimum aspirations of the poor, better nutrition might play an important, relatively fast-acting, and highly visible role. Better nutrition had a direct relationship to well-being and to some extent was within the means of India to provide.

Recognition of nutrition's vote-getting appeal was slow in coming, particularly among the political leadership, who were the followers rather than the leaders of the new nutrition interest. The prominent exception was

C. Subramaniam, minister of food and agriculture in the mid-1960s, act-ing president of the new wing of the Congress party after the split in 1968, minister of planning in 1971–72, and, throughout, a close adviser to Prime Minister Indira Gandhi. A panel he headed laid out a credo for the depart-ing faction of the Congress party. It called for a Socialist Charter for Chil-dren, noting that "the majority of our children do not have the benefit of a balanced diet . . . we are producing a generation of intellectually and physically stunted growth. Any talk of equality of opportunity for indi-viduals in [such] a society has no meaning . . . due to malnutrition." The theme was incorporated in the party's 1969 platform,* which called for a guaranteed minimum diet for 80 million preschool-aged children. A sug-gested 1 percent national cess on all taxes to raise the necessary revenues for the program was heralded in the local press.[22]

Beginning steps were taken to implement the "Childrens Charter" in 1970. Better nutrition became one of the major themes of the following year's campaign and an important plank in the Congress Party Manifesto.†

In her successful 1971 election campaign Mrs. Gandhi hammered away at themes she had enunciated earlier: "Just as economic strength is the true basis of national strength, adequate nutrition is essential for the individual personality to unfold. Without attention to nutrition, we shall be denying large sections of our people an opportunity to help themselves and to make their contribution to the country."[24] "Malnutrition being the 'mother of illness,' emphasis on India's food battle is one not only of quan-tity but of quality as well. Our Government attaches the greatest impor-tance to programmes which give protective foods to the needy—in par-ticular to children and to mothers."[25] "A nation realises its potentialities through its children, and is judged by what it does for its children."[26]

---

* Once the "New" wing of the party adopted nutrition as a major program, the opposition or "Old" wing introduced nutrition into its program: "While India cannot ensure socialist equality to the people here and now, our earnestness has to be shown in what we do for our children. The Congress, therefore, attaches the highest priority to the provision of nourishment, particularly high protein food, to all the children."[21]

† "Children are the wealth of the nation and their welfare is an essential invest-ment in economic, social and cultural development. It has been known for many years now that protein malnutrition is an important cause of infant mortality, stunted growth, low work output, premature aging and reduced life-span. The Congress has, therefore, accepted the provision of adequate nutrition to the pre-school children to improve the quality of the coming generation as an important national programme. The year 1970–71 marks a beginning in providing this service to pre-school children belonging to the vulnerable sections. The Congress is determined to enlarge this pro-gramme to cover all pre-school children."[23]

WHAT BEGAN as an experiment now forms the beginning of a national program—and is being looked on as a prototype by other nations. The Indian experience is significant for its scientific achievements and applications of technology. Perhaps more important are the underlying reasons the nutrition programs were taken up and the innovative approaches employed in implementing them. Their adoption reflects serious thought devoted to the developmental ramifications of malnutrition, to the economic dimensions of the problem, to the distribution of benefits of such programs, to the vote-getting appeal of nutrition in a democracy, and to sophisticated nutrition planning.

India's nutrition problems are by no means under control. The gains against them are significant—and cumulative—but must not be magnified out of proportion. Not all of the recently devised activities can be expected to evolve into viable projects; by definition, many were experiments. Also, the need is of such magnitude that even the best of government intentions may fall short. Massive logistical and cultural barriers stand in the way of reaching the neediest elements in the society. However, the possibility of reaching the targets of need has been strengthened by India's recent experience. The country's leaders recognize the problem and are committed to doing something about it. Although implementation of the commitment still poses many questions, a promising start has been made.

## CHAPTER TWELVE

# Policy Directions and Program Needs

Malnutrition in developing countries is a problem of huge proportions and wide-ranging implications. Combating malnutrition alone does not, of course, offer a simple solution to underdevelopment; on the contrary, nutrition is one of many interrelated determinants of human performance requiring advancement. Under some circumstances, however, better nutrition may be a precondition to the advancement of the other factors and a propellant to many forms of production. In short, not only is malnutrition a consequence of underdevelopment but it is a contributing factor, a drag on the potential from which better nutrition might be provided.

The problem is even more poignant in light of the development experience of the 1960s. Even fairly successful national growth, in conventional terms, has left out substantial fractions of the populations in low-income countries—some even ending up the decade in worse shape than they started. This has prompted redefinition of development objectives and increasing realization that greater attention must be directed to the improvement of life quality. In this context, malnutrition looms large.

Many people are incapable, both economically and educationally, of supplying by their own initiative the nutrients needed to meet the basic health requirements and the development of full mental and physical potentials of their children and often themselves. While most governments recognize the importance of an educated populace to development, and have provided substantial financial support for education systems, only a few realize that a well-nourished population is of comparable importance (as well as a significant factor in the effectiveness of the education system).[1] Presumably governments assume responsibility for education, offering free and sometimes compulsory schooling, in the belief that many parents are not equipped to provide it. The state of child nutrition in much of the world raises the doubt whether parents are any better equipped, for whatever reason, to provide adequate nutrition. If malnutrition is to be overcome, governments must intervene. Most short-cut solutions to bring help to the neediest will necessitate some kind of government action.

Although mass poverty is often the underlying cause of malnutrition, a general attack on poverty is not necessarily the best means of getting at malnutrition, especially among small children. Income increases and agricultural growth have a major positive effect on the problem of malnutrition and could have much more if nutrition were one dimension in the consideration of income and agriculture policies. (In addition to being examined for their impact on employment or on distribution of ownership, many programs in low-income countries could usefully be examined for their impact on malnutrition, just as legislative proposals in the United States are now scrutinized for their ecological consequences as well as their costs, manpower requirements, and so on.) But income and agricultural growth of themselves are often insufficient to meet nutritional needs within a satisfactory period of time. Complementary actions, especially to meet distributional and educational needs, are required.

Of the complementary actions available, those that avoid extensive administrative mechanisms—that is, those with a broad application—are especially attractive. Working, for example, through price policies, mass media, fortification, seed improvement, or distribution through normal marketing channels—perhaps with subsidy—is usually less costly, less cumbersome, and much quicker than the more common small-scale approaches to malnutrition. Specifications are difficult to designate, given the different needs and circumstances in different countries—clearly, nutrition programs must be custom made—but some highlights do emerge from the experience to date.

In many ways, fortification is the most attractive of all the complementary alternatives considered in this study. Where it is feasible, fortification offers a means through technical ingenuity of meeting a problem relatively quickly and at extraordinarily low cost. Perhaps more than any other solution, fortification points up the opportunity for very poor countries to provide better nutrition at an early stage of economic development and even in absence of broad national growth. India was able to achieve a fifty-year life expectancy in 1970 when its per capita national income was about $70; the United States, by contrast, did so when the comparable value of its income was twenty times as great. That was 1910, when the means of controlling traditional epidemics were not as effective, easy to administer, and low in cost as they are today. The same concepts may be applied to improving diets. Properly exploited, food fortification to control nutritional anemias and vitamin A-related blindness, for instance, could someday be the equivalent of a smallpox vaccination. When fortification of staples and weaning foods is an appropriate mechanism, governments should make it mandatory.

Also high on the list of activities deserving priority attention—for many of the same reasons that make fortification attractive—is the genetic improvement of seed varieties to obtain higher nutrient content. In the long run, perhaps the greatest contribution to nutrition betterment can be made in this way.

Neither fortification nor genetic improvement of seeds is likely to solve many of the problems of the vulnerable very young. Here the priority need is for a heavy dose of nutrition education with an aim toward encouraging breast feeding and then supplementary solid feeding at the appropriate age. Although nutrition education has been a dull, lackluster business, the introduction of mass media—with its commercial success in changing food habits—may be the key to getting the message to the mother.

Given limited resources, and the need to establish priorities, lesser emphasis in low-income countries may be appropriate on the development of new foods and ingredients for these foods, and greater emphasis on finding ways to reach those people in need with foods already known and available. Both the mass institutional feeding programs (under some circumstances they may be the only sure mechanism to reach specific groups of nutritional need) and the marketplace provide potential; but major changes in orientation will be required if the potential is to materialize. Meanwhile, an unquestioning "more of the same" posture for both vehicles would be ill-advised.

Similarly ill-advised in most countries would be investment, for nutrition reasons, in traditional animal protein products. Increases in production of meat, milk, and eggs seldom have direct impact on malnutrition among the very needy.

None of the above is intended to prejudge appropriate activities for any given setting. Clearly, one of the major needs is for more systematic analysis and planning, a point to be pursued later.*

---

* Some of the programs this study advocates are encouraged with as little evidence of impact as others that are rejected for the lack of evidence of impact. The former, however, are the promising activities that are too new to have had a fair chance at establishing a record while most of the latter have failed over a reasonably long span to make a mark (and some have had a chance to show their weaknesses).

## A Broad Commitment

The response to malnutrition in most countries is modest, fragmented, and lacking in operational orientation. This is partly explained by the evolution of nutrition activities. Interest in operational nutrition programs emerged from medical origins. For more than half a century, laboratory and clinical research in low-income countries has been directed to this problem; in some twenty of the larger of these countries, and several of the smaller ones, special nutrition institutes or nutrition wings of other medical research facilities have been established. A medically oriented response to malnutrition grew naturally from this base. Pediatric nutrition wards in hospitals, health centers, and, later, nutrition rehabilitation centers emphasizing curative rather than preventive efforts have reached only a small portion of the child population—probably less than 1 percent.

The need for more far-reaching efforts, especially nutritional supplements to a larger child audience, became clear in the emergencies during and following World War II. The response was institutional child feeding, now organized in over a hundred countries and reaching an estimated 125 million children at an approximate cost of three-quarters of a billion dollars a year. Although these programs rely mainly on foreign-donated foods, the receiving countries themselves contribute an estimated $250 million a year to meet administrative and logistical expenses and to buy local food. But do these programs reach the right children (commonly, fewer than 10 percent of the beneficiaries are of the vulnerable but difficult-to-reach preschool-aged group); do they benefit the economically neediest elements in the population; and might less cumbersome and costly ways be found to meet the same objectives?

Recognition that nutrition could in part be improved by better use of resources already or potentially available led to efforts in the 1950s to bring about conscious changes in food practices. Among the several forms of nutrition education attempted, the major one has been the village-level applied nutrition programs, or variations, now under way in some twenty countries. These programs have not been noteworthy for their success.

In the early 1960s, with an increased appreciation of the magnitude of malnutrition, attention moved to the cost and availability of existing nutrients, leading to the development of technologies aimed at providing low-cost solutions. New processes for soybean, cottonseed, groundnut, and other oilseeds have made possible large sources of protein seldom previously used in most countries for direct human consumption. Work has also advanced on fish protein concentrate and single cell protein. At least a dozen technological institutes have been established in developing countries to promote such work. The new nutrient sources have been used both to fortify existing food staples and in the formulation of new food forms. Several large-scale government fortification projects are currently operational, and new formulated foods are being produced in several developing countries, mostly for use in institutional feeding programs. Although industry has been courted and commercial distribution begun, industry's nutritional contribution has been insignificant, primarily because of economic reasons.

Nutrition needs were also consciously included in a few agricultural efforts in the 1960s, primarily in the move to develop cereal staples with higher nutrient content.

From the experience to date, several generalizations may be drawn: (1) Most activities have been ad hoc in conception, lacking integrated analysis that matches responses to need and compares options. (2) With the exception of institutional child feeding programs, nutrition activities have been limited mostly to experiments and pilot projects. (3) Nutrition investments (as interpreted by the countries themselves[2]) have seldom been directed specifically to the most vulnerable portions of the population. (4) Most programs whose objectives have been deliberately concerned with nutrition have concentrated on face-to-face health or education techniques. (5) The nutrition field has been the province of the medical scientist and the food technologist, whose contributions are largely responsible for the current level of knowledge and capacity for response to the nutrition problem. But these disciplines have not been able successfully to move the field into operational channels. (6) Most nutrition projects have been made possible by foreign food and financial grants.[3]

Given this picture, what needs must be met to increase nutrition programming to a significant level? A national nutrition program requires an awareness of the problem, a commitment to do something about it, and implementation. No matter where any particular country now stands on this scale, what most of them need is a different and broader conception of malnutrition and a quantum jump in the nature of their response. The problem is massive, and it has hardly been budged. Officials must not be seduced by minor achievements that are often peripheral to the central problem. The "every little bit helps" philosophy that characterizes much of the thinking in the nutrition field may even be counterproductive, since it diverts attention from more significant needs. A small success is meaningful only if it is a useful step on the way to a large success that can be achieved in a short time. The nutrition advocate should insist that nutrition activities be consequential.

To achieve a consequential scale requires totally changing the complexion of nutrition as practiced today. For nutrition to attain a place in the mainstream of development, attention must be directed to the form and scope of nutrition planning and programming, organizational needs, personnel requirements, and research orientation. All require radical change.

## A Systematic Approach

Comprehensive nutrition planning and analysis are sorely needed, and with an increased scope of nutrition activities envisioned, this need becomes even more critical. Projects now are generally adopted because someone comes along with an idea (the idea commonly reflecting the background of the advocate; thus the medical man sees solutions quite differently from the plant geneticist or the food industry official), with its costs, and with the mechanism to carry it out. In this way a little piece may get done—a commercial fabricated food, a fish protein concentrate, a chain of mothercraft centers. The project may or may not be useful in isolation; perhaps other simultaneous actions—extension work, credit provisions, marketing services, food regulations—must take place to make it effective. The activities that exist today in the field of nutrition are, more often than not, the result of the persistence and persuasiveness of the project advocate rather than of a thoughtful look at total needs and alternative ways of meeting them.

This need not be so. Today in other fields there are accepted planning approaches that can and should be adapted for nutrition purposes. The elements of a nutrition plan and a proposed framework to analyze nutritional needs and identify the most appropriate methods to fulfill them are laid out in Appendix D. Two important portions of that framework are the need for clearer objectives and a more systematic approach to identifying problem causes and solutions.

First, nutritional objectives and target groups need to be carefully defined. The imprecise coverage of current programs appears to result in waste of a portion of the resources invested in nutrition, or certainly in a far from maximum return.[4] In most countries it will be impractical to think of eradicating nutritional deficiencies among all portions of the population. To provide institutional feeding to all those in need in a country the size of Ethiopia would cost upwards of $130 million a year. All children in the vulnerable six-to-twenty-four-month-old group and women in the last trimester of pregnancy could be nourished for a more manageable $8 million–$9 million.

Second, malnutrition's close relationship to socioeconomic forces argues for a comprehensive and systematic approach to planning analysis. A disciplined, systematic search for causal factors and relations may expose useful points of intervention in the food-health complex that conventional nutrition planning would never encounter. What has been described in some places as a nutrition problem may from this view be identified as a transportation or storage problem.

Refrigerated vans, for example, might prove a worthy nutrition investment in Peru, where the largest per capita fish catch in the world rarely penetrates beyond the immediate fish-catching region.* Storage appears to be a critical problem in Korea, where common seasonal shortages of nutrients might disappear if facilities were available to store the kinds of foods that carry these nutrients.[5] Price incentives, which have proved effective for changing production patterns of masses of farmers, may show up to be a critical lever. It is conceivable that a shift in price policies on pulses could do more for the nutritional status of large numbers of children than the many current efforts to produce and distribute formulated foods; yet price incentives have seldom, if ever, been explored in relation to nutrition objectives beyond sheer increase in grain supply. Because of the relationship between malnutrition and parasitic and infectious diseases, under certain circumstances a mass immunization program or improvement of water supply may do more for nutrition than a better food supply, or perhaps a combination of one or both of these with food would prove most effective.

In some situations, the maintenance of a father's good health and productivity may be the best means of assuring nutritional adequacy among his young. In others, insuring adequate nutrition of the mother in her latter

---

* The major contribution to the solution of the regional famines in India appears to have been construction of the railroad. The project was not undertaken a hundred years ago with this in mind, but if a nutrition planning exercise had been undertaken in India it would have recognized that the existence of a transportation system that enables surplus areas to feed deficit areas is the most substantial contributor to alleviation of mortality and morbidity from malnourishment in India.

months of pregnancy may be the best way to achieve the objective of lowering malnutrition in youngsters. A description of the child's diet and the influences at work in that diet may suggest new foods, potential carriers for fortification, or potential mass media presentations designed to change food habits.


## Forceful Administration

Strong leadership in nutrition programming and a vigorous, goal-oriented organization with a clear mandate are essential. As things now stand, some of the major factors and policies influencing nutritional status —agriculture, income distribution, transport, and so on—are outside the interest and reach of those people and entities charged with looking after their country's nutrition, and those who formulate such policies do not specifically include nutrition needs as part of their planning equation. Moreover, most conscious nutrition efforts have serious implementation problems, greater even than those in other development fields because of the multifaceted nature of nutrition activities. If a strategy is to concentrate solely or primarily on a single project, such as legume production or school feeding, the program might well fall under the aegis of the ministry of agriculture or education. If, as is more likely, a nutrition program consists of several elements—agricultural, health, educational, industrial—the question is where to fix the responsibility.

*The interministerial body.* A commonly proposed solution to nutrition programming is the establishment of an interministerial council. There has, in fact, been such a fixation on this approach that insufficient attention has been directed to the inherent shortcomings of a council and to alternative mechanisms. Nutrition program direction via a hybrid council is attractive in theory but rarely works. Program management typically is passive (usually at best serving a review function), rather than offering dynamic and purposeful leadership. The council, once it is through the throat-clearing stage, tends to take on the complexion of the membership; for instance, the group may include medical nutritionists, food technologists, and industrialists, but lack voices representing the virtues of agricultural research, price policy shifts, or other broadly based nutritional interventions.

Because a council is the secondary responsibility of its participants, it receives only secondary organizational allegiances. Its activities are out of the mainstream of the functions and interests of the participating agencies.

Coordination is not a natural reflex; on the contrary, there is usually a magnetic pull toward greater bureaucratic autonomy. Moreover, nutrition councils are usually constituted at too low a level to make or even affect policy.

In short, successful direction by committee has historically been enormously difficult to achieve. The interministerial body most often dies or rests in a state of operational coma that is tantamount to the same thing. In Ethiopia, nutrition councils were set up twice; the first met once, the second not at all.[6] In Zambia, a coordinating body met twice between 1964 and 1966—its first and last meetings.*[7] In India, a long-standing National Nutrition Advisory Council has postponed more meetings than it has held; it has met on the average once every three years.

Recognizing the shortcomings of its nutrition council, India in 1968 established a streamlined version at the cabinet secretary level, chaired by a member of the Planning Commission. Although the move resulted in increased interest and activity, it too was limited by the committee approach to problem solving. Wrote the chairman of the group: "The more we try to coordinate the programmes here in the Planning Commission, the larger is our realization, on the one hand, of the tremendous potentialities of what has been undertaken and, on the other, of the immense difficulties and intricacies of actual implementation."†[8]

An interministerial body can even be an impediment to a nutrition pro-

---

* Although an executive committee of this group met eleven times during the eighteen months, the membership from the participating ministries changed completely three times, and the individual representative, on the average, attended only three meetings.

† Even were all the participating bodies in a nutrition committee agreed to common objectives, representatives would likely see quite different ways of meeting them, each from the perspective of his own agency. What will a policy or action mean to his organization's program, its staff, its budget, and its influence? Will it detract from the main mission?[9] The good bureaucrat, bound by the instinctive conviction that what is best for his agency is best for all, jealously protects his organization's vested authority. Unless one of the participating agencies dominates the bureaucratic in-fighting, little in the way of forceful direction emerges. The council likely will take an ambiguous posture, exacting little from the participating vested interests. Thus, hard choices will be left unmade and, for the most part, programs will run as they have in the past.[10]

gram. The first net effect of coordination is often reduced operational output. Additional clearances require additional time, and coordination can become a bottleneck rather than a facilitating device.

Coordination among government agencies as well as among nongovernment groups with a major stake in nutrition programming does, of course, have merits. A coordinating nutrition council, however, should be created with an understanding of what it can do and what it cannot. At best, it can serve as a forum for discussion and coordination of activities assigned to operational entities. It cannot provide the forceful leadership and entrepreneurial qualities that nutrition cries out for. The need in most countries is not so much for coordination as for a big push.

*An existing ministry.* Administration of nutrition programs can be placed in an existing ministry. Vesting operational responsibilities as well as coordination functions in an established administrative entity offers the advantage of centralization and the savings in time and cost that automatically result. Again, however, the approach looks better on paper than in practice. Where this approach has been tried, nutrition has invariably been assigned low priority and has been often buried deep in the ministerial bureaucracy—since, after all, nutrition is not the main mission of such a ministry. The government organization most commonly chosen is the health ministry, which in developing countries is usually among the weakest of the operational ministries. To the extent attention is directed to nutrition, activities generally adhere to those within the ministry's own interest, influence, and control. Health ministries have generally viewed malnutrition as a health problem and have treated it like other diseases; most nutrition budgeting is for curative rather than preventive activities. None charged with nutrition responsibility has become known for devoting its energies to the promotion of agricultural price policies advantageous to nutrition or to research in higher yielding legumes. The vested-interest ministry is unlikely either to give the support or to have the breadth necessary for an effective nutrition program.

The same is true of national nutrition institutes which in several countries serve as the cornerstones for nutrition programs, usually under the aegis of health ministries. Such institutes are primarily devoted to research and training, almost exclusively in health or food technology. Although theirs is an important contribution to nutrition goals, such organizations, as generally constituted, cannot provide leadership for broad operational activities.

Coordination by an assigned operative ministry also causes problems. Most specialist agencies are not very effective in coordinating the work of other specialists who, in turn, "resent and resist extraneous attempts to exercise initiative and leadership over their activities."[11]

*A separate entity.* One way to avoid such consequences, and to assign clear accountability for nutrition, is to establish an autonomous nutrition department or ministry (or perhaps more practicable, a food and nutrition ministry). It should represent the several strains of thought and approach that characterize a good nutrition program. If malnutrition is a problem of sufficient size and importance to merit large-scale policy and budgetary attention, it also merits consideration as a separate administrative entity. Administrative autonomy of course is a popular call among new claimants for bureaucratic attention, and a call for proliferation of agencies rarely falls with favor on the ears of legislators. In the case of nutrition, however, the potential political attractiveness of the subject is high, and the political value is partly contingent on the public attention that is drawn to the program. The case for a separate entity is stronger than normal because of the bastardized format of nutrition programs. Nutrition straddles a variety of disciplines and ministries. To force it into an existing administrative pattern will almost certainly inhibit performance.

Nutrition programming by a separate entity may seem impossible because of its heavy dependence on existing bureaucratic machinery. But analogous programs that engage more than one ministry and more than one discipline are centrally administered. The United States, for example, has established an autonomous agency responsible for problems of the environment, although portions of a program may be administered by traditional agencies.

The structure of a separate nutrition entity will depend on local circumstances. It may take the form of an operating ministry with responsibility for all nutrition operations. Or it may be designed to develop and monitor nutrition policy, serve as the nutrition voice in policy councils, and contract with existing ministries for operational implementation. Whatever the format, the nutrition entity must be given sufficient authority to achieve its objectives; this usually means that the agency head must report directly to the most important policy official.

The creation of such an entity requires the development of a new breed of professional, capable of dealing with nutrition programming issues in new and creative ways.

## A New Discipline

Nearly all countries need to distinguish the science of nutrition from the practice of nutrition. Both are now lumped together, so that any issue touching on nutrition generally involves the same people and the same institutions. The biochemists, pathologists, food technologists, pediatricians, and other nutritionists have been extraordinarily successful in identifying dietary needs and finding answers to them; given the many problems still to be solved, their role will continue to be important.

In a successful nutrition activity, however, the issues move beyond the clinic, laboratory, and experimental field project. Concern shifts to operations, communications, logistics, administration, and economics, and the need shifts to professional planners, programmers, and managers.

The officer responsible for nutrition must not only determine the extent of malnutrition and its effect on an area's development but go on to weigh the alternative means of meeting the shortage. Is the answer increased food production? If so, what are the implications for land use? Is the answer a reorientation of agricultural research, to put more emphasis on legumes, less on cereals? Is it a change in government pricing policy? A new distribution or marketing mechanism? Fortification? Large-scale child feeding programs? New foods? Should the government deliberately subsidize diets to correct consumers' errors in making decisions? If so, how and to what extent? Are the benefits of nutrition education worth the costs? What does the needy person already know about the relation between food intake and health, what motivates him, what messages get through, and which media under given circumstances can get them through?

When one or more of these steps merits pursuit, another important series of questions must be answered. If, for example, fortification appears to be a useful, economical, and feasible approach, what foods can be fortified with what nutrients at what cost? To narrow the selection, a battery of related issues must be resolved if a project is to succeed. In India, for example, a decision by the secretary of food to fortify ground wholewheat meal and *atta* led to twenty-five programming questions. Among them were: (1) Should the fortification be mandatory by government directive, or should it be voluntary? If the latter, how will the unfortified product be distinguished from the fortified one, assuming bulk packaging? (2) Should the increase in cost be passed on to the consumer, or should it be absorbed by the government via a subsidy? Will the prices of other commodities be affected by this price change? (3) Are the nutrients locally available in adequate quantities? (4) Should the nutrients be procured directly by the flour mills or through the government? Should ceiling prices be set for these nutrients? (5) Should loans be available to the flour mills for the purchase and storage of nutrients? (6) What standards should be set for the quality of the protein concentrate? How should these standards be checked and enforced? (7) What equipment will the flour mills need? Is the equipment locally available? If not, how can it be imported or locally manufactured? (8) What tests of acceptability should be run? (9) What changes in the food-standards regulations will be necessary? (10) Should the program be accompanied by explanatory promotions?

Beyond lie the operational responsibilities of procurement, movement, and storage of materials, the institution of regulatory procedures, surveillance, and so on.* These are obviously no longer matters of nutrition science, and personnel policies must be adjusted accordingly.

This all suggests a role for a new discipline or nutrition subdiscipline including professionals with planning and project design capabilities.† Nutrition programmers,[13] or "macronutritionists," are needed to convert the findings of the scientific community into large-scale action programs.

Without such a new discipline for nutrition, many issues either will not be addressed at all or will be assigned to the scientific community or, more likely, to professionals from other disciplines who lack the knowledge, interest, and commitment to assure success.

The nutrition programmer's role should not supplant but supplement existing work. Its importance is contingent on the work of the scientist, but the ultimate value of the scientist's work would hinge on the nutrition programmer's success in reaching the target population.‡

* An effective international network for exchanging information is needed to make managerial experience broadly available. Steps have been taken to provide retrieval systems for research findings in scientific aspects of nutrition and food technology.[12] Such a clearinghouse concept should be broadened to include planning and programming, so that advantage may be taken of the lessons, both good and bad, learned from other pioneers in this field.

† Although several countries and assistance agencies are beginning to recognize the importance of nutrition planning and are starting to staff to meet this need, little thought generally has been given to translating the plan into eventual projects. There is need to prepare people—these often with different experience, skills, and temperaments than planners—to design and prepare detailed nutrition project proposals that meet the requirements of appropriate financing bodies.

‡ The plant geneticist was instrumental to what happened in the green revolution, but the revolution would not have happened had it not been for the programmers— the extension work, the agricultural credit, and all the other components that made

The Indian experience suggests that there is an additional value in such a function: the programmer can provide liaison between government and the scientific community. Too often in the past, usually for lack of vision rather than deliberate oversight, programs affecting nutrition have been developed without the counsel of the nutritionist. The programmer may also be in a position to offer operational insight to assist the work of the scientific community.

Efforts must be undertaken to identify and encourage a cadre of young people to pioneer in this new discipline—and thought must be given to the establishment of training facilities and curricula to equip the cadre.[14] Because the need is immediate, thought should also be given to providing short-term training for officials now working in related fields.

## Mission-Oriented Research

Nutrition is a relatively new profession—most of the vitamins, for example, were discovered after 1930—and there are many unknowns. Some of these unknowns require biochemical and other forms of basic research. More urgent are the unknowns that call for mission-oriented research.

In the past, research interest centered on clinical and laboratory work, with little attention to testing for practical application and for linking findings to policy and program needs. Applied work has been regarded as low in sophistication and prestige value, especially among scientists trained in Western countries who sometimes conceive of research in terms of esoteric problems and shiny equipment. International funding agencies have often exacerbated this problem; a leading Nigerian scientist, for example, had no trouble obtaining funds for an amino acid analyzer but failed to procure help for a badly needed field survey. The former director general of the Indian Council of Medical Research has said that well-meaning foreign-funded research projects are often counterproductive because they outbid local resources for limited talent and facilities to do work that may not deserve high priority.[15] Such research is often more closely tied to the needs of the funding country than those of the host.

---

it work. The developers of contraceptives (Dr. Lippi, developer of the loop, for example) were of course critical in the family planning movement but could hardly have accomplished much without the help of programmers. This is not to suggest that the scientist could not in some cases fill the programmer's role, but he may not have the interest or the temperament to deal with administration, logistics, and painful bureaucratic processes. Should the scientist opt to work in such a position, he should be able to devote full time to it and should be appropriately trained for it.

As a result, good scientists are seldom attracted to applied research and, more important, scientists commonly are insulated from the policy maker by the nature of their research work. Seldom is nutrition research related to questions directly affecting policy and programs. "Applied" research is commonly interpreted to mean research as applied by doctors in hospitals or health centers—for example, curative techniques for nutritional disorders. If the value of nutrition-research investment in low-income countries were measured by the numbers of needy children who benefit, the conclusions would not be reassuring.[16]

The need for a mission-oriented approach to nutrition research in developing countries is clear. An appropriate strategy would aim at identifying and providing the information necessary to develop policies and programs.

Nutrition-related research—both past and current, and either local or foreign—that may provide portions of the needed information should be systematically cataloged. As gaps of knowledge are recognized, priorities should be established for filling these gaps, and available resources for research should be allocated in accord with the established priorities. (Funding bodies should solicit specific research projects related to these priorities rather than, as they commonly do, waiting for individual project proposals.) The resulting research projects should be monitored to assure they remain relevant to the problem. A conduit must be established to assure systematic flow of research findings to the authorities responsible for nutrition policy and programming.

The body responsible for establishing and supervising the nutrition research program should include policy and program officers as well as scientists; the latter may tend to be circumscribed by their training and to promote and perpetuate research in their own areas of interest and expertise.

This approach will require top-caliber work in a variety of applied research areas, and incentives will be necessary to upgrade the status of applied research and to attract competent researchers. Such incentives may include money, career opportunities, and recognition—awards and other honors of significance for applied nutrition research.

A large policy-oriented nutrition research program that engages both nutrition scientists and social scientists, as well as people with programming skills and operational experience, must be mounted. The effort should be well funded to support work of the highest quality. Such a need can be met both on the local, developing country level and through an international nutrition institute capable of major investment addressed to solving problems common to many countries.

THE CONSEQUENCES of malnutrition for national development are increasingly clear. Without improved nutrition in the less-favored two-thirds of the world, the development of human resources—and the development of the nations themselves—may well be retarded. It should be clear that we are talking not just of the quality of life, but of the quality of people. Unless the current levels of malnutrition are dramatically checked, they may be significantly detrimental to the performance, appearance, physical well-being, and perhaps even the mental capability of much of the world's population.

To prevent such scars will require new approaches, new research, new organizational entities, a new discipline, and most important, a new scale of concern about the problem and a concomitant new scale of action. Although a great deal of investigation clearly is needed to obtain more precise data and reduce the ranges of uncertainty, knowledge of nutrition—the problems as well as the techniques and technologies to meet them—is at a stage where much can be done. Enough information already is in hand to justify resource allocations for nutrition on a substantial scale. The token efforts of the past are an inadequate and thus unacceptable response. It is no longer sufficient to think of nutrition in terms of projects that are doing something good or useful; they must be aimed at doing something of consequence.

# Nutrition in Disasters:
# A Case Study

Much of the impetus for the nutrition program launched in India in the late 1960s came from the Bihar-centered famine of 1966–67. The Indian Ministry of Food and Agriculture described the famine as "a natural calamity of a magnitude unknown in recent times."[1] Yet, after the fact, it became known as "the disaster that never was," "the great grim famine that wasn't."[2] Not that the crisis evaporated. Instead, a catastrophe was prevented by "one of the biggest and most successful relief operations ever undertaken."[3]

Such disasters have profound nutritional implications, involving nutrition authorities in relief operations and in special kinds of planning and operational problems dealing with malnutrition.[4] This appendix examines the backdrop of the Indian crisis and activities that were attempted and evaluates results in terms of their applicability in disaster relief work elsewhere.

## The Background

Famine, of course, was no stranger to India. In 1769–70 an estimated one-third of Bengal's population of 30 million perished; in 1877–78 more than 5 million deaths were attributed to food shortage; and millions more died in other grim famines of the eighteenth and nineteenth centuries.[5] Improved transportation and more sophisticated communication did much to lessen the blow of famine in modern times, and this, in part, is why India was spared during the first four decades of this century. However, even these improvements did not prevent a peculiar set of circumstances from culminating in disaster. Still fresh in the minds of many adult Indians is the Bengal famine of 1943, when millions died and two-thirds of the 60 million inhabitants of Bengal were said to be destitute. "So many people collapsed on the sidewalks that, at times, the authorities despaired of being able to collect and cremate the bodies."[6] The victims, in a way, were casualties of World War II (the number of Indian dead was four times greater than the total number of Americans and Britons—civilians and military—who lost their lives as a result of enemy action, and probably higher than the number of Germans killed). The Japanese invasion of Burma had closed off the normal supply of imported rice, and domestic

211

production was cut 25 percent as a result of a cyclone, torrential rains, three tidal waves, a related crop fungus, and "root rot." From the limited food that was available, India was called upon to feed armies at home and abroad and to care for thousands of refugees from neighboring countries. Also, once Burma and Malaya fell, there was fear of invasion of India itself, and small farmers were reluctant to bring surplus crops to market. Hoarding became a major problem.

The famine of the mid-1960s was different. It was brought on by two successive years of drought, a phenomenon that may not have occurred more than once or twice in the last hundred years. In the crop year 1965–66, the drought was extensive, affecting seven states. The following year, some of the same states were again afflicted, with the drought in the eastern part of the country being of unprecedented intensity. A grain shortfall of nearly 30 million tons over the two-year period (from more than 88 million tons in 1964–65 to 72 million tons and 74 million tons during the two drought years) depleted food stocks of producers, traders, and consumers. Although the famine was a national disaster, it was most intense in the state of Bihar. It was here that the causes were most dramatically graphic and the relief activities were primarily centered and most successfully performed.

## The Setting

Bihar, though rich in mineral resources, is primarily an agricultural state— nearly nine-tenths of its 1966 population of 53 million were engaged in farming. Its population, the second largest among Indian states, was roughly equivalent to that of France. Population density of nearly 700 persons per square mile was double that of the rest of India.

Poverty was endemic in Bihar. Thirty-eight percent of the population belonged to scheduled castes (a euphemism for untouchables) and tribes. Of the 16 million agriculturists, more than a quarter were landless laborers. Three-quarters of those who worked the land owned only 1 percent of it. Four-fifths of all land holdings were under five acres.

The per capita income of $27 a year was India's lowest. Even in the best of times, Bihar was a deficit state in food grains. The reasons for this are not hard to find: of the 27 million acres sown to crops, less than a fifth were irrigated, and only a third of these—or 7 percent of total cultivation—were irrigated from assured sources, and thus invulnerable to a poor monsoon. A promising tubewell development program that got under way after independence was halted in less than a decade, despite the fact that much of Bihar sits atop one of the world's largest reservoirs of ground water. Irrigation schemes had been so delayed that irrigated acreage probably had declined during the two decades since 1947. An ancient, elaborate irrigation system had been the responsibility of the zamindars, and when this landlord institution (started as a control device by the East India Company in the late 1700s) was nationalized, the irrigation system was not properly kept up.

The official Bihari administration of the 1960s could never have been mistaken for a model of efficiency. Indian newspapers in the early days of the famine described the state administration as "incompetent," "bungling," "unimaginative," and "unresponsive." In addition, the state's capacity to withstand drought had been weakened by the drought of the previous year. Reserves of food grains, necessary for seeding as well as for food, had by and large been consumed. The fall crop was one-fourth the normal yield, and in some areas almost a complete failure. The important February-March rains did not arrive with sufficient force in south Bihar, resulting in a winter-spring crop of half the norm. By cruel contrast the plains in north Bihar were hit with heavy, crop-destroying floods toward the end of August.

In short, Bihar seemed singularly unprepared to cope with the situation it faced. Its cupboard was bare. Its administrative apparatus was less sophisticated than those of most Indian states. It was one of the few states that did not have a large child feeding program that could be used as a base for a relief effort, and a base is not easily or quickly built in a state with 70,000 villages. The commonly expressed conclusion in the fall of 1966 was that a tragedy of major proportions was unfolding.

There were, however, unexpected assets on the balance sheet. Because of the previous year's drought, the federal or center government had fresh experience in establishing relief machinery, setting up fair price shops, transporting mass quantities of grain, and streamlining the port capacity to handle grain. Similarly, the larger voluntary agencies had picked up useful experience in hurriedly developing extensive feeding programs in other states. Also, by good fortune, considerable quantities of food were already en route to India—partly, delayed shipments from the previous year and, partly, shipments for regularly scheduled child feeding programs.

For all its backwardness, Bihar had a basic administrative structure on which famine relief operations could be built. Transport and storage were adequate. The existence of the Education Department network and its capacity to adapt to famine relief programming turned out to be a crucial element. Finally, Bihar had a prepared, published, and well-distributed famine code that specified appropriate actions to be taken under differing conditions as they developed.

The picture in the fall of 1966, however, in balance was bleak. As the central government in New Delhi began receiving reports in September and October of the impending starvation, interministerial survey teams were dispatched to the field for first-hand observation. Their reports were increasingly disturbing. In November Prime Minister Indira Gandhi, after touring the drought areas of eastern India, reported to the nation, "There is hunger and distress in millions of homes."[7]

## The Response

The major need, of course, was food, and the prime objective of the Indian government's relief program was to obtain sufficient supplies of food and to dispense it equitably to those in want. The distribution system followed the traditional Indian plan for meeting scarcity conditions. The basic outlet was the fair price shop—twenty thousand of them were established in Bihar—through which nearly a million and a half tons of grain were distributed at fixed subsidized prices. To provide purchasing power to buy food at the fair price shops, relief works schemes were authorized; they not only provided badly needed employment to millions of Indians, but served also to check migration. Most of these projects required heavy manual labor, such as earth moving by agricultural laborers. A second food distribution program permitted nearly a million aged and infirm to obtain ten ounces of free grain a day, and a third, the child feeding program, at the famine peak provided approximately six million children and mothers with one free meal a day. There were also a number of free-food kitchens run by local voluntary agencies; the number of beneficiaries is not clear but was probably in the hundreds of thousands.

Throughout the relief effort several nutrition specialists attempted to concern government authorities with the nutritional dimensions of the famine in both its human and national development aspects. Many officials were vaguely aware that malnutrition was linked to the high Indian death rate. But the famine increased their understanding of some of the broader implications of inadequate nutrition. Officials traveling in the famine areas began noticing evidence previously ignored, and the apathetic eyes of the youngsters apparently left their mark. A special survey of the famine area for Mrs. Gandhi reported: "It is quite common to be told that the people are lazy, indolent, stupid. Angry words, but true—and the result of malnutrition over several generations. ... The economic cost to the nation of the consequent human inefficiency has never been calculated. It must run to hundreds of crores of rupees each year."[8]

The new attitudes were reflected in policies and relief programs favoring children. The new concern led, for example, to the hurried development and production of the cereal-based high protein food for children that became Bal Ahar. In early 1967 the Food Ministry decided "to include all expectant and nursing mothers and all children between two and fourteen years of age in a program of distribution of Bal Ahar."[9] The product was industrially processed and packaged and then distributed by the government. The product that was developed to meet the famine need was not without problems, such as poor quality control in manufacturing. Subsequent improvements resulted in a reformulated Bal Ahar that received high marks for acceptability.[10]

Famines usually connote the need for food. The need for water is often as great, and in parts of Bihar it sometimes became the more critical. Although estimates vary, approximately 13 million people in more than 18,000 villages were without an assured drinking water source within 1 mile of their residences. The scarcity of water posed health hazards, especially in the hottest months of the year (temperatures of 120 degrees Fahrenheit are not uncommon in the Bihar plains). It also threatened the food distribution system; if lack of drinking water caused the migration of large numbers of villagers, the delicate food distribution apparatus might collapse.

To provide each person a minimum of two gallons of water daily, the government developed a two-pronged program of well drilling and water transport. The core of the program was the hand-digging of small mud wells (known as *kutcha*) and the conversion of the *kutcha* wells to *pukka* (good, solid wells) by lining them with brick. Without lining, the wells could be expected to cave in with the next heavy rains, but even as temporary devices, each provided drinking water and irrigated half an acre of land until May and June, the driest period of summer. (Indications are that half a million *kutcha* wells were dug in Bihar, and perhaps another 10,000 were converted to *pukka* wells. Some 25,000 tubewells were sunk or deepened during the drought period.)

The water needs not met by the well program were covered by an elaborate water carriage system: by truck and rail, water was shipped daily to storage centers, from which it was transported further by large army water tankers and a fleet of bullock carts. People were assured that at given spots on certain days they could pick up water, just as milk delivery is carried out in other countries.*

Frequently famine is accompanied by widespread disease and, in some cases, deaths from such epidemics outnumber deaths from starvation. During the Bengal famine in 1943, cholera, smallpox, and malaria all took a major toll. Although the latter had by 1966 largely been eradicated from India, much concern about the other two remained. Since the incidence of cholera is related to malnutrition, there was cause for fear. Similarly, an abnormally high number of smallpox cases led some journalists to suggest the beginnings of an epidemic. Inoculations and well disinfectant treatments were extensively carried out, and epidemics never developed. In fact, no doubt partly as a result of these efforts, the number of cholera cases was substantially lower during 1966–67 than the two years before or after. Smallpox also declined from predrought figures.

Need for accurate, timely information was recognized as essential for successful control measures, and a team of management systems specialists designed an information reporting system to improve the flow of data. Techniques were instituted to communicate in days messages that normally took months to move through layers of bureaucracy. In some important instances the data were communicated in hours and minutes—via telegraph and long distance telephone, otherwise infrequently used mediums for conducting local government business. Radio was employed for regular famine bulletins to keep field workers abreast of the rapidly changing situation. In a master control room, data were collected and charted concerning food stocks, disease rates, deaths, water levels, crime rates, food prices, and numbers of people participating in relief work activities. If, for example, the water level in an area was reported to be reaching bottom, appropriate actions could be taken in anticipation that people might soon be on the move. The number of people attending free kitchens and work projects also reflected the degree of need. Similarly, the rate of food looting provided a measure of the local condition.

Finally, there was the problem of maintaining some semblance of economic

---

* Although the water program undoubtedly was of value, the critical Bihar drinking water situation probably was alleviated more by the fortuitous arrival of unseasonal rains in the spring of 1967, which enabled Bihar to survive the cruel months through mid-June.

stability. At the height of the famine, Bihar was prostrate. Seed had been consumed, many farm animals had succumbed, and money for agricultural necessities was unavailable because of the crop failure. Prices of food grains in some places had doubled and tripled, and certain development projects were stopped in midconstruction. Recognizing that any chance of crops for 1967–68 required revitalization of the rural economy, the government provided Biharis $32 million in loans ($85 million throughout India) to purchase seeds, fertilizers, animals, and pesticides.

## The Effects

To some, the government's concern and response was slow in developing. The Indian bureaucracy, like most, is a cumbersome piece of machinery that does not maneuver into position overnight. When it does, however, it has the capacity to move effectively, as it demonstrated in this case.

In 1966–67 more than 20 million tons of food grain were moved into drought areas of India, much of this from abroad, but also much from elsewhere in India. (The latter was not without problems. Reallocation of domestic supplies was cause for several serious confrontations between state and federal governments.) During the crisis, the Indian government loaded and moved an average of 7 trains a day—50 cars per train—an average of 550 miles. By the end of 1967, 153,000 fair price shops were operating in the country (20,000 in Bihar, benefiting 47 million Biharis) and 6 million people were involved in relief works projects (700,000 in Bihar). Programs for youngsters and destitutes reached nearly 20 million (7 million in Bihar) during the two years. The cost of all this: somewhere in the vicinity of $700 million (perhaps $200 million of it spent in Bihar). Help came from many foreign quarters, but the major flow came from the United States which provided one-fifth of its wheat crop. This unprecedented movement of food from one country to another required an armada of some 600 ships. Ships docked at a rate of three a day, depositing an average of 2 billion pounds a month. Sixty million Indians are estimated to have been sustained for two years solely by these shipments.*[11]

What was the result of this extraordinary effort? Foremost, large-scale deaths from starvation were prevented. Some died, although the number probably is not large and certainly nowhere near the millions predicted in the early days of the crisis.† The discrepancy is not due to ill-founded predictions but to the substantial program that prevented tragedy on a large scale.

The major and most direct reason for success was the food distribution pro-

---

* The U.S. aid, however, was not without a good deal of anxiety and controversy, most of it centering around attitudes and policies of President Johnson.[12]

† The number that died is not clear. Charges and refutations of starvation deaths appeared regularly in the Indian press. Few, however, were reported formally. (The official figures for 1966—released March 15, 1970—were 219 starvation deaths nationwide, 7 of these in Bihar.) Local officials were personally held responsible for starvation in their jurisdictions, and thus any report from them of a death would reflect their own inability to prevent it. As a result, deaths were sometimes attributed to other causes. There may have been hundreds, or by high estimates several thousand, deaths caused by the famine.

grams. Although not without problems, these programs generally were effective, many so much so that "the state of children's health was much better than at any other time."[13] Wrote George Verghese:

For the poorest sections of the society, 1967, the Year of the Famine, will long be remembered as a bonus year when millions of people, especially children, probably for the first time were assured of a decent meal a day . . . in a "normal year," these people hover on the bread line. They are beyond the pale, nobody's concern, they starve. In a famine year, they eat. Their health is better and the children are gaining weight. For them this is a year of great blessing. This is the deep irony, the grim tragedy of the situation.[14]

There was probably more milk in Bihar in 1967 than there had ever been before and, in the judgment of one local official, may ever be again. A CARE officer calculated that more than a ton of nutritional iron was ingested by the traditionally anemic population, along with substantial quantities of proteins and other nutrients.[15] Also, the famine was directly responsible for the production of Bal Ahar, which might never have come into existence had there not been this extraordinary need. (By 1971, the annual Bal Ahar production was three times larger than the total production of all similar blended foods in all other developing countries; the specifications devised for Bal Ahar later were accepted as international standards for blended foods by the Protein Advisory Group of the United Nations.) The many nutrition undertakings undoubtedly had an impact on the health and well-being of millions of young Biharis.

The famine and the emergency program dramatized the importance of nutrition to the government. The famine led to interest and in some cases emotional commitment, which in turn led to a variety of programs, a national nutrition policy, and a chapter on nutrition for the first time in the Five Year Plan. Mrs. Gandhi herself was visibly moved by the severely malnourished youngsters she observed in her several trips into famine areas.*

The famine left a nutrition imprint on other senior officials as well. Minister of Food and Agriculture C. Subramaniam, later serving as acting president of the New Congress party, was responsible for the formulation and adoption of the Children's Charter as a major plank of the party platform. (In 1971 Mr. Subramaniam was named by UN Secretary General U Thant to chair a special commission to study ways for the United Nations to play a more active and effective role in nutrition.) Secretary of Food A. L. Dias, who was in large part responsible for the success of the relief program, soon after the famine became the key government advocate for a national nutrition program. George Verghese, information adviser to the prime minister during the famine, became the nutrition movement's spokesman as editor of the *Hindustan Times* with his frequent editorials calling for action. I. Mahadaven, personal secretary to Minister Subramaniam, was made managing director of Modern Bakeries and was responsible for introducing India to fully fortified bread, special nutri-

---

* In her first radio broadcast following the 1967 national elections, the prime minister said: "Although we are immediately confronted with a critical shortage of foodgrains, I do not believe we can afford to ignore the long-term and equally basic problem of malnutrition, which affects the health, physique and stamina of the mass of our people. . . . I think it is necessary and possible to draw up a forward-looking charter . . . to improve the nutritional standards of the people."[16] This was the first reference to what later became known as the Children's Charter (see Chapter 11).

tious products for the needy, and a national nutrition education campaign. Kalyan Bagchi, the Health Ministry's representative to the famine survey teams, became the leading force in his ministry on nutrition matters. He was later responsible for the first comprehensive nutrition plan, a forerunner to the systems approach to nutrition subsequently examined in various international quarters. N. P. Sen, managing director of the Food Corporation of India, which produced Bal Ahar for the famine relief effort, was instrumental in the formation of the Protein Foods Association of India.

The Bihar relief program stimulated other developmental progress. During the two years of the famine as many wells were dug as during the three previous five-year plans, and three times as many were energized. There were projects for field leveling, embankments, drainage, and restoration of old water tanks and irrigation ditches that had fallen into disrepair. Farmers displayed an increased interest in purchasing fertilizers, pesticides, and new seed varieties, much of this the result of the increased irrigation and the stepped up agricultural extension work that went along with it.

The famine also brought into prominence the role of the voluntary agencies. As in other countries, the motives of voluntary agencies in India—both foreign and local—sometimes were suspect. With rare exception (when accusations were made that relief food was being used for proselytization) the impressive responses of the agencies during the famine dispelled these suspicions. Planning Adviser P. K. J. Menon said in April: "If Bihar is saved, it will be the result of voluntary agency feeding programs." The prime minister, in a meeting after the relief effort concluded, said the impact of the agencies not only convinced the Indian government of their contribution in emergencies, but also of the importance of using emergencies to attain broader developmental objectives.

## The Lessons

What, then, are the lessons to be learned from the Indian famine experience?

1. The Bihar famine proved there is no substitute for strong leadership in relief operations. Some have recommended that famine assistance activities be directed via a committee of the many interested ministries and organizations. Although coordination by committee is theoretically desirable, it is not the best forum for decision making. Especially in a rapidly changing situation, officials must have the authority—and the willingness to use the authority—to make on-the-spot decisions.* There was no reluctance, for example, on the part of the government's relief head to pick up the phone and force actions that normally take many meetings, many files, and many months to achieve. The same need applies to state officials at all levels.

2. The frequency with which disaster visits a land mass the size of south Asia is unfortunate—but, in fact, can be anticipated. In the past, with each disaster, people in most countries awoke with surprise and began pulling together an organizational structure to begin anew. As a result of the famine,

---

* Some civil servants may be reluctant to accept unfamiliar authority. With the powers must come assurances that careers will not be jeopardized if mistakes are made in the fast action required in disaster relief.

India recognized the need and established a permanent entity to anticipate disasters, to monitor them as they unfold, and then to conduct the necessary relief operations.

Although it is difficult to budget for disaster, the need for funds should not come as a surprise. Rather than annually withhold funds from budgets of national development programs, a country might consider the feasibility of including, as India now does, a provision in the national budget for relief contingency purposes.

Similarly, a predetermined plan or manual of relief operation can save much time in the early organization of a program. India's *Famine Code*, a thoughtful and detailed guide to local officials, was useful and surprisingly relevant, considering it had been written decades earlier.

The Indian government was especially effective in conducting activities in which it was long experienced, such as standard food distribution projects and conventional work relief schemes. The record is less impressive in its handling of new measures such as water development programs.

3. What foods should be provided in time of disaster? Most critical among the criteria is that the food be available. This seems obvious. However, much time was devoted to obtaining commodities of high nutritional value when, in fact, the greatest need was simply for something to eat. The food should be simple, easy to cook, and require a minimum of utensils. Fuel and water requirements must be considered. Acceptability is an important factor, even under the most traumatic conditions; therefore, if possible, the food should be a familiar part of the existing diet. It should have a shelf-life that can withstand the conditions of the environment it will face; it should be easily transportable under the most harrowing of circumstances; and, if possible, it should not have an attractive black market value. Finally, the selection of a commodity or commodities should include nutritional considerations based on needs of the local group—which may vary considerably from one situation to another.

4. The Bihar experience demonstrated that as a general operating rule in time of crisis, it is better to capitalize on existing institutions—for instance, school or health systems—rather than build new ones. Even though the existing entity may lack desired efficiency, energies should be devoted to grafting the necessary innovations onto them to make them work. (Schools in Bihar proved to be the best outlet for mass distribution to both school and preschool-aged children; they placed a burden on the education system, however, and classes in many areas came to a standstill.)

Although the famine dramatized the significance of voluntary agencies, such organizations vary in their capability. Just as it turned out to be best to use existing institutions rather than build new ones, it became clear that it is best to channel resources through established voluntary agencies rather than through organizations that are formed for the purpose of helping in the disaster. For example, CARE was able to move in quickly with a large and well-trained staff, and as a result conducted the largest and most successful of the relief programs. The religious agencies worked well where resident missionaries were able to build on years of familiarity with local habits and confidence of the local people. It is questionable whether the eventual contribution of certain agencies justified the time of the busy, often harassed, government officials who were required to deal with them. Also, though there was reasonably good cooperation among the many agencies in the field, cooperation was not synonymous with coordination. There were well-intentioned efforts to sort out the many activities and make maximum use of the limited resources, but it was a rare district officer who could impart a sense of order. In general the operations worked only because there was so much to be done in so many places that there was little room for conflict or overlap. In any subsequent relief operation, governments should give thought to direct assignments to the voluntary agencies. Groups could be made responsible for a particular type of project—feeding, public works, water, health—and projects further specified by geographic area and age group.

5. The Bihar experience proved that it is possible to design a relief work program that is not the commonly practiced "make work" activity, but a development program that would help prevent the need for such relief operations in the future. (Many of the relief projects were related to water development, and there is no reason why future activities could not also include projects such as construction of food storage facilities and central kitchens.) What might have been a major disaster was, in fact, an incentive for more development in Bihar than probably took place in any other comparable period in history. There is an important psychological dimension to this. The famine, which was dramatic and created attention, was parlayed and effectively used for agricultural, nutritional, and other developmental objectives. It is doubtful, even with a sufficient budget, that such activities would have taken place in the absence of the trauma created by the famine.

6. The relief effort also clearly demonstrated the need for a communications system to provide officials with decision-making information. Trained, objective, interdisciplinary groups are essential for initial surveys, and surveillance must continue since the picture in a disaster is apt to change frequently. Although the information system in Bihar was implemented too late to play a major role during peak need, it was used sufficiently to establish the value of a system of this nature for future operations.

Another information requirement is a program designed to keep the general public apprised of what is happening and what facilities and programs are available to them. Just knowing of official efforts to cope with the problem is psychologically important to those waiting out a disaster.

7. For foreign assistance agencies attempting to help local governments in time of disaster, certain points also emerged from this experience. The major need is for the delegation of authority to field personnel. Time is critical and the usual delays of intercontinental communication dilute effectiveness. Though it seems obvious that an agency can be severely handicapped by lack of adequate personnel, it is difficult from afar to know the man-hour requirements for rerouting ships, for transferring food, and for doing the paper work entailed in an operation of this magnitude. In sustained emergencies, efficient, experienced staffing should receive highest priority.

8. The crisis conditions under which relief is carried out require reevaluation of standards and values. Resources are inadequate. Inefficiencies exist. Graft and profiteering are common in disasters. The need is to recognize the reality and try to strike a balance of reasonable efficiency, productive use of limited resources, and social justice, even if it means letting the latter slip a bit to get things done.

9. Nutritionally, studies of the Bihar famine, while noting serious deficiencies, also pointed to unexpectedly good nutritional status among children, resulting undoubtedly from the relief programs.[17] Among specific nutritional findings of the Bihar experience are:[18]

Heavy manual labor schemes should not be encouraged when available food supplies are inadequate. Although the dole concept runs against the grain of fundamental principles of development, it may be preferable to burning up energy when calories are in extremely limited supply.

Nutritionally deficient people could be rehabilitated by the intelligent use of unsophisticated basic foodstuffs.

Provision of protein and calories as relief measures did not have maximal effect, without simultaneously attacking anemia, tuberculosis, and other health problems commonly found in the malnourished.

Distribution of standard multivitamin tablets appeared to be of little value.

10. Finally, it was seen that for all the many difficulties, democratic institutions can respond quickly enough and with sufficient force to meet a disaster of major proportions. Some observers had recommended greater involvement by the army or a complete takeover by the center government. But local officials, splendidly supported by New Delhi, responded more effectively than anyone had envisioned. By any measure, it was a remarkable achievement. Help came from many sources but, in the final analysis, the victory clearly was that of the government of India and the local officials. The Bihar-centered episode may have been the first time in modern history that a government declared war on large-scale famine—and won.

"THE FAMINE," wrote Verghese in 1967, "has been a revelation, a trial, a shame; but also an opportunity and an awakening. It has transformed some of the inertia of the past into energy."[19]

By 1969, parts of Bihar had reverted to old form. Some of the inertia had returned and the delays and sluggishness in project implementation had again become part of daily life. But, also, much had changed. In the year following the drought, Bihar's food grain production achieved an all-time high, nearly double that of the drought year, and a 7.6 percent increase over the last pre-drought year. In 1968–69, production increased by another 10.5 percent. Although Bihar was still one of the least developed of Indian states, there were improvements of land, of body, and of frame of mind. As one Bihari official said, things can never be the same.

# Statistical Tables

TABLE B-1. *Child Mortality Rates in Selected Countries, 1970*

| Country | Percent in age group who die each year | | Percent that die before 5th birthday | Age at which same percent as in col. 3 die in | |
|---|---|---|---|---|---|
| | Under 1ᵃ (1) | 1–4 (2) | (3) | Taiwan (4) | United States (5) |
| India | 13.9 | 4.40 | 28.1 | 61 | 63 |
| Pakistan | 14.2 | 5.30 | 31.0 | 63 | 66 |
| Egypt | 11.7 | 3.93 | 24.8 | 60 | 61 |
| Guinea | 21.6 | 5.20 | 36.7 | 66 | 68 |
| Cameroon | 13.7 | 3.93 | 26.5 | 61 | 62 |
| Guatemala | 8.9 | 2.75 | 18.5 | 55 | 57 |
| Taiwan | 2.0 | 0.43 | 3.6 | 5 | 20 |
| Japan | 1.5 | 0.14 | 1.9 | 1 | 1 |
| United States | 2.1 | 0.10 | 2.5 | 2 | 5 |
| Sweden | 1.3 | 0.07 | 1.7 | 1 | 1 |

Sources: UN, *Demographic Yearbook, 1963, 1967, 1969,* and *1970;* Population Reference Bureau, "1970 World Population Data Sheet" (Washington: Population Reference Bureau).
a. Live births.

TABLE B-2. *Changes in Number of Childhood Deaths in Selected Countries If 1970 Mortality Rates of India, Taiwan, Japan, and Sweden Are Applied*
In thousands of deaths

| Country | Deaths of infants under 1[a] | | | | | Deaths of children 1 to 4 | | | | | Deaths of children under 5 | | | | |
|---|---|---|---|---|---|---|---|---|---|---|---|---|---|---|---|
| | At country's own rate | Difference at rate of[b] | | | | At country's own rate | Difference at rate of[b] | | | | At country's own rate | Difference at rate of[b] | | | |
| | | India | Taiwan | Japan | Sweden | | India | Taiwan | Japan | Sweden | | India | Taiwan | Japan | Sweden |
| India | 3,238 | 0 | −2,772 | −2,888 | −2,935 | 2,928 | 0 | −2,643 | −2,841 | −2,881 | 6,166 | 0 | −5,598 | −5,854 | −5,925 |
| Pakistan | 972 | −21 | −835 | −869 | −884 | 1,059 | −180 | −973 | −1,033 | −1,045 | 2,031 | −75 | −1,851 | −1,932 | −1,954 |
| Egypt | 171 | +32 | −142 | −149 | −152 | 173 | +21 | −154 | −167 | −170 | 344 | +166 | −297 | −318 | −324 |
| Guinea | 41 | −14 | −38 | −38 | −39 | 29 | −4 | −27 | −28 | −29 | 70 | −5 | −64 | −67 | −67 |
| Cameroon | 40 | 0 | −34 | −35 | −36 | 36 | +4 | −32 | −35 | −35 | 76 | +28 | −66 | −71 | −72 |
| Guatemala | 21 | +12 | −16 | −17 | −18 | 20 | +12 | −17 | −19 | −19 | 41 | +41 | −33 | −37 | −38 |
| Taiwan | 9 | +48 | 0 | −2 | −3 | 7 | +63 | 0 | −5 | −6 | 16 | +158 | 0 | −7 | −9 |
| Japan | 30 | +244 | +10 | 0 | −4 | 9 | +274 | +20 | 0 | −4 | 39 | +809 | +39 | 0 | −9 |
| United States | 77 | +425 | −4 | −22 | −30 | 15 | +645 | +48 | +6 | −4 | 92 | +1,509 | +53 | −18 | −37 |
| Sweden | 2 | +19 | +1 | * | 0 | * | +21 | +2 | +1 | 0 | 2 | +50 | +3 | +1 | 0 |

Sources: UN, *Demographic Yearbook, 1970;* and Population Reference Bureau, "1971 World Population Data Sheet."
* Less than 1,000.
a. Live births.
b. Negative numbers represent lives that would be saved at projected rate; positive numbers reflect additional number of deaths at projected rate.

223

TABLE B-3. Childhood Deaths Due to Causes Commonly Related to Malnutrition, in Selected Countries, by Age Group, 1967[a]

Percent due to

| Country | Gastritis and enteritis[b] | | | Pneumonia and influenza | | | Measles | | | Bronchitis | | | Whooping cough | | | All five causes | | |
|---|---|---|---|---|---|---|---|---|---|---|---|---|---|---|---|---|---|---|
| | Under 1 year | 1–4 years | Under 5 years | Under 1 year | 1–4 years | Under 5 years | Under 1 year | 1–4 years | Under 5 years | Under 1 year | 1–4 years | Under 5 years | Under 1 year | 1–4 years | Under 5 years | Under 1 year | 1–4 years | Under 5 years |
| Chile | 14.9 | 11.4 | 14.5 | 26.2 | 30.3 | 26.8 | 2.2 | 11.6 | 3.5 | * | * | * | * | * | * | 43.3 | 53.3 | 44.8 |
| Colombia | 20.2 | 26.4 | 22.6 | 10.2 | 12.1 | 10.9 | 0.9 | 4.7 | 2.3 | 10.1 | 9.7 | 9.9 | 0.0 | 0.0 | 0.0 | 41.4 | 52.9 | 45.7 |
| Ecuador | 14.5 | 15.8 | 15.0 | 7.5 | 8.6 | 7.9 | 1.7 | 7.8 | 4.0 | 16.7 | 13.5 | 15.5 | 8.4 | 11.1 | 9.4 | 48.8 | 56.8 | 51.8 |
| Guatemala | 13.2 | 20.8 | 17.0 | 18.0 | 21.0 | 19.5 | 2.7 | 9.5 | 6.1 | * | * | * | 6.8 | 10.4 | 8.6 | 40.7 | 61.7 | 51.2 |
| Mexico | 18.1 | 19.2 | 18.5 | 19.8 | 20.8 | 20.1 | 0.9 | 6.9 | 2.8 | 5.6 | 3.8 | 5.1 | 1.3 | 5.3 | 2.6 | 45.7 | 56.0 | 49.1 |
| Nicaragua | 25.4 | 19.4 | 23.4 | 5.6 | 6.4 | 5.9 | 0.6 | 3.3 | 1.4 | * | * | * | 1.3 | 3.8 | 2.1 | 32.9 | 32.9 | 32.9 |
| Peru | 11.0 | 13.7 | 11.9 | 20.5 | 22.0 | 21.0 | * | * | * | 9.6 | 8.4 | 9.2 | 7.4 | 10.3 | 8.4 | 48.5 | 54.4 | 50.5 |
| Egypt | 53.1 | 62.2 | 57.1 | 2.8 | 5.0 | 3.7 | 0.6 | 3.0 | 1.7 | 10.7 | 17.9 | 13.9 | * | * | * | 67.2 | 88.1 | 76.4 |
| Angola | 21.5 | 23.2 | 22.2 | 8.3 | 11.8 | 9.8 | * | * | * | * | * | * | * | * | * | 29.8 | 35.0 | 32.0 |
| Nigeria | 11.3 | 5.6 | 7.6 | 23.8 | 11.6 | 15.9 | 4.5 | 4.9 | 4.8 | * | * | * | * | * | * | 39.6 | 22.1 | 28.3 |
| Mauritius | 31.5 | 44.9 | 35.6 | 5.3 | 5.9 | 5.4 | * | * | * | 4.0 | 5.6 | 4.5 | * | * | * | 40.8 | 56.4 | 45.5 |
| Philippines | 8.0 | 15.3 | 10.9 | 17.6 | 33.1 | 24.8 | 1.0 | 4.2 | 2.3 | 6.9 | 11.4 | 8.7 | 0.1 | 0.1 | 0.1 | 33.6 | 64.1 | 46.8 |
| Average of the above twelve | 20.2 | 23.2 | 21.4 | 13.8 | 15.7 | 14.3 | 1.3 | 4.6 | 2.4 | 5.3 | 5.9 | 5.6 | 2.1 | 3.4 | 2.6 | 42.7 | 52.8 | 46.3 |
| Japan | 4.0 | 4.8 | 4.1 | 9.3 | 11.2 | 9.7 | 0.3 | 1.2 | 0.5 | 0.8 | 1.3 | 0.9 | * | * | * | 14.4 | 18.5 | 15.2 |
| United States | 1.3 | 2.2 | 1.4 | 7.2 | 10.7 | 7.7 | * | * | * | * | * | * | * | * | * | 8.5 | 12.9 | 9.1 |
| Canada | 1.3 | 2.2 | 1.5 | 8.2 | 9.4 | 8.4 | * | * | * | * | 0.8 | * | * | * | * | 9.5 | 12.4 | 9.9 |
| Sweden | 0.6 | 1.2 | 0.7 | 2.2 | 7.6 | 2.9 | 0.8 | 3.2 | 1.1 | * | * | 0.1 | * | * | * | 3.6 | 12.0 | 4.7 |

Sources: PAHO, Health Conditions in the Americas 1965–68, Scientific Publication No. 207 (Washington: PAHO, 1970), Table 12; UN, Demographic Yearbook, 1967, Table 25; World Health Organization, World Health Statistics, 1967 (Geneva: WHO, 1970), Tables 2, 4.1, 5.1.

* Less than 0.05 percent.

a. In Nigeria in 1963, Egypt in 1964, Angola in 1965, Guatemala and Nicaragua in 1966, and Canada in 1968.

b. Includes all gastrointestinal diseases.

224

TABLE B-4. *Malnutrition as Primary or Associated Cause in Deaths of Children under Five, in Selected Areas, 1971*

| Area | Percent of deaths in which malnutrition is associated cause | | | | | Percent of deaths caused by malnutrition | | |
| --- | --- | --- | --- | --- | --- | --- | --- | --- |
| | Measles | Diarrhea | Other infective or parasitic cause | Respiratory cause | Other cause | Primary cause | Associated cause | Primary or associated cause |
| Argentina | | | | | | | | |
| San Juan Province | | | | | | | | |
| San Juan | n.a. | 68 | n.a. | 8 | 33 | 3 | 37 | 40 |
| Suburban | 36 | 62 | 48 | 35 | 33 | 9 | 39 | 48 |
| Rural | 36 | 53 | 57 | 39 | 30 | 8 | 39 | 47 |
| Chaco Province | | | | | | | | |
| Resistencia | 67 | 67 | 71 | 50 | 47 | 7 | 57 | 64 |
| Rural | 54 | 67 | 48 | 25 | 20 | 3 | 48 | 51 |
| Brazil | | | | | | | | |
| Recife | 74 | 70 | 64 | 51 | 34 | 6 | 60 | 66 |
| São Paulo | 52 | 63 | 50 | 33 | 41 | 6 | 45 | 51 |
| Ribeirão Prêto area | | | | | | | | |
| Ribeirão Prêto | 71 | 75 | 90 | 56 | 54 | 2 | 67 | 69 |
| Franca (small town) | n.a. | 69 | n.a. | 46 | 28 | 9 | 49 | 58 |
| Colombia | | | | | | | | |
| Cali | 65 | 51 | 47 | 40 | 35 | 16 | 40 | 56 |
| Cartagena | 94 | 64 | 67 | 36 | 33 | 15 | 44 | 59 |
| Medellín | 84 | 62 | 74 | 29 | 45 | 11 | 51 | 62 |
| Jamaica: Kingston | n.a. | 41 | 36 | 24 | 31 | 6 | 32 | 38 |
| Bolivia: La Paz | 50 | 67 | 53 | 25 | 11 | 4 | 41 | 45 |
| Mexico: Monterrey | 74 | 70 | 64 | 51 | 34 | 4 | 48 | 52 |
| Chile: Santiago | n.a. | 52 | 52 | 31 | 38 | 6 | 39 | 45 |
| El Salvador | | | | | | | | |
| San Salvador area | | | | | | | | |
| San Salvador | 69 | 48 | 60 | 29 | 29 | 9 | 49 | 58 |
| Rural | 78 | 55 | 50 | 40 | 24 | 14 | 44 | 58 |
| Average of all areas | 65 | 61 | 58 | 36 | 33 | 8 | 46 | 54 |

Source: Data in PAHO, *Inter-American Investigation of Mortality in Childhood, First year of Investigation, Provisional Report* (Washington: PAHO, 1971).
n.a. Not available.

225

TABLE B-5. *Male Life Expectancy at Specified Ages in Selected Countries*[a]

| | Expected years remaining at age | | | | | |
|---|---|---|---|---|---|---|
| Country | 0 | 1 | 5 | 10 | 15 | 20 |
| Cameroon | 34 | 40 | 42 | 41 | 38 | 35 |
| Central African Republic | 33 | 40 | 41 | 38 | n.a. | 31 |
| Chad | 29 | 34 | 34 | 31 | n.a. | 26 |
| Colombia | 44 | 50 | 52 | 48 | 44 | 40 |
| Egypt | 52 | 56 | 61 | 57 | 52 | 48 |
| Gabon | 25 | 34 | 38 | 36 | n.a. | 29 |
| Guinea | 26 | 33 | 35 | 32 | n.a. | 29 |
| India | 42 | 48 | 49 | 45 | 41 | 37 |
| Japan | 69 | 69 | 66 | 61 | 55 | 51 |
| Mexico | 61 | 62 | 60 | 56 | 52 | 47 |
| Nigeria | 37 | 45 | 49 | 47 | 43 | 39 |
| Sweden | 72 | 72 | 68 | 63 | 58 | 53 |
| Taiwan | 66 | 67 | 64 | 59 | 54 | 49 |
| United States | 67 | 67 | 64 | 59 | 54 | 49 |

Source: Data in UN, *Demographic Yearbook, 1968* and *1970.* Data are for various years in the 1950s and 1960s.

n.a. Not available.

a. Number of years of life remaining.

TABLE B-6. *Production and Yield of the Seven Major Edible Oilseeds, 1970*

| Oilseed | Production, thousands of tons | | | Increase over 1960 production, percent | Oilseed yield, percent[a] | | Price per ton, dollars | | |
|---|---|---|---|---|---|---|---|---|---|
| | *Oilseed* | *Oil* | *Meal* | | *Oil* | *Meal* | *Oilseed* | *Oil* | *Meal* |
| Soy bean | 46,521 | 5,960 | 26,810 | 70 | 19 | 79.0 | 102 | 263 | 87 |
| Cotton seed | 22,066 | 2,385 | 6,900 | 10 | 13 | 55.0 | 119 | 240 | 78 |
| Groundnut (in shell) | 18,144 | 3,230 | 4,020 | 30 | 28 | 39.0 | 229 | 364 | 112 |
| Sunflower seed | 9,653 | 3,780 | 3,700 | 58 | 26 | 26.0 | 66 | 332 | 87 |
| Rapeseed | 6,502 | 1,855 | 2,920 | 71 | 38 | 60.0 | 137 | 262 | 115 |
| Copra | 3,395 | 2,110 | 1,140 | (−3) | 65 | 7.5 | 204 | 343 | n.a. |
| Sesame seed | 1,866 | 595 | 800 | 23 | 40 | 58.0 | 267 | n.a. | n.a. |

Sources: Data in FAO, *Production Yearbook, 1970*; and Alan Holz, "Price Patterns for Oilseeds and Products," *Foreign Agriculture*, Dec. 31, 1971, p. 14.

n.a. Not available.

a. Oilseeds yield meal, oil, and waste. Indian extraction rates are used wherever possible.

TABLE B-7. *Price and Protein Content of Protein Products, 1971–72*

| Product | Price per kilogram of product, dollars | Protein content, percent[a] | Price per kilogram of protein, dollars[b] | Annual cost to meet one-third of protein needs of a country of 10 million people, millions of dollars[c] |
|---|---|---|---|---|
| Oilseeds | | | | |
| *Soybean*[d] | | | | |
| Flour | 0.13 | 50 | 0.26 | 21.0 |
| Concentrate | 0.48 | 70 | 0.69 | 54.6 |
| Isolate | 0.83 | 90 | 0.92 | 73.9 |
| *Cottonseed* | | | | |
| Flour | 0.36 | 55 | 0.67 | 53.8 |
| Concentrate | 0.36 | 65 | 0.55 | 43.8 |
| *Groundnut* | | | | |
| Flour | 0.11 | 50 | 0.22 | 17.7 |
| Isolate | 0.77 | 90 | 0.86 | 69.1 |
| *Coconut* | | | | |
| Flour | 0.44 | 25 | 1.76 | 141.3 |
| Concentrate | 1.75 | 70 | 2.50 | 197.7 |
| *Sesame seed* | | | | |
| Flour | 0.88 | 65 | 1.35 | 107.7 |
| Grain concentrates | | | | |
| *Wheat* | 0.11 | 23 | 0.48 | 38.0 |
| *Rice* | 0.11 | 16 | 0.69 | 54.4 |
| Single cell protein | | | | |
| *Yeast* | 0.30 | 50 | 0.60 | 48.2 |
| *Bacteria* | 0.44 | 65 | 0.68 | 54.6 |
| *Algae* | 0.84 | 65 | 1.29 | 103.6 |
| Fish protein concentrate | 0.48 | 80 | 0.60 | 47.4 |
| Leaf protein concentrate | 1.00 | 50 | 2.00 | 158.2 |
| Synthetics | | | | |
| *Lysine* | 2.20 | e | e | e |
| *Methionine* | 2.20 | e | e | e |

Source: Standard prices and protein content data of companies producing the products. Prices for products not yet commercially produced are estimates of commercial and university research groups. Commercial prices fluctuate with the market, so figures can differ considerably by time and locale.

a. Grams of protein per 100 grams of product. Data based on such qualitative measures of protein content as biological value, protein efficiency ratio, or net utilizable protein are not available.

b. Price includes the carbohydrate and fat values of the product since these values are not available in all cases.

c. Assumes the average adult requires 65 grams per day.

d. The price of soybeans in 1972 nearly doubled. The demand for soybeans increased largely because the supply of fish meal decreased due to an extraordinarily poor fish catch off the west coast of South America.

e. Synthetic amino acids serve only as supplements to improve the protein of existing foods.

# Methodology for Computing the Value of Human Milk

The value of breast milk can be determined from the cost of securing an equivalent amount of nutrients through commercial milks. Assuming that mother's milk alone supplies an adequate diet during the first six months and thereafter serves as a supplement, it is possible to estimate the economic contribution of the nursing mother to her child's nourishment.

Calculations in this appendix of the volume of breast milk that the average nursing mother produces are based on studies by Gopalan[1] and McKigney.[2] The volume of fresh cow's milk and of whole powdered milk formula necessary to feed an infant in its first six months is based on the recommended average daily allowance computed by McKigney. The value of breast milk is derived from the cost of providing the equivalent nourishment through cow's milk at $145.40 per ton or whole powdered milk formula at $240.00 per ton. The average mother's production of breast milk and the costs of substitutes are given in Table C-1. The cost would be smaller if it reflected the cost of supplementing the lactating mother's diet and greater if it included the equipment and other extra costs involved in bottle feeding.

The losses to governments due to the decrease in breast feeding are reflected in Tables C-2–C-6. They are derived by applying the equivalent value of mother's milk production to the percentages of mothers breast feeding at various times. Those percentages represent the difference between the number of new mothers and that number reduced by a weaning rate. The weaning rate used in the calculations is the percentage of mothers who have completely ceased breast feeding during a particular time frame.

TABLE C-1. *Average Mother's Production of Milk and Costs of Substitutes*

| Baby's age bracket, in months | Mother's milk production | | | Fresh cow's milk equivalent | | Whole powdered milk formula equivalent | |
|---|---|---|---|---|---|---|---|
| | Milli-liters per day | Calories per day | Total liters | Liters | Cost, in dollars | Kilo-grams | Cost, in dollars |
| 0–6 | 850.0 | 600 | 155.5 | 183 | 27 | 24.6 | 59.0 |
| 7–12 | 500.0 | 385 | 91.5 | 105 | 16 | 14.0 | 33.5 |
| 13–18 | 500.0 | 385 | 91.5 | 105 | 16 | 14.0 | 33.5 |
| 19–24 | 200.0 | 154 | 36.5 | 42 | 6 | 5.7 | 13.7 |
| 0–24 | 512.5 | 381 | 375.0 | 437 | 65 | 58.3 | 139.7 |

TABLE C-2. *Losses Due to Decreases in Breast Feeding in Chile, 1951 and 1970*

| Babies' age and year of data | Number of babies, in thousands | | Breast milk production, in thousands of tons | | |
|---|---|---|---|---|---|
| | Total | Breast-fed | Potential | Actual | Loss |
| Up to 1 year | | | | | |
| 1951 | 206.6[a] | 196.2 | [b] | [b] | [b] |
| 1970 | 333.2[a] | 27.8 | [b] | [b] | [b] |
| 1–2 years[c] | | | | | |
| 1951 | 176.0 | 167.2 | 57.7 | 54.8 | 2.9 |
| 1970 | 302.5 | 18.2 | 93.2 | 14.6 | 78.6 |

Source: F. B. Mönckeberg, "The Effect of Malnutrition and Environment on Mental Development," *Proceedings of Western Hemisphere Nutrition Congress II, San Juan, Puerto Rico, August 1968* (1969).

a. First year total is actual number of births.

b. Included in figures for 1–2 years; separate figures not available for first year.

c. Figured from total births reduced by number of infant deaths.

TABLE C-3. *Value of Breast Feeding Losses in Calcutta, 1971*

| Babies' age bracket, in months | Number of babies, in thousands | | Value of breast milk, in thousands of dollars[a] | | |
|---|---|---|---|---|---|
| | Total | Breast-fed | Potential | Actual | Loss |
| 0–6 | 360.7[b] | 349.9 | 8,581.0 | 8,323.5 | 257.5 |
| 6–12 | [b] | 317.4 | 4,963.2 | 4,368.0 | 595.2 |
| 12–24 | 310.5[c] | 180.1 | 5,971.2 | 3,463.3 | 2,507.9 |
| 0–24 | 671.2 | 847.4 | 19,515.4 | 16,154.8 | 3,360.6 |

Source: Data in UN, *Demographic Yearbook, 1970;* and Hindustan Thompson Ltd., *Food Habits Survey* (Calcutta: Hindustan Thompson, 1971).
a. Based on cost of fresh cow's milk furnishing equivalent number of calories.
b. Total for 0–6 months includes 6–12 months; it is the actual number of births.
c. Figured from total births reduced by number of infant deaths.


TABLE C-4. *Trends in Breast Feeding in Singapore, 1951–60*

| Babies' age, in months | Breast-fed babies | | | | Percent decline, 1951–60 |
|---|---|---|---|---|---|
| | Number, in thousands | | Percent of all babies | | |
| | 1951 | 1960 | 1951 | 1960 | |
| 1 | 41 | 40 | 84 | 63 | 23 |
| 2 | 38 | 31 | 78 | 50 | 36 |
| 3 | 35 | 27 | 71 | 42 | 41 |
| 4 | 33 | 22 | 67 | 35 | 48 |
| 5 | 33 | 20 | 67 | 32 | 52 |
| 6 | 31 | 17 | 62 | 27 | 56 |
| 7 | 27 | 15 | 54 | 23 | 57 |
| 8 | 22 | 13 | 46 | 21 | 54 |
| 9 | 21 | 11 | 42 | 17 | 60 |
| 10 | 17 | 11 | 35 | 17 | 51 |
| 11 | 16 | 8 | 33 | 13 | 61 |
| 12 | 14 | 8 | 28 | 13 | 54 |

Source: Wong Hock Boon, K. Paramathypathy, and Tham Ngiap Boo, "Breastfeeding among Lower Income Mothers in Singapore," *Journal of the Singapore Pediatric Society*, October 1963, pp. 89–93. Data are restricted to Chinese population; breast feeding is even less common among Malays and Indians.

TABLE C-5. *Value of Breast Feeding Losses for Babies under One Year Old in Singapore, 1951 and 1960*

| | Value of breast milk, in thousands of dollars[a] | | | | |
|---|---|---|---|---|---|
| | Actual | | Potential, | | Loss as |
| | First 6 | Second 6 | first 12 | | percent of |
| Year | months | months | months | Loss | potential |
| 1951 | 950 | 305 | 2,100 | 845 | 40 |
| 1960 | 706 | 171 | 2,692 | 1,815 | 67 |

a. Based on cost of fresh cow's milk furnishing equivalent number of calories.

TABLE C-6. *Value of Breast Feeding Losses in the Philippines, 1908, 1958, and 1968*

| | Breast-fed babies | | Value of breast milk, in thousands of dollars[a] | | | Loss as |
|---|---|---|---|---|---|---|
| Babies' age and year of data | Number, in thousands | Percent of all babies | Actual | Potential | Loss | percent of potential |
| Up to 1 year | | | | | | |
| 1908 | 287 | 100 | 12,237 | [b] | [b] | [b] |
| 1958 | 490 | 64 | 20,873 | [b] | [b] | [b] |
| 1968 | 406 | 44 | 17,294 | [b] | [b] | [b] |
| 1–2 years | | | | | | |
| 1908 | 242 | 100 | 5,285 | 17,522 | 0 | 0 |
| 1958 | 451 | 64 | 9,823 | 47,750 | 17,054 | 36 |
| 1968 | 377 | 44 | 8,218 | 58,247 | 32,735 | 56 |

Source: Ma Linda Gabucan-Dulay, "Current Feeding Patterns as Observed among 1,000 Filipino Infants," *Philippine Journal of Pediatrics,* April 1970, pp. 95–103. Values may be underestimated by as much as 50 percent because calculations are based on birthrates that probably were grossly underestimated.

a. Based on cost of fresh cow's milk furnishing equivalent number of calories.

b. Included in figure for 1–2 years old; separate figures not available for first year.

# Nutrition Program Planning: An Approach

In response to the need to broaden understanding of malnutrition and improve planning for its alleviation, this appendix attempts to lay out a systematic approach and a framework for analyzing the nutrition problem and identifying the most appropriate methods of attacking the problem. Essentially this is an adaptation of established planning techniques. It begins with the assumption that the decision maker recognizes the problem, is aware of its relationship to broad national objectives, accepts the notion that good nutrition can be an investment in human capital analogous to education, and has decided to give increased attention to the nutrition sector. Moreover, it is based on the premises that malnutrition will not be alleviated widely or quickly under current development policies and trends, that important shifts in policies and practices may be required to effect changes, and that the scope of such shifts may involve many people, activities, and entities not now regarded as part of the nutrition universe.

## The Nutrition Planning Sequence

As with other forms of planning, the nutrition planning sequence starts with a definition of the nature, scope, and trends of the problem, this leading to a preliminary statement of broad objectives. It next moves through a description of the environment in which the nutritional condition arises. As causes are traced, programs and policies that are relevant to the objectives are sorted out, and then, in a comparison of the alternatives, an interrelated nutrition program is constructed. Final selection of objectives, programs, and projects emerges after a budgetary and political process in which programs to attack malnutrition are pitted against competing claims on resources and, if necessary, redesigned to fit actual budget allocations. The last step is evaluation of the programs' effects, with the conclusions fed back into subsequent rounds of the planning sequence.*

* The approach has many variations; some have five steps, some have ten, but all begin with problem identification and end with evaluation.

233

In practice, planning does not simply follow a series of textbook steps, but is rather an iterative process that resembles more the tango—four steps forward, three steps back, with an occasional turn-around. Objectives, for example, are not settled on early in the game. As various proposals are developed, the worth of one objective is judged against the worth of another. Having modified his objectives, the planner reexamines program proposals in a continual process of testing the desirable against the practical.

### Identifying the Problem

Step one in the planning process is problem description. What are the specific nutritional deficiencies? How severe are they? Who is affected, and where are they? What are the trends? For the most part, this step consists of a straightforward collection of already available or easily obtainable hard data through a variety of established techniques. Four standard methods are used for measuring the nature and extent of malnutrition: food balance sheets, consumer expenditure surveys, food consumption surveys, and direct medical nutrition surveys.

*Food balance sheets.* A measurement technique developed in great statistical detail by the UN Food and Agriculture Organization is the food balance sheet. Estimated supplies of different foods within a country (or region) are translated into calories and nutrients, from which the per capita amounts available for human consumption are computed after taking account of losses and other uses. Availabilities can be compared with recommended standards for that country, to arrive at an estimate of the aggregate nutritional gap. Possible changes in this gap can be projected to conform to future changes in population, food output, and other variables. This aggregate measure conceals individual features of the complex reality it describes; it fails to take into account the dispersion of the income distribution within the population, regional variations, intrafamily food distribution mores, or seasonal hunger.[1] Thus, it does not yield an estimate of how many actually are suffering from malnutrition or give a profile of who they are. To strike an average as a means of ascertaining collective need for additional nutrients may be worse than meaningless; it can be dangerously misleading.*

*Consumer expenditure surveys.* In combination with income distribution data, consumer expenditure surveys of the amount and kind of food purchased at specified levels of income or expenditure can yield estimates of the numbers of people consuming different levels of nutrients. These findings can then be compared to minimum nutritional requirements. Depending on the reliability and detail of the data, such surveys can give a picture of the overall magnitude of nutritional deficits, the distribution of the deficits among areas and certain

---

* A positive food balance does not indicate absence of a problem where an aggregate surplus exists, as best seen in countries showing large surpluses of nutrients on the food balance sheets but still facing malnutrition. When a country has anything less than a moderate surplus, it almost is certain that a serious problem exists within individual regions or social classes.

broadly defined population groups, and the apparent consumption levels of different nutrients. Although this technique provides a closer look than the balance sheet approach, it still omits important factors affecting nutrition such as the impact of cooking methods on the nutrient content of food, distribution habits within families, and the incidence of parasites or other health problems that reduce food utilization.

*Food consumption surveys.* In the food consumption survey, data are gathered on the kinds and quantities of food consumed in selected households which represent the sociological, demographic, and economic patterns of the general population. By calculating the nutritive value of diets and comparing the value with nutritional requirements, deficiencies can be estimated. This method is not without problems. Precision is required to determine the actual quantity and quality of food eaten by the various members of the household. Answers given may reflect errors in judgment as well as a manipulation of the facts to present a favorable image by the family being questioned. Special influences on dietary patterns—such as season of the year, periods of the month and week, paydays and holidays—must be accounted for. Food reported as "consumed" may in fact have been wasted in cooking or left on the plate. Nutrients may have been lost because of malabsorption.

*Medical nutrition survey.* The direct nutrition survey involves a field examination of the nutritional status of a sample of the population. For the specific group studied, this is the most accurate of the four measures but also the most costly, the most time consuming, and the most difficult. By necessity, the samples are small, and thus not necessarily representative of the whole population. If various direct surveys are compared to project a broader picture, they often suffer from a lack of standardization of clinical and biochemical definitions, uneven representativeness of the materials, and methodological problems such as failure to make allowances for seasonal variations.

*Shortcomings of analytical methods.* Each of the analytical methods has shortcomings, but together they can present a reliable picture. All four would benefit measurably if the surveys were oriented toward policy issues. What appears on the surface as a potentially rich mine of data is often of limited usefulness to the planner; usually the survey is designed without regard to unanswered (and generally unstated) policy questions and without regard to how the data would eventually be used.

*Secondary-source survey.* A less formal, and less imposing, technique is capable of providing quick, generalized conclusions if direct studies are not available—and can add a helpful dimension even if they are. This is the secondary-source survey based on available vital statistics; collective impressions obtained from interviews with nutrition experts as well as with a sampling of public health officials and others on the local scene constantly exposed to the problem; and a compilation and analysis of earlier studies—including village work of cultural anthropologists and medical surveys conducted for other purposes—which, when patched together, may present the outlines of a distinctive pattern. The secondary-source survey technique lacks the desired precision for later detailed quantification and therefore should not be considered a substitute for a more comprehensive search. In most countries, however, it offers a prompt means of gaining a useful first perspective of the problem.[2] For many planning situations, a partial answer today is worth a great deal more than a complete answer three years from now.

*The problem identified.* In the process of identification, the planner pinpoints the need. He now recognizes the specific maladies (for example, protein-calorie malnutrition, iron-deficiency anemia, vitamin A deficiency) and he is able to quantify roughly the extent of the problem (for example, a 25 percent consumption shortfall in meeting minimum protein or vitamin A requirements). This may then be translated into specific nutrient requirements.*

### Nutrition Objectives

With an adequate description in hand of the scope and nature of the nutritional problem and the victims, the next step is to begin identification of possible objectives. Lack of attention to this seemingly most obvious step in the planning process has caused many nutrition programs to flounder. Government officials, often incorrectly assuming that the objectives are understood, give little if any time to formulating them. In neglecting this step, they risk setting forth a program of little consequence.

The first look at objectives is a general one, emerging from some kind of interaction between the decision maker and the planner. The nature of the interaction will vary. In some countries there may be an explicit dialogue between planner and decision maker; in others, the communication will be much less direct. (The distinction between decision maker and planner should be clear. The planner may be in a position to advise, but not to establish objectives. No amount of planning analysis substitutes for the kind of moral and political value judgments that enter into policy decisions.) The early discussions block out the desired aims, such as preservation of life, reduction of deficiency diseases, freedom from infection, and development closer to genetic potential. Also, they raise such concerns as whether the program is developmental or humanitarian; whether it is looking for immediate results or concentrating on long-term improvements; and whether it should aim to appease hunger or raise nutritional standards.

One of the planner's early analytic strategy concerns is the determination of proper scope for analysis. He wants to reach as far as possible but within the bounds of realistic attainment. He recognizes that the narrowness of nutrition activities to date may in part reflect the nutrition advocate's assumption that only token resources would be available, which has resulted in a "pilot project here, research activity there," often missing the real determinants of nutrition status. So the first look at alternate objectives should be ambitious—usefully realistic, but ambitious. Adjustments can be made later as the planner begins to match need against resources, but at the outset he should not restrict thinking by automatically closing off imaginative avenues of intervention. Even if cer-

* In estimating quantities of gross requirements, allowance needs to be made for nutrient losses that can be anticipated from vomiting, diarrhea, administrative mishaps, and so on.

tain programs later prove beyond the reach of limited resources, the exploration of such avenues may yield insights leading to otherwise unidentified possibilities.

An important element in objective making is selection of targets, based on findings of the earlier problem identification.[3] Should the program be directed to the infant? The preschool-aged child? The schoolchild? The pregnant woman? The nursing mother? The breadwinner? Or, more realistically, what combinations of these groups? The sick or the well? The pros and cons of various targets including relative growth dividends deserve considered attention, the issue generally not being as simple as suggested on the surface.[4] For example, the nutritionally vulnerable young child—especially the already severely malnourished young child—would seem to deserve primary attention. Yet, a hospital bed for a severely malnourished youngster may cost as much as food supplements for thirty other needy children, who without supplements may themselves soon fall into the queues for hospitalization.

With the target in mind, the responsible officers might begin formulating tentative but specific nutrition objectives. For example: By 1978, to achieve in country $x$ the provision of adequate protective foods and services in types and quantities required to reduce from 30 percent to 10 percent the number of six- to twenty-four-month-old children suffering third degree and second degree protein-calorie malnutrition.

Three things are important to any meaningful, "plannable" nutrition objective, and they will affect the planning and budgeting process at different points as it progresses. First, compared with broad national goals like "eradication of malnutrition" or "improvement in the quality of life," the objective must cite a specific deficiency and a numerical target, or final output, as a benchmark for estimating the needed resource inputs. (At this stage the objective is still illustrative. Its formulation helps point the way for the kinds of analyses needed, but without the attendant data on costs—specifically, the relation between increasing inputs and higher levels of benefits—it is impossible to know how much it would cost to reach any proposed target or whether having achieved, say, the reduction to 10 percent it would take a great deal more money, or perhaps only a very small increment, to reach 5 percent or virtually zero.)

Second, the objective must have a time frame that requires a definite sequence of action for attaining the objective by a given date and specification of resources to be allocated at each step in that sequence to achieve the objective of defined magnitude.

Third, the resources the program will require must be calculated. Their provision will become subobjectives, marking paths of the programs and conditions that will have to be created along the way toward the specific target. For example, increased production capacity for certain foods or food products might be required. Or reduction of associated health and environmental problems. Or an understanding by legislators or other policy makers of the significance of a particular program. Thus, a subobjective may be to create sufficient awareness of the implications of a problem to provide a receptive climate for required legislation and appropriation. Subobjectives also should be translated into a program quantified and positioned in a time frame.

In short, as objectives are stated with increasing precision, the planner becomes increasingly able (and aware of the need) to develop a systematic program of inquiry and action.

### Anatomy of the Problem

Most studies of nutrition have concentrated on identifying the nature and scope of the problem. Less attention has been directed to the root causes, often perhaps because the causes seem too obvious to merit serious attention. Surface conclusions, however, can be misleading and poor analysis here may lead nutrition advocates astray in the quest for solutions.

For purposes of useful discussion, one can distinguish three strata of causes of malnutrition. The most proximate causes, from the medical point of view, are insufficient nutrient intake, poor utilization of nutrients from the food ingested, and the heightened nutritional needs caused by bouts of nutrition-related illnesses. At the other extreme are such factors as general inadequacy of national resources, rapid population growth, and the entire constellation of causes that together constitute underdevelopment. In between, and the area in which a nutrition planning analysis should concentrate, are those socioeconomic factors directly influencing diet and utilization that can possibly be manipulated to improve nutritional status. Here belong such causes as low family income, local ecological deficiencies, distribution shortcomings, price relationships, food waste, and errors of consumer behavior. The understanding of such causal factors lags far behind the medical nutritionist's knowledge of physiological causal connections.

*A systems approach.* There has been growing recognition that because malnutrition is a problem deeply imbedded in the surrounding socioeconomic environment, a more comprehensive and systematic or "systems" approach could provide a powerful analytic and programming tool. First attempts to apply systems techniques to the nutrition problem have mapped out the ground, but the results have been too broad for practical usefulness. Systems practitioners tend to produce flow charts reflecting the relationships of everything to everything, the result being something more akin to a Jackson Pollock canvas than to a useful planning chart. Comprehensiveness is desirable, but it becomes counterproductive if it focuses time and attention on tertiary variables or strives for precision that may be spurious because of limited and inaccurate data.

A practical systems approach to nutrition should yield guidance for decision makers within a reasonable time period, identify and analyze not the entire complex of causes but those major determinants of nutritional status in particular malnourished populations, and be subject to policy levers. Exposing this system even in a limited form should have more than explanatory value. It should show which of the many causes are the major factors and how they operate. It should reveal, thereby, points where interventions might effect desirable changes and result in improvements in nutritional status.

The basic difference between the systems approach and the conventional means of nutrition planning is in their focus. In the latter, the analysis and solutions focus on the most immediate determinants of the problem, and generally the identification of a nutrition deficiency prompts reflex responses such as proposals for new formulated foods or for health center activities. A systems approach, instead of jumping forward from problem to solution, moves backward to a study of the complex, interacting forces of the environment within which the malnutrition arises.

In attacking protein deficiencies among children under two years of age, for instance, the prime determinants—food intake and health—would be examined separately. Each would be subdivided: food intake, for example, into family food purchases, family food production, family food habits, food provided through institutional feeding programs, and food provided from the mother's breast. Subdividing still further, the planner would try to isolate at each stage the most important or potentially important influences. Whenever possible, he would quantify his answers. The same line of inquiry would be posed for the health determinant; infection is a more significant determinant of nutritional status in some situations than is nutrition intake.

The analytical process of drawing out the system and of pressing for causal factors and relations constitutes a disciplined systematic search for relevant factors. In following one problem as well as each indication of what may be an important contributing element, the nutrition planner picks his way through the connecting paths of the system that have been exposed in the process of describing the problem in its fullness.

Thinking through such a system is a first step to understanding the causes of and potential solutions to the nutrition problem. Even if no further analysis were undertaken, this would represent an improvement over the impressionistic or unstructured nutrition planning that is generally prevalent. However, for appreciation of the total system, more data often will be required, as will a clearer understanding of the interrelationships of the many factors in the system. Where sufficient data exist, or can easily be generated, it is conceivable that simulation models of the interrelated systems could be constructed to test the impact of different interventions, thereby increasing the likelihood of selecting the most effective ones.

*The Tamil Nadu systems study.* A prototype activity, in the Indian state of Tamil Nadu (formerly Madras), gives some insight into how a nutrition planning system might be approached.[5] The Tamil Nadu systems project was designed to identify the determinants of diet of children under age five and pregnant and lactating women, and to expose the relationships between variables in such a way as to make evident some promising points of intervention. To simplify the analysis, the nutrition system was divided into three subsystems: agricultural production, processing and distribution, and the consumer.

Approaching the problem as one of agricultural production, the inquiry looked at price relationships among agricultural commodities, the nutrition implications of existing agricultural policies in general and in particular of the agricultural subsidy system, the workings of agricultural credit (primarily to see whether it was discriminatory to certain crops), infrastructure investments and how much they shaped cropping decisions, and so on. From a processing and distribution viewpoint, the study examined nine different food delivery systems and the costs associated with each, as well as margins of profit at each stage of the distribution system, the nature and coverage of the food processing industry, the role of cooperatives as a potential delivery system, the costs to transport certain foods, and so on. The consumer habits subsystem study looked at food expenditure patterns, intrafamily food distribution, food taboos, and so forth. In twenty-five hundred households, four interviews—to detect seasonal variations—of two and a half hours each were scheduled.

Interwoven in all of the analyses was a study of government's role: amounts, availability, acceptability, and effectiveness of existing services (for example, child feeding programs, health activities, nutrition education), and budget analysis of existing programs. It was found, for instance, that Tamil Nadu health officers prided themselves on one of India's largest and best health delivery systems, and yet there was little satisfaction with the system's ability to lower death rates among children. This raised questions about possible reallocation of resources and possible consolidation of delivery systems.

The collected data were to produce a nutrition model that would establish the relationship of diet to family income, to religion, to caste, to morbidity and income, to mortality and income, to education level of parents, to use of health services, to presence of nonnuclear family member (like grandparent), to occupation, to size of family and per capita food expenditure, to maternal employment (outside of household), to consumption of convenience foods, to safety of water supply (and other environmental hygiene factors), to outside eating, to awareness of "nutrition," to practice of family planning. From established relationships, further multiple correlations could be attempted.

The ultimate aim of the study was to develop a nutrition model—a completely open data bank that would permit testing of alternative nutrition intervention programs—and to examine tradeoffs between solutions; to initiate activities (the state wanted to build in demonstration projects at an early stage); and to move on to devise a comprehensive nutrition program.*

For many countries the planning apparatus, to be workable, must be more modest than that in Tamil Nadu. Generally the funds, data, trained planners, and administrative talent are limited and a complex nutrition planning undertaking could be counterproductive. Obviously the degree of complexity of any planning effort needs to be scaled to existing capabilities. Systematic nutrition planning need not be—in many cases should not be—designed to produce a highly sophisticated computerized model, requiring extensive investment of time, talent, and money. Rather, it should be regarded as a conceptual approach, a systematic way of looking at a problem to sharpen decision making.†

---

* Similar studies have been undertaken in Colombia, Ecuador, and the Brazilian state of São Paulo.

† Complex techniques are not a prerequisite to good planning. In the experience of Charles Hitch, one of the pioneers of systems planning, "what distinguishes the useful and productive analyst is his ability to formulate (or design) the problem; to choose appropriate objectives; to define the relevant, important environments or situations in which to test the alternatives; to judge the reliability of his cost and other data; and finally, and not least, his ingenuity in inventing new systems or alternatives to evaluate."[6]

*Identification and Comparison of Alternative Interventions*

Once the determining factors and their relative importance are identified, the nutrition planner has a basis for judging the relevance and relative effectiveness of the kinds of interventions the nutritionist often recommends—nutrition education, fortification, maternal-child health facilities, blended foods, and so on—and for developing new or particular interventions suggested by the particular anatomy of a country's nutrition problems—for example, interventions relevant to regional storage and distribution, opportunities for income supplements, or price policies.

*Nutritional profiles.* The attractiveness of any intervention will, of course, depend on the nutritional problem at issue, the particular population group comprising the target, the factors that determine the nutritional status of that group, and the intrinsic characteristics of the intervention. For any one population group, the systems description would provide information for a nutritional profile, which would characterize the group by the important variables defining and determining its nutritional status. Such a profile would serve as a kind of litmus paper against which any of the standard nutrition intervention programs could be tested. Characteristics of population groups that typify profiles found in many parts of the world include:

NONMONETIZED SUBSISTENCE GROUPS: Very low real income. Regional or local ecologically determined nutritional deficiencies. High incidence of infectious diseases aggravated by malnutrition. Deleterious food preparation habits. Low food productivity combined with substantial spoilage and losses. Illiteracy.

LOW-INCOME SMALL FARMERS, PARTIALLY MONETIZED: Substantial portion of diet comprises local staple, locally milled every day or so. Small expenditures on processed products such as salt, sugar, tea, and condiments. Poor food habits and low productivity. Limited access to commercial distribution channels and certain basic mass media. Low functional literacy. (Small tenant farmers probably less responsive to price system and productivity-raising programs because of insecurity of tenure and rental arrangements.)

LOW-INCOME LANDLESS AGRICULTURAL LABORERS: Same as low-income farmers but also socially disadvantaged and less well served by government agencies at the local level. Limited benefits from general economic progress because of seasonal underemployment.

LOW-INCOME URBAN MIGRANTS: Deleterious food habits. Slightly higher income often spent on nutritionally inferior forms of processed foods. High mass communications exposure. Declining breast feeding, and high incidence of infant disease from unsterile feeding procedures.

In the simple process of matching previously identified alternatives to the profiles,[7] many preconceived notions will have to be discarded. This does not mean that a single project must meet the test of practicality for all groups, but at least this filtering process clarifies the potential impact and limitations of a given project. A cereal fortification alternative obviously would be meaningless to a group whose food is not centrally processed. Price policies would have little impact on nonmonetized segments of the population. Nutrition education is of little use if needed nutrients are not available.

## Comparing the Alternatives

Once remedial measures have been screened for their probable success, alternatives need to be compared in terms of their costs and relative effectiveness, their impact on other activities, and certain practicalities not easily accounted for in economic analysis.

*Costs and benefits.* Of course, most important is the nutritional impact (and economic and social benefits) of interventions relative to their costs. At this stage, little is known about the impacts of various approaches. A common mistake is failure to take all costs into consideration. For example, in the case of mass fortification projects, per capita cost of effective intervention must be computed in terms of total outlay, including the cost of reaching those who do not need the extra nutrients as well as those who do.

Among the questions to be raised in evaluating a potential livestock project would be: Who will consume the products emerging from the project? (If planned for domestic consumption, what income groups, age groups, geographic and cultural groups? If planned for export, who are the beneficiaries of the project income?) What impact will this have on calorie and protein consumption of the poor? How is the land necessary for the project now used? (If for crops, what crops, and who consumes them—by income and age group? Is the land for the project suitable for agriculture?) What will be the income implications of livestock projects on the nutritionally needy? For example, how labor intensive is the project compared to the activity (if any) it will replace? Will it generate related employment (for example, meat processing, shipping)? Will it change the land tenure structure? What will be the effects of the project on the price of meat and grain? Finally, what will be projected protein and calorie consumption patterns when taking all of the above into account—and how does this compare to current intake?

In the battery of standard considerations included in project analysis are the questions whether the project will be self-sustaining (After the initial investment, will the project pay for itself? Examples would be incentives to encourage the launching of low-cost commercial foods or fortification projects in which the costs could eventually be borne by the consumers); what kinds of costs are involved; and from what sources the costs can be met. Some activities, such as nutritional education, might be supported by local moneys. Others, such as production of soy isolate, may have significant foreign exchange costs. The costs of some proposed strategies, such as institutional feeding programs, can be covered partly with food commodities readily available and free of charge from international sources. Similarly, technical and capital foreign assistance may be more easily available for certain projects than for others. This is not to suggest that foreign assistance in nutrition is without its costs—financial, administrative, political, and even psychic. Properly handled foreign aid can be useful in reducing the country's burden, but such considerations must be brought into the cost equation.

To restrict benefit calculations to those factors that are measurable also would be a distortion. Good nutrition may improve labor efficiency by preventing blindness or by reducing anemia, and the resulting increased productivity is measurable. But to stop there would ignore the main benefit: the increased well-being—mental and physical—of those involved. In short, the benefit-cost analysis would not have been carried out in terms of actual benefits but of those benefits that happen to be easy to measure.[8] Thus, some interventions do not lend themselves to standard quantification of costs and benefits, in part because of severe limitations of data and in part because of the quantification difficulties inherent in programs designed to change human behavior. The planner's contribution here is to narrow down as much as possible what is known about the potential costs and benefits of such interventions and to make clear what is conjecture. Decisions in such instances often must be left to common sense judgments, which will be easier if the planner is honest about assumptions and uncertainties.

*Impact on nonnutrition sectors.* Nutritional activities affect nonnutritional sectors in ways that need to be taken explicitly into account. The significance of second-order consequences of nutrition interventions can vary widely. A large nutrition education activity can be viewed in greater isolation than a new policy designed to shift crops. The former will impinge on administrative time and resources otherwise available for other programs, but the latter might necessitate reallocations of foreign exchange.

Some nutrition interventions may strengthen other development efforts. Free food supplements may, for instance, draw young mothers to a family planning clinic or improve student well-being and school attendance rates.

*Constraints.* Besides standard questions of feasibility (availability of equipment and other inputs, legal requirements, and so on), a number of practical constraints are important to decisions. These are worth singling out for special attention because they have often hampered nutrition activities in practice. Good management is such a scarce resource that preference should be given to interventions requiring minimum dependence on an administrative structure. For example, a nutrition policy depending on a health center–oriented operation may require a huge staff, a shift in price policy virtually none. An education program leaning heavily on face-to-face techniques requires thousands of extension workers in a large country whereas a mass media effort designed to achieve the same end may require only a few dozen employees. The management requirements of extensive feeding programs may pose serious obstacles, even where existing school, health, and other institutions are used. If these entities are fully employed, the added feeding function may appear to have no incremental cost besides provision of the food; but it will incur real costs in terms of reduced time devoted to the primary functions of the existing institutions. For intervention programs not tied to an existing infrastructure, a heavily administered program also means a claim on limited talent affecting costs of attaining other national goals.

Another factor to be carefully weighed is replicability. If the project's success depends on multiplying the impact of an isolated success that is dependent on the personal initiative and vitality of the initiator—for example, a pilot village applied nutrition program—the chances of success are more limited than for broad, sweeping policies creating the same nutritional impact without going through the replication effort. Too often a successful pilot project loses its impact in the process of bureaucratization.

Time is an important consideration, especially with respect to protein-calorie malnutrition among young children. The criticality of early periods of growth for subsequent mental and physical capacity requires the planner to heavily discount those options that will begin to affect a nation's nutritional status only after a long time. For those children passing out of the critical months impaired by protein-calorie malnutrition, the effects of these delayed benefits will be very small. Formulated foods, cereal fortification, shifts in price policies can pay off very quickly. Activities still in the basic research stage—work on single cell protein or fish protein concentrate—may not, even if technically successful, produce a significant nutrition impact for years. Between these extremes are successful laboratory projects that still require field testing—for example, the fortification of salt in India and of sugar in Guatemala. Thus, alongside his project options, the planner should plot a separate track indicating the time span implied. A strategy might do well to stress measures with immediate impact, with an eye toward development of better substitutes to gradually replace the initial measures over time.

Finally, such practical bureaucratic questions of the capabilities, commitment, and forcefulness of the people in charge of proposed programs, and of the number of officials and the time involved in the clearance procedure, combine with the other factors that help to predict program success or failure. As these considerations are superimposed on the purely technical judgments, a shorter list of program opportunities emerges and the final shape of the program begins to take more distinct form.

The planning analysis thus far will help determine which set of inputs, or which program, would be likely to achieve the desired target, within the desired time frame, for the least cost. However, the total cost commonly turns out higher than the resources eventually provided through the budgetary process. After the financial availabilities and policy framework are set,* it is usually necessary to return to the drawing board. Some realignment of objectives, time frame, and the mix of projects will have to be made, within the limits of the resources actually budgeted. Objective-making is an iterative process, involving frequent adjustment throughout the various planning stages. As data are collected and analyzed, the planner's notions may change about the nature of the problem and costs to overcome it. Flexibility to alter objectives is essential to the entire process.

While adjusting objectives it is important for the planner to return to the original analysis. In scaling down an objective, it may turn out that what passed the cost-effectiveness test in the context of an ambitious national program may not be the best way to reach more modest numbers.

---

* The matter of funding generally comes to a head during the annual upheaval called the budget process, and, in many countries, every four or five years during formulation of the development plan. The difficulty of getting new moneys out of treasuries is legend, all developing countries suffering from some form of financial anemia. Those interested in promoting nutrition programs should carefully distinguish between costs that show up in the nutrition budget and those that do not. Any new request for a large budgetary appropriation on already overstrained budgets can be expected to encounter resistance.

*The Decision*

Throughout the planning sequence the nutrition planner, in an attempt to keep his efforts relevant, tries to get guidance or at least clues indicating areas and scope of interest of the policy makers. Now he places before the decision maker the options, alternate objectives, alternate strategies, and, most important, the potential programs and consequences of alternate strategies.* The executive probably is a political figure, and he will add—if it is not there already—a political dimension to the analysis. First, is the overall concept politically attractive? And if so, is it sufficiently visible? How long will it take to see results? Within the specific program and project options, there may be greater political attractiveness attached to one proposal than to another. A massive child feeding program offers high visibility and many potential votes. A shift in cropping pattern to achieve the same end may go undetected by the electorate; indeed, it may offend some commodity interest groups, many of which are notoriously efficient in influencing policy to meet their ends.

Also, since most nutrition programs are forms of income redistribution, certain approaches may be more politically palatable than others. Taxation to feed hungry children is less likely to arouse resistance in those being taxed than a direct money transfer to the poor. There are political considerations when other countries are involved in the program. For example, the executive must weigh the cost of potential political embarrassments should they arise.

Decisions finally result from a complex debate and adversary process among various interest groups, the legislative body, and the executive, involving political values and judgments based on emotion, intuition, or the desire to protect a bureaucratic position. The planner thus becomes only marginally influential in the final decision-making stage. He has, however, been able to systematically analyze and articulate the options. Clearly when the executive has some indication of the consequences of various actions, he is in a position to make up his mind more intelligently. As Alice Rivlin notes on the merits of the planning process: (1) It is better to have some idea where you are going than to fly blind, and (2) it is better to be orderly than haphazard about decision making.[9]

Now the planner has presented the alternatives to the executive and selection has been made. The decision should reflect a mix of immediate, intermediate, and long-term payoffs, blending action and research components, with greater emphasis on action.

*Evaluation*

After decisions have been made, policies formulated, programs adopted, manned, and put into operation, the final step is to determine whether the hypothesis has worked out, with the ultimate measure of activities being their contribution to achievement of the broad objective. (One of the common mistakes of food programmers is the assumption that achievement of the subobjectives—for example, distribution of $x$ tons of food through $y$ schools—

* Complicating the life of the planner is the common absence of an individual who is *the* decision maker. Decisions often result from a far more diffuse process than the "centralized decision making" that organization charts imply.

implies success.) Evaluation measures the actual performance; it informs the planner of weaknesses needing adjustment, assumptions needing alteration or further research, and how costs and benefits are developing under actual operating conditions. Evaluation feeds these important judgments back into the planning process, connecting one planning cycle with the next. For the sake of objectivity, the evaluation should be conducted by someone (or some entity) other than the program's planner or implementer.

Evaluation is the element of the nutrition planning process that generally receives the least amount of effort.[10] In principle no one is opposed to evaluation; in practice it is rarely undertaken. (Perhaps one reason funds for evaluation are not included in project budgets is that administrators are reluctant to ask; a request may be interpreted as admission of doubt of the program's effectiveness and therefore may hamper basic funding for the project. Another is that findings of a poorly managed program supported by outside assistance may inhibit future funding from the same aid source in other sectors.)[11] When evaluation does take place, results often are vulnerable to methodological attack: data may have been collected erroneously, the sample improperly drawn, or interpretations made unsatisfactorily. At the outset, programs must be systematically designed in a way that will generate data for measuring the program's effectiveness.

## The Planning Process in Perspective

Although the planning process has earned an enviable reputation in the development business, in practice it is not without its limitations. Asok Mitra, secretary of India's Planning Commission, once wrote that the planning process is similar to elephants' love-making: "It takes the best part of a year to learn the way about it; the moment of love can be painful and rather hazardous; and anyway there's an eighteen-month wait for the result."[12] In addition to program constraints, there are analytical constraints. Conclusions depend heavily either on available data, often of uncertain quality, or on personal judgments which themselves are subject to human error. A common shortcoming is inadequate recognition of the discrepancy between what logically makes sense and what is operationally realistic.

Also, in quest for the perfect model, planning can be overdone, to the point it becomes a prison or straightjacket to operational movement. (In one of the larger development agencies, the lengthy and cumbersome planning procedures prompted one food programmer to retort: "Let them eat plans.") In the beginning, the important thing is not that the bear walk straight but that he walk at all. Clearly there have been instances in which the promise of planning techniques has been greater than the delivery[13] and instances in which complicated methodological devices have fallen of their own weight. Even though there is now common agreement that "the new planning" has passed the point in its development "which medicine passed in the nineteenth century where it begins to do more good than harm,"[14] it is still a fairly new and not yet totally refined art. False starts and blind alleys can be expected as part of the occupational hazards.

Properly scaled to local capabilities and properly action oriented, the planning process can serve a highly useful function for those concerned with better nutrition. If the problem has been clearly defined, the objectives precisely stated, and interventions adequately analyzed, this approach serves as a systematic means of producing what will probably be the best possible range of program solutions.

The making of a nutrition plan could take years—or weeks. Clearly, some good indications of desirable direction are obtainable without elaborately detailed studies. When a government endorses a detailed nutrition planning undertaking, it should not be at the cost of operational delay. Ongoing projects should not be derailed; new actions can be initiated on the basis of preliminary analysis and best judgments while more elaborate studies are under way. In most instances it is far easier to study and report on the consequences of an operation than to predict those consequences in the abstract.

# References

CHAPTER 1

1. George Orwell, *The Road to Wigan Pier* (London: Victor Gollancz, 1937), p. 91.

2. See UN Secretariat, Department of Economic and Social Affairs, "Strategy statement on action to alert the protein crises in the developing countries," Report of the Panel of Experts on the Protein Problem Confronting Developing Countries, ST/ECA/144 E/5018/Rev. 1, May 1971; Robert S. McNamara, Address to Board of Governors, International Bank for Reconstruction and Development, Washington, Sept. 27, 1971, and Address to UN Economic and Social Council, New York, Oct. 28, 1971; and Alan Berg, Nevin Scrimshaw, and David Call (eds.), *Nutrition, National Development and Planning* (MIT Press, forthcoming).

3. It is symptomatic of nutrition's obscurity that it was not included among the 41 variables selected as the most important indicators of social, political, and economic development by I. Adelman and C. T. Morris in *Society, Politics and Economic Development: A Quantitative Approach* (Johns Hopkins Press, 1967).

4. Abraham Horwitz, "The Physician's View of Nutritional Needs in the Western Hemisphere," in *Proceedings of the Western Hemisphere Nutrition Congress, Nov. 8–11, 1965* (American Medical Association, 1966), pp. 3–6.

5. As reported in interview, Henry Sebrell, 1968.

6. Food and Agriculture Organization (FAO), *Lives in Peril: Protein and the Child* (Rome: FAO, 1970), p. 25.

7. Pan American Health Organization (PAHO), *The Inter-American Investigation of Mortality in Childhood*, Provisional Report (PAHO, September 1971).

8. FAO, *Lives in Peril*, p. 7.

9. UN Protein Advisory Group, "Statement on the Nature and Magnitude of the Protein Problem," Statement No. 3 (Oct. 27, 1969).

10. World Health Organization, "WHO Activities in the Field of Protein (-Calorie) Malnutrition," Nutr/70.1, agenda item 8.10 (UN Protein Advisory Group Meeting, New York, 1970), p. 2.

11. FAO, *Lives in Peril*, p. 5.

12. Philip Sartwell (ed.), *Maxcy-Roseneau Preventative Medicine and Public Health* (9th ed., Appleton-Century-Crofts, 1971); and John Bryant, *Health and the Developing World* (Cornell University Press, 1969).

13. Joint FAO-WHO Expert Committee Reports, 1954 to present; Derrick B. Jelliffe, *Infant Nutrition in the Subtropics and Tropics*, WHO Monograph No. 29 (2nd ed., 1968); National Academy of Sciences–National Research Council, *Pre-School Child Malnutrition: Primary Deterrent to Human Progress*, Publication 1282 (NAS–NRC, 1966).

248

CHAPTER 2

1. F. Mönckeberg, "Nutrition and Mental Development" (paper presented at Conference on Nutrition and Human Development, East Lansing, Michigan, 1969).

2. Pedro Rosso, Julia Hormazabal, and Myron Winick, "Changes in Brain Weight, Cholesterol, Phospholid, and DNA Content in Marasmic Children," *American Journal of Clinical Nutrition*, October 1970, pp. 1275–79. Letter to the author from Myron Winick, Jan. 19, 1972.

3. Nevin S. Scrimshaw and John E. Gordon (eds.), *Malnutrition, Learning and Behavior, Proceedings of an International Conference, 1967* (MIT Press, 1968); Salvador Armendares, Fabio Salamanca, and Silvestre Frenk, "Chromosome Abnormalities in Severe Protein Calorie Malnutrition," *Nature*, Vol. 232 (July 23, 1971), pp. 271–73; Merrill S. Read, "Human Studies on Nutrition and Mental Development: Problems, Pitfalls and Progress" (paper presented at Symposium on Malnutrition and Behavior, Prague, Czechoslovakia, September 1969; processed).

4. J. Cravioto, E. R. DeLicardie, and H. G. Birch, "Nutrition, Growth and Neurointegrative Development: An Experimental Ecological Study," *Pediatrics,* Supplement, August 1966, pp. 319–72.

5. J. Cravioto and E. R. DeLicardie, "The Long-Term Consequences of Protein Calorie Malnutrition," *Nutrition Reviews,* May 1971, p. 111.

6. Joaquin Cravioto and Elsa R. DeLicardie, "The Effect of Malnutrition on the Individual," in Alan Berg, Nevin Scrimshaw, and David Call (eds.), *Nutrition, National Development and Planning* (MIT Press, forthcoming). Also see Fernando Mönckeberg and others, "Malnutrition and Mental Development," *American Journal of Clinical Nutrition*, Vol. 25 (August 1972), pp. 766–72.

7. Summarized in David Coursin, "Report of the Sub-committee on Nutrition, Brain Development and Behavior" (paper presented to Committee on International Nutrition, Food and Nutrition Board, National Academy of Sciences, 1972; processed).

8. Myron Winick, "Malnutrition and Brain Development," *Journal of Pediatrics,* May 1969.

9. Hector Correa, "Nutrition, Health, and Education" (Tulane University, n.d.; processed).

10. Alfred Picasso de Oyagüe, "Scientific Study of Malnutrition as a Limiting Factor in the Development of Education," UNESCO Doc. NS/ROU/212 Rev., Feb. 15, 1971.

11. J. M. Bengoa, "Recent Trends in the Public Health Aspects of Protein-Calorie Malnutrition," *WHO Chronicle*, December 1970, p. 559.

12. Picasso de Oyagüe, "Scientific Study of Malnutrition."

13. A. R. Kamat, "Primary Education: Participation and Wastage," *Economic and Political Weekly* (India), April 27, 1972, p. 877.

14. Bo Vahlquist, "Problems of Human Malnutrition" (paper presented at Dag Hammarskjöld Seminar on Nutrition as a Priority in African Development, Uppsala, Sweden, July 1971); W. W. Greulich, "A Comparison of the Physical Growth and Development of American-born and Native Japanese Children," *American Journal of Anthropology*, Vol. 15 (1957), p. 489; T. C. Tung, paper presented at 12th Pacific Science Congress, Canberra, Australia, August 1971; and William Insull Jau, Toshio Oiso, and Kenzaburo Tsuchiy, "Diet and Nutritional Status of Japanese," *American Journal of Clinical Nutrition*, July 1968, pp. 753–77.

15. Rose Frisch and Roger Revelle, "Variations in Body Weights Among Different Populations," in *World Food Problem, Report of the President's Science Ad-*

*visory Commission* (1967), Vol. 3 (Harvard Center for Population Studies Reprint, 1967).

16. J. M. Bengoa, "Priorities in Public Health Nutrition Problems," in *Proceedings of the Seventh International Congress of Nutrition*, Vol. 4: *Problems of World Nutrition* (Hamburg, Germany: Pergamon Press, 1967).

17. Food and Agriculture Organization, *Lives in Peril: Protein and the Child* (Rome: FAO, 1970), p. 9.

18. C. Gopalan, "Health Problems in Preschool Children III—World-wide Experience: Special Problems and Preventative Programmes, (1) India," *Journal of Tropical Pediatrics*, December 1958, p. 229.

19. Elinor F. Downs, "Nutritional Dwarfing: A Syndrome of Early Protein-Calorie Malnutrition," *American Journal of Clinical Nutrition*, November 1964, pp. 275–81. Similar observations have been made in Mexico (see Cravioto, DeLicardie, and Birch, "Nutrition, Growth, and Neurointegrative Development," p. 36; and "Influencia de la desnutrición en la capacidad de aprendizaje del niño escolar," in *Boletín Médico del hospital infantil* (Mexico), Vol. 24 (1967), p. 217.

20. J. M. Bengoa, "Significance of Malnutrition and Priorities for Its Prevention," in Berg, Scrimshaw, and Call, *Nutrition, National Development and Planning*.

21. Ancel Keys and others, *The Biology of Human Starvation* (University of Minnesota Press, 1950). Also see Joseph Brozek, "Food as an Essential: Experimental Studies on Behavioral Fitness," in Seymour Farber and others, *Food and Civilization* (Charles C. Howe, 1966), pp. 29–60; R. B. Bradfield (ed.), "Assessment of Typical Daily Energy Expenditure," Symposium, *American Journal of Clinical Nutrition*, December 1971, pp. 1403–93; Maurice E. Shils, "Food and Nutrition Relating to Work and Environmental Stress," in Michael Gershon Wohl and R. S. Goodhard (eds.), *Modern Nutrition in Health and Disease* (4th ed., Lea, 1968), pp. 1014–44; Josef Brožek, "Nutrition and Behavior: Psychological Changes in Acute Starvation with Hard Physical Work," *Journal of the American Dietetic Association*, July 1955, pp. 703–7; W. D. Keller and H. A. Kraut, "Work and Nutrition," in Geoffrey H. Bourne, *World Review of Nutrition and Dietetics* (Hafner, 1962), Vol. 3, pp. 69–81; Robert McCarrison, *Nutrition and National Health* (London: Faber and Faber, 1944), pp. 18–25; Robert McCarrison, *Work*, ed. H. M. Sinclair (London: Faber and Faber, 1953), pp. 265–70, 299; *Nutrition and Physical Activity: Symposium of the Swedish Nutrition Foundation* (Uppsala, Sweden: Swedish Nutrition Foundation, 1967); F. E. Viteri and O. Pineda, "Effects of Starvation on the Individual: Effects on Body Composition and Body Function, Psychological Effects," in Gunnar Blix, Yngve Hofvander, and Bo Vahlquist (eds.), *Famine: Nutrition and Relief Operations in Times of Disaster* (Uppsala, Sweden: Almqvist and Wiksells, 1971), pp. 25–40.

22. H. Kraut and others, in *Arbeitsphysiologie*, Vol. 14 (1950), p. 147; F. W. Lowenstein, *Nutrition and Working Efficiency*, Special Paper No. 3 (FAO, WHO, and Organization of African Unity, Scientific, Technical and Research Commission, May 1968); W. H. Forbes, "The Effects of Hard Work upon Nutritional Requirements," *Milbank Memorial Fund Quarterly*, January 1945, pp. 89–96; P. S. V. Ramamurthy and R. Dakshaljane, "Energy Intake and Expenditure in Stone Cutters," *Indian Journal of Medical Research*, September 1962, pp. 804–9; P. S. V. Ramamurthy and Bhavani Belvady, "Energy Expenditure and Requirement in Agricultural Labourers," *Indian Journal of Medical Research*, October 1966, pp. 977–79; John V. G. A. Durnin and R. Passmore, *Energy, Work and Leisure* (London: Heinemann Educational Books, 1967).

23. Henry Borsook, "Nutritional Status of Aircraft Workers in Southern California," *Milbank Memorial Fund Quarterly*, April 1945, pp. 99–185; National Research Council, *The Food and Nutrition of Industrial Workers in Wartime, Report of the Committee on Nutrition in Industry* (NRC, 1942); NRC, *The Nutrition of Industrial Workers, Second Report of the Committee on Industrial Workers* (NRC, 1945); T. A. Lloyd Davies, "Nutrition in Industry," in *Proceedings of the Sixth International Congress of Nutrition* (Edinburgh: Livingstone, 1964), pp. 24–27; T. Bedford, *The Health of the Industrial Worker in India,* Report of the Industrial Health Research Board of the Medical Research Council in the United Kingdom, Department of Health, Government of India, Simla, India (1946); Magnus Pyke, *Industrial Nutrition* (London: MacDonald and Evans, 1950); *Report of the Subcommittee of the Nutrition Advisory Committee on Nutritional Requirements of Working Class Families* (Faridabad: Government of India, 1965); Bhavani Belvady, "Nutrition and Efficiency in Agricultural Labourers," *Indian Journal of Medical Research*, October 1966, pp. 971–76; N. H. Areskog, Ruth Selinus, and B. Vahlquist, "Physical Work Capacity and Nutritional Status in Ethiopian Male Children and Young Adults," *American Journal of Clinical Nutrition*, April 1969, pp. 471–79.

24. Gilberto Freyre, *The Masters and the Slaves* (Knopf, 1946), pp. 65–66.

25. "Management of Slaves, &c," *Farmers' Register*, No. 1 (1837), p. 32. See also, Ulrich Bonnell Phillips, *American Negro Slavery: A Survey of the Supply of Employment and Control of Negro Labor as Determined by the Plantation Regime* (Appleton, 1918); Eugene D. Genovese, *The Political Economy of Slavery* (Pantheon, 1965); Robert S. Starobin, *Industrial Slavery in the Old South* (New York: Oxford University Press, 1970); Joseph C. Goulden, *The Money Givers* (Random House, 1971); Lewis Cecil Gray, *History of Agriculture in the Southern United States in 1860* (Peter Smith, 1958), Vol. 1; Kenneth M. Stampp, *The Peculiar Institution: Slavery in the Ante-Bellum South* (Knopf, 1963); letter from Robert Leckie to the Commissioner of Public Buildings, the Marble Quaries, May 16, 1817 (National Archives, Record Group No. 42, Letters Received, Vol. 24).

26. Nevin Scrimshaw, Carl E. Taylor, and John E. Gordon, *Interactions of Nutrition and Infection*, Monograph Series No. 57 (Geneva: World Health Organization [WHO], 1968).

27. Bengoa, "Significance of Malnutrition."

28. C. Gopalan and K. Vijaya Raghavan, *Nutrition Atlas of India* (Hyderabad: National Institute of Nutrition, Indian Council on Medical Research, 1969), pp. 2–3. Also see Pan American Health Organization, "Proposals of Change and Strategies of Health for the Decade 1971–1980" (paper prepared for meeting of Ministers of Health of the Americas, Santiago, Chile, October 1972; processed); and WHO, *Nutritional Anemias*, Technical Report No. 405 (Geneva: WHO, 1968).

29. Gopalan and Raghavan, *Nutrition Atlas*, pp. 64–65.

30. Nutrition Society of India, *Report of the Study on Nutritional Anemia* (Hyderabad: Nutrition Research Laboratories, July 1968).

31. Bo Vahlquist, "Occurrence of Nutritional Anemias in Children," and S. K. Sood, L. Baherji, and V. Ramalingaswami, "Occurrence of Nutritional Anemias in Tropical Countries," in Gunnar Blix (ed.), *Occurrence, Causes and Prevention of Nutritional Anemias, Symposia of the Swedish Nutrition Foundation, VI* (Stockholm, Sweden: Almqvist and Wiksell, 1968), pp. 36–46, 66–71.

32. F. E. Viteri and others, "Dietary Intake, Energy Cost of Work, Total Caloric Expenditure and Caloric Balance in Two Agricultural Labourer Populations of Guatemala" (processed).

33. Gopalan, "Health Problems in Preschool Children," pp. 228–32.

34. H. A. P. C. Oomen, D. S. McLaren, and H. Escapini, "Epidemiology and Public Health: Aspects of Hypovitaminosis A," *Tropical and Geographical Medicine*, 1964, pp. 271–315.

35. C. Gopalan, "Nutrition Needs of the Young," *Illustrated Weekly of India*, Oct. 15, 1967, p. 51, and "Malnutrition in the Tropics," *British Medical Journal*, Dec. 9, 1967, pp. 603–7.

36. Theodore W. Schultz, "Investment in Human Capital," *American Economic Review*, March 1961, p. 1. Also see Theodore W. Schultz, "Investment in Human Capital in Poor Countries," in Paul D. Zook (ed.), *Foreign Trade and Human Capital* (Southern Methodist Press, 1962), pp. 1–15; and G. S. Becker, *Human Capital* (Columbia University Press for National Bureau of Economic Research, 1964).

37. Edward F. Denison, *Why Growth Rates Differ* (Brookings Institution, 1967).

38. Hector Correa, *The Economics of Human Resources* (Amsterdam: North Holland Publishing Co., 1963), "Nutrition, Working Capacity, Productivity and Economic Growth," *Proceedings of Western Hemisphere Nutrition Congress II, San Juan, Puerto Rico, August 1968* (Chicago: American Medical Association, 1969), pp. 188–91, and "Sources of Economic Growth in Latin America," *Southern Economic Journal*, July 1970, pp. 17–31. Also see Hector Correa and Gaylord Cummins, "Contribution of Nutrition to Economic Growth," *American Journal of Clinical Nutrition*, May 1970, pp. 560–65; Vincent Taylor, *How Much Is Good Health Worth?* (Santa Monica, Calif.: Rand Corp., July 1969); Selma Mushkin, "Health as an Investment," *Journal of Political Economy*, October 1962, pp. 129–57; John J. Hanlon, *Principles of Public Health Administration* (C. V. Mosby, 1964); Herbert E. Klarman, *The Economics of Health* (Columbia University Press, 1965); H. E. Klarman (ed.), *Empirical Studies in Health Economics* (Johns Hopkins Press, 1970); E. A. Winslow, *The Cost of Sickness and the Price of Health* (Geneva: WHO, 1951); and D. P. Rice, *Estimating the Cost of Illness*, Health Economics No. 6 (GPO, 1966).

39. Hector Correa, "The Contribution of Better Nutrition and Health to Economic Development: A Comparative Study of Eighteen Countries" (Tulane University, n.d.; processed).

40. Monroe Berkowitz and William G. Johnson, "Towards an Economics of Disability: The Magnitude and Structure of Transfer Costs," *Journal of Human Resources*, Summer 1970, pp. 271–97.

41. J. I. McKigney, "Economic Aspects of Infant Feeding Practices in the West Indies," *Journal of Tropical Pediatrics*, June 1968, pp. 55–58.

42. J. M. Bengoa, "Curative Aspects of Malnutrition and Rehabilitation of the Malnourished Child" (paper presented at the United Nations Children's Fund [UNICEF] Eastern Mediterranean Region Food and Nutrition Seminar, Beirut, Jan. 26–29, 1970; processed), p. 6.

43. Ibid., pp. 6–7, 15.

44. *Young Child Nutrition Programmes: Review and Guidelines* (proceedings of the Zagreb Meeting on Young Child Nutrition Programmes, 1971; processed), p. 36; and Gopalan, "Health Problems in Preschool Children."

45. *The Economics of Human Resources*. His estimates of national shortfalls in working capacity are projections of individual shortfalls calculated by Gunther Lehmann, Erich A. Miller, and Helmut Spilzer, in "Der Calorienbedarf Bei Gewerblicher Arbeit," *Arbeitsphysiologie*, Vol. 14 (1950), pp. 166–235.

46. National Academy of Sciences, *Rapid Population Growth: Consequences and Policy Implications* (Johns Hopkins Press, 1971).

47. P. Rosenstein-Rodan, "Disguised Unemployment and Underemployment in Agriculture," *Monthly Bulletin of Agriculture Economics and Statistics*, July/August 1957, pp. 1–7; and Robert d'A. Shaw, *Jobs and Agricultural Development* (Overseas Development Council, 1970).

48. International Labour Organization (ILO), *Nutrition in Industry*, International Labour Office Studies, New Series, No. 4 (ILO, 1946). Also see reference 23 of this chapter.

49. David Turnham, *The Employment Problem in Less Developed Countries* (Paris: Organization for Economic Cooperation and Development, 1971).

50. Martin J. Forman, "Supplemental Feeding for the Preschool Children," and John E. Canham, "Relationship of Physical Performance to Nutrition Status," both in *Proceedings of the Third Far East Symposium on Nutrition, Manila, Feb. 14–22, 1967* (GPO, 1967); Morris Janowitz (ed), *The New Military: Changing Patterns of Organization* (Russell Sage Foundation, 1946); E. R. Buskirk, "Standard Work Tests in Man: Some Illustrative Results," and Josef Brozek, "Assessment of Performance Capacity: An Epilogue," both in Harry Spector, Josef Brozek, and Martin S. Peterson (eds.), *Performance Capacity, Symposium Conducted by the Nutrition Branch, Food Division, Quartermaster Food and Container Institute for the Armed Forces and Environmental Protection Research Division, Quartermaster Research— Engineering Center, Chicago, April 12–13, 1957* (National Academy of Sciences, 1961), pp. 115–31, 243–57; Josef Brozek, "Research on Diet and Behavior" (paper presented at Symposium on Feeding the Military Man, U.S. Army Natick Laboratories, Natick, Mass., Oct. 20–22, 1969).

51. A. Picasso de Oyagüe, "Malnutrition as a Limiting Factor in the Development of Education" (paper presented at UN Protein Advisory Group meeting, Paris, June 1972).

52. William J. Baumol, "On the Social Rate of Discount," *American Economic Review*, September 1968, pp. 788–802.

53. Marcelo Selowsky, "Infant Malnutrition and Human Capital Formation" (paper presented at the Research Workshop on Problems of Agricultural Development in Latin America, Caracas, May 1971). Selowsky does not attempt to carry the analysis further by adjusting rates of return for unemployment or specifying other conditions that might be necessary for the higher productivity potential to be realized.

54. Maureen Woodhall, *The Use of Cost-Benefit Analysis as a Guide to Resource Allocation in Education: A Case Study on India* (Paris: International Institute for Educational Planning, 1969).

55. Cyril Hunnikin, "The Iodization of Crude Salt for the Prophylaxis of Goiter," *Food Technology*, October 1964, pp. 40–43. Also see F. C. Kelly and W. W. Snedden, *Endemic Goiter*, WHO Monograph No. 44 (Geneva: WHO, 1960).

56. F. A. Arnold, Jr., "The Use of Fluoride Compounds for the Prevention of Dental Caries," *International Dental Journal*, Vol. 7 (1957), p. 56; and H. Trendley Dean and others, "Studies of Mass Control of Dental Caries Through Fluoridation of the Public Water Supply," *Public Health Report*, Oct. 27, 1950, pp. 1403–8.

## CHAPTER 3

1. Frances Gulick, "A Suggested Approach Toward a Related Nutrition and Family Planning Strategy and Program in India" (staff memorandum, U.S. Agency for International Development, New Delhi, May 13, 1969; processed).

2. A. S. David (ed.), *Infant and Child Mortality and Fertility Behavior, Con-*

*ference Held at Research Triangle Park, North Carolina* (Research Triangle Institute, Feb. 17, 1971).

3. Carl E. Taylor, "Population Trends in an Indian Village," *Scientific American,* July 1970, p. 114.

4. Thomas Poffenberger, "Age of Wives and Numbers of Living Children of a Sample of Men Who Had Vasectomy in Meerut District, U.P.," *Journal of Family Welfare* (India), Vol. 13 (June 1967), pp. 48–51.

5. Thomas Poffenberger, *Husband-Wife Communication and Motivational Aspects of Population Control in an Indian Village* (Gujarat: Department of Child Development, University of Baroda, 1968), pp. 45–46.

6. Carl E. Taylor and Marie Françoise Hall, "Health, Population and Economic Development," *Science,* Aug. 11, 1967, p. 4.

7. John B. Wyon and John E. Gordon, *The Khanna Study* (Harvard University Press, 1971), p. 161.

8. Ibid., p. 205.

9. David A. May and David M. Heer, "Son Survivorship Motivation and Family Size in India: A Computer Simulation," *Population Studies,* July 1968, pp. 199–210.

10. N. W. Pirie, "Orthodox and Unorthodox Methods of Meeting World Food Needs," *Scientific American,* February 1967, p. 27; and Antonia Fraser, *Mary Queen of Scots* (Dell Publishing, 1971), p. 641.

11. Harald Frederikson, "Determinants and Consequences of Mortality and Fertility Trends," *Public Health Reports,* August 1966, pp. 715–27. Also see *The World Food Problem, A Report of the President's Science Advisory Committee* (1967), pp. 34–36; Carl E. Taylor, "Health and Population," *Foreign Affairs,* April 1965, pp. 475–86; S. Hassan, "Influence of Child Mortality on Fertility" (paper presented at annual meeting of Population Association of America, New York, April 1966; processed); Walsh McDermott, "Modern Medicine and the Demographic Disease Pattern of Overly-Traditional Societies: A Technologic Misfit" (paper presented at Institute on International Medical Education of Association of American Medical Colleges, Washington, Mar. 28, 1966; processed); World Health Organization, *The Organization of Mother and Child Health Services,* Technical Report No. 428 (Geneva: WHO, 1969); and H. M. Wallace, E. M. Gold, and S. Dooley, "Relationship between Family Planning and Maternal and Child Health" (paper presented at American Public Health Association meeting, Detroit, 1968).

12. Wyon and Gordon, *Khanna Study,* pp. 205–6.

13. Michael V. E. Rulison, *Report on Topical Investigation and Analysis of Nutritional Supplements in Family Planning Programs in India and Pakistan* (Research Triangle Institute, 1970), p. 23. Also see Taylor and Hall, "Health, Population and Economic Development."

14. B. A. Cooper, G. S. D. Cantlie, and L. Brunton, "The Case for Folic Acid Supplements During Pregnancy," *American Journal of Clinical Nutrition,* June 1970, pp. 848–54; and C. Gopalan, "Effect of Nutrition on Pregnancy and Lactation," *Bulletin of the World Health Organization,* Vol. 26 (1962), pp. 203–11; David J. Kallen, "Nutrition and Society," *Journal of the American Medical Association,* Vol. 215 (January 1971), pp. 94–100.

15. Letter to the author from Carl Taylor, May 29, 1969. Also see Taylor's "Population Trends in an Indian Village," *Scientific American,* July 1970, p. 106; and *An Appraisal of the Population Project of the Rural Health Research Center at Narangwal, India: The Integration of Family Planning and Rural Health Services at the Village Level* (Research Triangle Institute, 1971).

16. Taylor and Hall, "Health, Population and Economic Development."

17. "The Family Planning Movement in India," Baroda Lecture No. 2 (Gujarat University, 1971; processed), p. 16.

18. "An Appraisal of the Impact of the Population and Family Planning Programs on Health Services in Countries Receiving AID Assistance" (report to the Agency for International Development, March 27, 1969; processed), p. 8.

19. K. Visweswara Rao and C. Gopalan, "Nutrition and Family Size," *Journal of Nutrition and Dietetics* (India), Vol. 6 (1969), pp. 258–66; and Wyon and Gordon, *Khanna Study*, pp. 197–98.

20. J. M. Tanner, "Earlier Maturation in Man," *Scientific American*, January 1968, p. 27.

21. S. M. Wishik, "Nutrition, Family Planning and Fertility," Doc. 1.29/1 (paper presented at UN Protein Advisory Group meeting, Paris, June 1972).

22. Kamala Rao, "Rehabilitation of the Loop in India—An Appraisal for Developing a New Approach" (Carolina Population Center, Oct. 13, 1971; processed); Hale C. Sweeny, *Report on Topical Investigation and Analysis of Rehabilitating the IUD in South Asia* (Research Triangle Institute, 1970), p. 18.

23. G. B. Simmons, S. J. Ward, and E. Weiss, "The Use of the Intra-Uterine Device in Karnal and Rohtak Districts of Haryana" (Berkeley: University of California, Sept. 13, 1968; processed).

24. Robert E. Hodges, "Nutrition and 'The Pill'," *Journal of the American Dietetic Association*, September 1971, pp. 212–17; D. L. Yeung and C. Gillis, "Oral Contraceptive and Vitamin A" (paper presented at meeting of International Nutrition Congress, Mexico City, September 1972).

25. Joginder G. Chopra and others, "Maternal Nutrition and Family Planning," *American Journal of Clinical Nutrition*, August 1970, pp. 1043–58.

26. G. B. Searle and Co., Physicians' Product Brochure No. 67 (1967), p. 33; and J. W. Goldzieher and E. R. Rice-Way, *Oral Contraception: Mechanism and Management* (C. C. Thomas, 1966).

CHAPTER 4

1. F. James Levinson, "The Effect of Income Change on Food Consumption in South India and Ceylon" (Cornell University, May 1970; processed), p. 6.

2. Robert S. McNamara, *Address to the United Nations Conference on Trade and Development, Santiago, Chile, April 14, 1972* (International Bank for Reconstruction and Development, 1972); and David Turnham, *The Employment Problem in Less Developed Countries* (Paris: Organization for Economic Cooperation and Development, 1971).

3. Frances Gulick, "Nutrition Data Reported by State Nutrition Surveys in India, 1963–65: A Summary Note" (memorandum, U.S. Agency for International Development, India, May 10, 1969; processed).

4. Max F. Millikan, "Population, Food Supply and Economic Development," *Technology Review*, February 1970, p. 57. See also Patrick J. François, "Effects of Income Projection on the Protein Structure of the Diet," *Nutrition Newsletter* (Food and Agriculture Organization [FAO], October–December 1969), p. 12; and Hans Wilbrandt, "The Special Feature of the Protein Problem in Low-income Countries" (University of Göttingen, March 1970; processed).

5. McKim Marriott, *Village India* (University of Chicago Press, 1955).

6. See, for examples, Parvaghi K. Rao, "Socio-Cultural Factors and Malnutrition in Telengana Region of Andhra Pradesh," *Proceedings of the Nutrition Society of India*, No. 6 (1968), p. 62; and Operations Research Group, *Food Habits Survey* (Bombay: Protein Foods Association of India, 1969), pp. 153, 252.

7. See, for examples, I. Kelly, "An Approach to the Improvement of Diet" (background paper for Conference on Malnutrition and Food Habits, Cuernavaca, Mexico, 1960; processed); Anne Burgess and R. F. A. Dean (eds.), *Malnutrition and Food Habits* (London: Tavistock Publications, 1962), p. 54; J. Yudkin, "The Need for Change," in J. Yudkin and J. C. McKenzie (eds.), *Changing Food Habits* (London: MacGibbon and Kee, 1964), p. 22; and J. Périssé, F. Sizaret, and P. François, "The Effect of Income on the Structure of the Diet," *Nutrition Newsletter*, July–September 1969, p. 5.

8. See, for examples, R. P. Devadas, "Better Food Utilization and Changing the Food Habits," *Indian Journal of Home Science*, January 1968, pp. 1–8, and "Social and Cultural Factors Influencing Malnutrition," *Proceedings of the Nutrition Society of India*, No. 6 (1968), p. 6; W. H. Sebrell, "Health in the Perspective of Nutrition," in Iago Galdston (ed.), *Human Nutrition, Historic and Scientific* (New York: International Universities Press, 1960), p. 20; James Trager, *Foodbook* (Grossman, 1970), p. 320; M. O. L. Klein Hutheesing, *The Sociology of Food Consumption Patterns in Some Asian Countries: A Critical Survey of the Literature* (Delhi: Asian Research Centre, 1968), pp. 14–15; P. G. Bailey, *Caste and Economic Frontier* (Oxford University Press, 1958), p. 188; and M. N. Srinivas, "Sociological Aspects of Indian Diet" (paper presented at Symposium on Freedom from Hunger Campaign, New Delhi, Jan. 10, 1964; processed).

9. Operations Research Group, *Food Habits Survey*, p. 142.

10. Calculations based on R. O. Whyte and M. C. Mathur, *The Planning of Milk Production in India* (London: Orient Longmans, 1968), p. 69; and C. Gopalan, "Nutritional Problems of Mother and Child" (Hyderabad, India: National Institute of Nutrition, 1969; processed), p. 42.

11. FAO, Paper Presented at Conference of Malnutrition and Food Habits, Cuernavaca, Mexico, 1960.

12. "Symposium Proceedings," *Proceedings of the Nutrition Society of India*, No. 8 (May 1970), p. 156.

13. FAO, *Lives in Peril: Protein and the Child* (Rome: FAO, 1970), p. 29.

14. U.S., Interagency Commission on Nutrition for National Defense (ICNND), *Nutrition Survey, Federation of Malaya* (GPO, 1964); R. C. Burgess, *Report on Indonesia* (February 1956); and Derrick B. Jelliffe, *Infant Nutrition in the Subtropics and Tropics*, Monograph Series No. 29 (2nd ed., Geneva: World Health Organization [WHO], 1968), p. 36.

15. See, for examples, S. G. Srikantia, "Food Fads and Community Nutrition," in *Nutrition* (Hyderabad, India: National Institute of Nutrition, 1969), pp. 24–30; Jelliffe, *Infant Nutrition*, pp. 36, 76; H. Trant, "Food Taboos in Africa," *Lancet*, October 1964, pp. 703–5; Mo Sumi, "A Study of Food Taboos in Agricultural Villages in Korea," *Journal of Korean Home Economics Association*, Vol. 5 (1966), pp. 15–22; R. Tichauer, *Journal of Pediatrics*, Vol. 62 (1963), p. 399; Anna M. Hlalele, "Report on Nutrition in Lesotho," and Y. H. Misomali, "Report on Nutrition in Malawi," *Proceedings of the Eastern African Conference on Nutrition and Child Feeding* (GPO, 1969), pp. 56–68 and 69–79; and Floy Eugenia Whitehead, "Nutrition Education Research Project" (U.S. Agency for International Development, Iowa City, Iowa, Oct. 20, 1970; processed), p. 55.

16. Rao, "Socio-Cultural Factors and Malnutrition," p. 62; R. Rajalakshmi, *Applied Nutrition* (Baroda, India: R. Rajalakshmi, 1969), p. 299; Margaret Mead, *Cultural Patterns and Technical Change* (Geneva: UN Educational, Scientific, and Cultural Organization, 1963), p. 210; and Florence E. Dovlo, "Consumers' Opinion on Malnutrition in Africa," *Nutrition Bulletin*, No. 7 (July 1969).

17. See F. A. Thompson, in *Royal Society of Tropical Medicine and Hygiene Transactions*, Vol. 42 (1949), p. 487; and J. Delon, in *Algérie Médicale*, Vol. 57 (1953), p. 553.

18. ICNND, Transactions of a Far East Symposium on Nutrition, Saigon, March 1962; ICNND, *Nutrition Survey, Republic of Vietnam* (GPO, 1960); S. C. Dube, *India's Changing Village* (London: Routledge, 1958); Indira Mahadevan, "Belief Systems in Food of the Telugu-Speaking People of the Telengana Region," *Indian Journal of Social Work*, March 1961; and Jelliffe, *Infant Nutrition*, p. 48.

19. See Mahadevan, "Belief Systems"; Yadav Dhillon, "Dietary Habits and Beliefs during Pregnancy and Lactation in Rural Bengal" (n.d.; processed); Jelliffe, *Infant Nutrition*, p. 48; Misomali, "Report on Nutrition in Malawi," pp. 75–76; and Mary Jo Bartholomew and Frances E. Poston, "Effect of Food Taboos on Prenatal Nutrition," *Journal of Nutrition Education*, Summer 1970, pp. 15–17.

20. See, for examples, Christine S. Wilson, "Food Beliefs Affect Nutritional Status of Malay Fisher-Folk," *Journal of Nutrition Education*, Winter 1971, pp. 96–98; Dr. Poorwo, quoted in Burgess and Dean, *Malnutrition and Food Habits*, p. 48; Ritchie, *Learning Better Nutrition*, p. 37; M. Freedman, *A Report on Some Aspects of Food, Health and Society in Indonesia* (WHO, 1954); Trant, "Food Taboos in East Africa," pp. 703–5; J. A. Ojiambo, "Background Study of Food Habits of the Abasamia of Busia District–Western Province, Kenya," *Nutrition*, 1967, pp. 216–21; ICNND, *Nutrition Survey, Federation of Malay* (GPO, 1964); Rajalakshmi, *Applied Nutrition*, p. 298; and Mahadevan, "Belief Systems," pp. 39–40.

## CHAPTER 5

1. Nevin Scrimshaw and Vernon Young, "Protein Calorie Relationships in Man" (report prepared for AID under Contract No. AID/CSd-2808 with MIT, 1972; processed).

2. *World War on Hunger*, Hearings before the House Committee on Agriculture, 89 Cong. 2 sess. (1966), Serial W, Pts. 1–3; William Paddock and Paul Paddock, *Famine 1975* (London: Weidenfeld and Nicholson, 1967).

3. Dana G. Dalrymple, *Imports and Plantings of High Yielding Varieties of Wheat and Rice in the Less Developed Nations*, Foreign Economic Development Report 14 (U.S. Department of Agriculture [USDA], 1972).

4. Dana G. Dalrymple, "The Green Revolution and Protein Levels in Grain" (USDA, Economic Research Service [ERS], International Development Center, Apr. 26, 1972; processed).

5. Robert Shaw, "The Social Impact of the Green Revolution," *International Conciliation*, January 1971, p. 44; Dana G. Dalrymple, *New Cereal Varieties: Wheat and Corn in Mexico*, AID Spring Review (USDA, International Development, Foreign Agricultural Service, May 1969); Wolf Ladejinsky, "Ironies of India's Green Revolution," *Foreign Affairs*, July 1970, p. 758; M. Schluter and John W. Mellor, "New Seed Varieties and the Small Farmer," *Review of Agriculture* (India), March 1972, pp. A-31–A-38; and Francine R. Frankel and Karl von Vorys, *The*

*Political Challenge of the Green Revolution: Shifting Patterns of Peasant Participation in India and Pakistan,* Policy Memorandum No. 38 (Center for International Studies, Woodrow Wilson School of Public and International Affairs, Princeton University, March 1972), pp. 16, 30.

6. Gunvant M. Desai and V. R. Gaikwad, *Applied Nutrition Programme: An Evaluation Study* (Ahmedabad, India: Center for Management in Agriculture, Indian Institute of Management, 1971).

7. Partap C. Arggarwal, "Impact of Green Revolution on Landless Labour," *Economic and Political Weekly* (India), Nov. 20, 1971, pp. 2363–65.

8. John B. Wyon and John E. Gordon, *The Khanna Study* (Harvard University Press, 1971), p. 304.

9. Based on Martin Forman and Byron Berntson, "The Green Revolution and Nutrition in the Developing World" (December 1971; processed); and reports of James Boulware to USDA, Foreign Agricultural Service.

10. Susan K. Alfano, "The Pakistan Experiment: Chronicle of a Nutrition Programmer's Internship" (master's thesis, MIT, 1972).

11. Summarized in W. R. Aykroyd and Joyce Doughty, *Legumes in Human Nutrition,* FAO Nutritional Studies No. 19 (Rome: Food and Agriculture Organization [FAO], 1964), pp. 80–85.

12. Dharm Narain, "Growth and Imbalance in Indian Agriculture," *Review of Agriculture* (India), March 1972, pp. A-2–A-4.

13. A. Pradilla and D. Harpstead, in *Proceedings of the Nutrition Society of India,* No. 8 (May 1970), p. 21.

14. Judy Fowler, "Triticale, a Wheat-Rye Grain, Is Deemed Revolutionary by Some, a Flop by Others," *Wall Street Journal,* March 1, 1971, p. 18.

15. Norman Borlaug, "Genetic Improvement of Crop Foods," *Nutrition Today,* January–February 1972, pp. 20–21, 24–25.

16. P. H. van Schaik, "Pulse Production, Status and Potential," in *Improving the Nutrient Quality of Cereals* (AID, June 1971), pp. A-9–A-24.

17. Ibid., p. A-23.

18. Lyle P. Schertz, *Economics of Protein Improvement Programs in the Lower Income Countries,* No. FEDR-11 (USDA, July 1971), p. 5.

19. Harold Rabinowitz, "Brazil Still Faces Beef Shortage in Spite of Government Action," *Foreign Agriculture,* March 20, 1972, pp. 9–10.

20. D. B. Jelliffe, "Parallel Food Classifications in Developing and Industrialized Countries," *American Journal of Clinical Nutrition,* Vol. 20 (1967), p. 279.

21. Noshir N. Dastur, "Direction and Scope of Dairy Development in the 70's," *National Food Congress* (India), 1970.

22. R. O. Whyte, "Dairy Development in Rural Asia," *Netherlands Milk Dairy Association,* Vol. 24 (1970), p. 126; K. S. Rao and others, "Protein Malnutrition in South India," *Bulletin of the World Health Organization,* Vol. 20 (1959), pp. 603–39; Derrick Jelliffe, "Social Culture and Nutrition," *Pediatrics,* Vol. 20 (July 1957), p. 135; and Operations Research Group, "Deductions from Tamil Nadu Food Habits Survey" (Baroda, India, 1972; processed).

23. UN Protein Advisory Group, "Report on the PAG ad hoc Working Group Meeting on Milk Intolerance—Nutritional Implications," Doc. 1.27/g (Nov. 22, 1971); and Michael Latham, "Background Information on Lactose Intolerance" (report to Committee on International Nutrition Programs, Food and Nutrition Board, National Research Council, 1971; processed).

24. G. S. Aurora, "Towards a Sociology of Foods and Nutrition in India," *Proceedings of the Nutrition Society of India*, No. 6 (1968), p. 25.

25. D. A. Alverson, A. R. Longhurst, and J. A. Gullard, "How Much Food from the Sea?" *Science*, April 24, 1970, pp. 503–5; *The World Food Problem . . . , A Report of the President's Science Advisory Committee* (GPO, 1967), pp. 345–47; J. H. Ryther, *Science*, Vol. 166 (1968), p. 72; Paul R. Erlich and Ann E. Erlich, "The Food-from-the-Sea Myth," *Saturday Review*, April 4, 1970, p. 53; and Lucian M. Sprague and John H. Arnold, "Trends in Use and Prospects Resources" (International Center for Marine Resources, University of Rhode Island, n.d.; processed).

26. *World Food Problem*, pp. 350–55.

27. S. V. Pingale, "Prevention of Losses in Storage," *National Food Congress* (India), 1970; H. A. B. Parpia, "Food Technology Problems in India and Other Developing Countries," *Food Technology*, January 1968, pp. 62–63; and UN Protein Advisory Group Meeting Report, Doc. 3.14/5 (Geneva, Sept. 1969), pp. 17–18.

28. FAO, *Food Losses—The Tragedy and Some Solutions*, Doc. E/3/3000 (FAO, 1970), p. 10; Joseph H. Hulse, "Increasing Food by Reducing Waste" (Canadian International Development Agency, n.d.; processed); *World Food Problem*, p. 554; and *International Action to Avert the Impending Protein Crisis*, Report to the Economic and Social Council of the Advisory Committee on the Application of Science and Technology to Development (United Nations, 1968).

29. Lester Brown, "Point of View," *New York Times*, Jan. 24, 1972, p. 45.

30. Carl Taylor, "Nutrition and Population," in Alan Berg, Nevin Scrimshaw, and David Call (eds.), *Nutrition, National Development and Planning* (MIT Press, forthcoming).

## CHAPTER 6

1. C. D. Williams, *Lancet*, Vol. 1 (1954).

2. J. E. de Oliveira, "Development of Protein Foods in Brazil," Doc. 19/3 (UN Protein Advisory Group meeting, New York, October 1967).

3. Letter to the author from A. P. Vamoer, June 30, 1971.

4. J. C. Likimani, "Report on Nutrition in Kenya," in *Proceedings of the Eastern African Conference on Nutrition and Child Feeding* (GPO, 1969), pp. 41–55.

5. Marjorie Scott Van Veen, "Some Ecological Considerations of Nutrition Problems on Java," *Ecology of Food and Nutrition*, Vol. 1 (1971), p. 30; Rajammal P. Devadas and Parvathi Easwaran, "Eating Habits of School Children in a Village Community," *Indian Journal of Home Science*, January 1968, p. 14; F. James Levinson, *Morinda* (Cornell University Press, forthcoming); and U. Rao and S. R. Mudambi, "Distribution of Protein-Rich Foods within the Family" (paper presented at meeting of International Nutrition Congress, Mexico City, September 1972).

6. See, for example, letter to the author from I. G. Patel, Secretary, Ministry of Finance, Government of India, Nov. 27, 1970.

7. Margaret Mead, "Cultural Change in Relation to Nutrition," in Anne Burgess and R. F. A. Dean (eds.), *Malnutrition and Food Habits* (London: Tavistock Publications, 1962), p. 53.

8. J. Stoetzel, "The Social Psychology of Food Habits," in Burgess and Dean, *Malnutrition and Food Habits*, p. 76.

9. Gunvant M. Desai and V. R. Gaikwad, *Applied Nutrition Programme: An Evaluation Study* (Ahmedabad, India: Center for Management in Agriculture,

Indian Institute of Management, 1971). For other applied nutrition program critiques see "Nutrition Programme a Flop" (Indian) *National Herald*, March 7, 1969; "Punjab Nutrition Plan Makes Poor Progress" (Indian) *Economic Times*, March 16, 1969; James M. Hundley, "Assessment of Applied Nutrition Programmes in India" (paper prepared for UN Children's Education Fund [UNICEF], April 1966); and C. R. Rathee, "Unsatisfactory Working of Applied Nutrition Scheme in Haryana" (Bombay) *Financial Express*, March 3, 1968.

10. UN Economic and Social Council, UNICEF, "General Progress Report of the Executive Director," E/ICEF/616, Part II, March 1, 1972, p. 16.

11. W. H. Sebrell and K. W. King, "The Role of Community Mothercraft Centers in Combating Malnutrition," in Paul György and O. L. Kline (eds.), *Malnutrition Is a Problem of Ecology* (S. Karger, 1970).

12. Michelini Beaudry-Darisme and Michael C. Latham, "Evaluation of Nutritional Rehabilitation Centers: An Evaluation of Their Performance," Doc. 1.23/2 (UN Protein Advisory Group Meeting, Geneva, Nov. 23, 1971).

13. V. Ramalingaswami, "Unfulfilled Expectations and the Third Approach," *British Journal of Medical Education*, December 1968, p. 247.

14. Patty Hostetter, "Women's Training Program," *Peace Corps Digest* (India), January 1969, pp. 4–6.

15. Desai and Gaikwad, *Applied Nutrition Programme*.

16. Memorandum to the author from F. James Levinson, Jan. 18, 1969.

17. Portions of this section are based on Richard K. Manoff, "A Mass Communications Campaign on Nutrition Education for the Government of India" (New Delhi, January 1970; processed).

18. Andreas Fuglesang, *Communication with Illiterates, A Pilot Study of the Problem of Social Communication in Developing Countries*, Pt. I (Lusaka, Zambia: National Food and Nutrition Commission, 1969).

19. "Nutrition Education in Medical Faculties," *American Journal of Clinical Nutrition*, December 1971, pp. 1399–1400.

20. L. E. Lloyd, "Nutrition Education as Presently Offered," *Journal of The Canadian Dietetic Association*, March 1970, p. 32.

21. Nevin Scrimshaw, quoted by Burgess and Dean, *Malnutrition and Food Habits*, p. 155.

22. R. Cook, "Is Hospital the Place for the Treatment of Malnourished Children?" *Journal of Tropical Pediatrics and Environmental Child Health*, March 1971, p. 22.

23. Sarah Bavley, "Changes in Food Habits in Israel," *Journal of the American Dietetic Association*, June 1966, p. 488.

24. Letter to the author from Gerson da Cunha, Feb. 18, 1968.

25. Sylvester da Cunha, Presentation for Operation Marketing Workshop, Protein Foods for National Development Conference, New Delhi, December 1969.

26. M. G. Kamath, "The Role of Mass Media in Agricultural Development," in *Proceedings of National Food Congress, 1970, New Delhi*, pp. 1–4.

27. P. R. Krishnaswami and Shyamal Ghose, "A Pilot Study" (Bombay) *Commerce*, July 24, 1971.

28. Jean A. S. Ritchie, *Learning Better Nutrition*, FAO Nutrition Studies No. 20 (Rome: Food and Agriculture Organization [FAO], 1967), p. 36; M. O. L. Klein Hutheesing, *The Sociology of Food Consumption Patterns in Some Asian Countries: A Critical Survey of the Literature* (Delhi: Asian Research Center, 1968), pp. 16,

18–19; Richard B. Mazess, "Hot-Cold Food Beliefs among Andean Peasants," *Journal of the American Dietetic Association* (August 1968), pp. 109–13; and M. McArthur, "Report on an assignment in Malaya" (Manila: World Health Organization [WHO], 1962; processed), p. 36.

29. P. S. V. Ramamurthy, "Physiological Effects of 'Hot' and 'Cold' Foods in Human Subjects," *Journal of Nutrition and Dietetics* (India), 1969, pp. 187–91; and Mazess, "Hot-Cold Food Beliefs."

30. Sylvester da Cunha, Presentation for Operation Marketing Workshop.

31. Derrick B. Jelliffe, *Infant Nutrition in the Subtropics and Tropics,* WHO Monograph Series No. 29 (Geneva: WHO, 1968), p. 158.

33. Sylvester da Cunha, "Proposals for Bal Ahar" (paper prepared for U.S. Agency for International Development, India, 1967; processed).

34. Interview, Uwe Kracht, Sept. 17, 1969.

35. Protein Foods Association of India, "A Mass Media Nutrition Programme" (Bombay, 1971; processed); and letter to the author from Shyamal Ghose, March 8, 1972.


CHAPTER 7

1. C. Gopalan, "Studies on Lactation in Poor Indian Communities," *Journal of Tropical Pediatrics,* December 1958, p. 92.

2. Ibid., pp. 91–92. Also see D. B. Jelliffe, "Approaches to Village Level Infant Feeding," *Journal of Tropical Pediatrics,* September 1967, p. 118; K. S. Rao and others, in *Bulletin of the World Health Organization,* 1959, p. 603; H. A. P. C. Oomen and S. H. Malcolm, "Nutrition and the Papuan Child," South Pacific Commission Technical Paper No. 118 (Noumea, New Caledonia, n.d.; processed); and P. S. Venkatachalam, "A Study of the Diet, Nutrition and Health of the People of the Chimbu Area, New Guinea Highlands," Monograph No. 4 (Department of Public Health, Territory of Papua and New Guinea, n.d.; processed).

3. D. B. Jelliffe, "Breast Milk and the World Protein Gap," *Clinical Pediatrics,* February 1968, p. 97.

4. Fernando B. Mönckeberg, "The Effect of Malnutrition and Environment on Mental Development," *Proceedings of Western Hemisphere Nutrition Congress II, San Juan, Puerto Rico, August 1968* (Chicago: American Medical Association, 1969), pp. 216–20.

5. Wong Hock Boon, K. Paramathypathy, and Tham Ngiap Boo, "Breastfeeding among Lower Income Mothers in Singapore," *Journal of the Singapore Pediatric Society,* October 1963, pp. 89–93.

6. Ma[ria] Linda Gabucan-Dulay, "Current Feeding Patterns as Observed among 1,000 Filipino Infants," *Philippine Journal of Pediatrics,* April 1970, pp. 95–103.

7. J. Paez-Franco, "Infant Feeding Practices and Availability of Vegetable Protein Mixtures in Colombia" (paper presented at Pan American Health Organization [PAHO] meeting, Bogotá, November 1970), Annex 4, p. 5; *FAO Trade Yearbook, 1970* (Rome: Food and Agriculture Organization, 1971).

8. A. M. Thompson, F. E. Hytten, and W. Z. Billewicz, "The Energy Cost of Human Lactation," *British Journal of Nutrition,* Vol. 24 (1970), pp. 565–71; PAHO, *Maternal Nutrition and Family Planning in the Americas,* Scientific Publication No. 204 (Washington: PAHO, 1970), pp. 4–5.

9. Operations Research Group, *Food Habits Survey* (Bombay: Protein Foods Association of India, December 1969), pp. 34, 50.

10. C. Gopalan and others, *Diet Atlas of India* (Hyderabad: National Institute of Nutrition, 1969), pp. 54–55.

11. Derrick B. Jelliffe, *Infant Nutrition in the Tropics and Subtropics*, Monograph Series No. 29 (2nd ed., Geneva: WHO, 1968), p. 163; Gopalan, "Studies on Lactation," p. 97; F. Faulkner and others, "Some International Comparisons of Physical Growth in the First Two Years of Life," *Courrier*, Vol. 8 (1958), p. 1; H. Gounelle and M. Demarchi, "Nutritional Status of Infants and Very Young Children in Bagdad, Iraq," *Journal of the Royal Faculty of Medicine* (Iraq), Vol. 17 (1953), p. 42; J. Millis, "The Feeding of Chinese, Indian and Malayan Infants in Singapore," *Quarterly Review of Pediatrics*, Vol. 14 (1959), p. 42; J. Sénécal, "Alimentation de L'enfant dans les Pays Tropicaux et Subtropicaux," *Courrier*, Vol. 9 (1959), p. 1; and H. F. Welbourn, "Bottle Feeding: A Problem of Modern Civilization," *Journal of Tropical Pediatrics*, Vol. 4 (1958), p. 157.

12. "New Urban Families" (Conclusions and Recommendations of a Workshop on Nutrition, International Pediatric Association, Vienna, Austria, Aug. 28, 1971); John B. Wyon and John E. Gordon, *The Khanna Study* (Harvard University Press, 1971), p. 158; *Nutritional Problems of Mother and Child* (Seminar on Nutritional Problems of Mother and Child in Developing Countries, Hyderabad, India, Jan. 16–23, 1967); Hindustan Thompson, Ltd., *Food Habits Survey* (Calcutta: Hindustan Thompson, 1971); K. C. Chaudhuri, "Observations on Human Milk and Cow's Milk in Infant Nutrition," *Indian Journal of Pediatrics*, Vol. 31 (1964), p. 105; C. Gopalan, "Nutritional Needs of the Young," *Illustrated Weekly of India*, Oct. 15, 1967; and Operations Research Group, *Food Habits Survey*, p. 231.

13. Nancie L. Soleim de Gonzáles, "Breast Feeding, Weaning and Acculturation," *Tropical Pediatrics*, April 1963, pp. 578–79; and letters to the author from Darwin Karjadi, Nutrition Research Institute, Bogor, Indonesia, May 22, 1971; C. C. Chen, U.S. Embassy, Taipei, Taiwan, October 1971; and G. T. Roberts, Education Office, Bathurst, Gambia, Aug. 17, 1971.

14. J. L. Pérez-Navarrette and others, "Estudio Longitudinal de un Grupa de Niños a los que se Siguió Durante su Primo Año de Vida en la Villa de Tlaltizapán," *Boletín Médico del hospital infantil*, Vol. 17 (1960), p. 282; and Sarah L. M. Morrow, "A Study of the Food and Feeding Habits of Young Children in a Mexican Village" (master's thesis, Cornell University, 1960), p. 31.

15. Letter to the author from Michael Latham, Feb. 28, 1972.

16. See Karl Eric Knutsson and Tore Mellbin, "Breast Feeding Habits and Cultural Context," *Journal of Tropical Pediatrics*, June 1969, p. 48; Jamal K. Harfouche, "The Importance of Breastfeeding," *Journal of Tropical Pediatrics*, Monograph No. 10 (September 1970), pp. 151–52; Robert G. Potter and others, "Applications of Field Studies to Research on the Physiology of Human Reproduction," *Journal of Chronic Disease*, November 1965, pp. 1125–40; Anru K. Jain and others, "Demographic Aspects of Lactation and Post-partum Amenorrhea," *Demography*, May 1970, pp. 255–71; Christopher Tetze, "The Effect of Breastfeeding on the Rate of Conception," *Proceedings of the International Population Conference, New York, 1971*, pp. 129–40; Michael Newton, "Mammary Effects," *American Journal of Clinical Nutrition*, August 1971, pp. 987–90; D. B. Jelliffe and E. F. P. Jelliffe, "Lactation, Conception and the Nursing Mother and Child," *Journal of Pediatrics*, Vol. 81 (1972), p. 829; J. W. B. Douglas, "Extent of Breast Feeding in Great Britain in 1946, with Special Reference to Health and Survival of Children," *Journal of Obstetrics*

*and Gynecology of the British Empire*, Vol. 57 (1950), p. 335; R. Gioisa, in *American Journal of Obstetrical Gynecology*, Vol. 70 (1955), p. 162; and John Knodel, in *Population Studies*, No. 212 (1967), p. 109.

17. M. F. El-Minawi and M. S. Foda, "Post-partum Lactation Amenorrhea." *American Journal of Obstetrics and Gynecology*, Vol. 3 (1970), p. 19; D. B. Jelliffe and E. F. P. Jelliffe, "An Overview," *American Journal of Clinical Nutrition*, August 1971, pp. 1013–24; Otto Schaefer, "When the Eskimo Comes to Town," *Nutrition Today*, November–December 1971, pp. 8–16; and "Relation Between Lactation and Ovulation" (bibliography of LaLeche League International, July 1971; processed), Reprint No. 22; I. Forsyth, "The Role of Primate Prolactation and Placental Lactogens in Lactogenesis," in *Lactogenesis: The Initiation of Milk Secretion Parturition* (University of Pennsylvania Press, 1969), p. 195; Jelliffe and Jelliffe. "Lactation, Conception and the Nursing Mother"; and T. McKeown and J. R. Gibson, "A Note on Menstruation and Conception during Lactation," *Journal of Obstetrics and Gynecology of the British Empire*, Vol. 61 (1954), p. 824.

18. Jain and others, "Demographic Aspects of Lactation," p. 269.

19. See Jelliffe, *Infant Nutrition*, pp. 60–61, 75, 78, 157, 169; Frank Lorimer, *Culture and Human Fertility* (Zurich: UN Educational, Scientific, and Cultural Organization [UNESCO], 1954); and L. Longmore, in *South African Medical Journal*, Vol. 28 (1954), p. 295.

20. Potter and others, "Applications of Field Studies," p. 1137.

21. Jelliffe, *Infant Nutrition*, pp. 44–45.

22. Fernando Mönckeberg, "Factors Conditioning Malnutrition in Latin America with Special Reference to Chile: Advices for a Volunteers Action," in Paul György and O. L. Kline (eds.), *Malnutrition Is a Problem of Ecology* (S. Karger, 1970), p. 30.

23. Letter to the author from Abdullah Kanawati, Nutrition Research Program, American University of Beirut, June 9, 1971.

24. Letter to the author from Darwin Karjadi, Nutrition Research Institute, Bogor, Indonesia, May 22, 1971.

25. Fernando Mönckeberg, "Programs for Combatting Malnutrition in the Preschool Child in Chile," in *Preschool Child Malnutrition: Primary Deterrent to Human Progress*, Publication No. 1282 (National Academy of Sciences–National Research Council, 1966), p. 172.

26. Harfouche, "Importance of Breastfeeding," pp. 146–47.

27. Joaquin Cravioto, quoted in Mönckeberg, "Factors Conditioning Malnutrition," p. 33; and M. Robinson, "Infant Morbidity and Mortality, A Study of 3,266 Infants," *Lancet*, Vol. 1 (1951), pp. 788–94.

28. See U.S. Department of Labor, Children's Bureau, *Infant Mortality*, Publication No. 68 (1920), p. 114, Publication No. 72 (1920), p. 118, and Publication No. 112 (1923), p. 122; Robinson, "Infant Morbidity"; E. Mannheimer, "Mortality of Breastfed and Bottlefed Infants," *Actae Genetica Medicae*, Vol. 5 (1955), pp. 134–63; PAHO, "Progress Report of the Inter-American Investigation of Mortality in Childhood" (report presented to 9th meeting of Advisory Committee on Medical Research, June 15, 1970), and *Maternal Nutrition and Family Planning in the Americas*, Scientific Publication No. 204 (PAHO, 1970), pp. 20–21.

29. D. S. McLaren, in *Lancet*, 1966, p. 485.

30. D. B. Jelliffe, quoted in Anne Burgess and R. F. A. Dean (eds.), *Malnutrition and Food Habits* (London: Tavistock Publications, 1962), p. 31.

31. H. R. Zimmer, *Hindu Medicine* (Johns Hopkins Press, 1948), p. 107.

32. D. Anand and A. Rama Rao, "Feeding Practices of Infants and Toddlers in Najafgarh Area," *Indian Journal of Medicine*, Vol. 11 (1962), pp. 172–81.

33. Indira Mahadevan, "Belief Systems in Food of the Telugu-Speaking People of the Telengana Region," *Indian Journal of Social Work*, March 1961, pp. 30–40.

34. See J. Feldman, *Principles of Antenatal and Postnatal Child Hygiene* (John Bale and Sons, 1927); Geoffrey Goer, "Burmese Personality" (New York Institute for International Studies, 1943; processed); and J. F. Brock and M. Autret, *Kwashiorkor in Africa*, Monograph Series No. 8 (Geneva: WHO, 1952), pp. 29–30.

35. N. Pralhad Rao, Darshan Singh, and M. C. Swaminathan, "Nutritional Status of Preschool Children of Rural Community Near Hyderabad City," *Indian Journal of Medical Research*, November 1969, p. 5.

36. WHO, Maternal-Child Health Team Report (Lahore, Pakistan: WHO, 1953; processed); and K. Someswara Rao and others, in *Bulletin of the World Health Organization*, Vol. 20 (1959), pp. 603–39.

37. William D. Davidson, "A Brief History of Infant Feeding," *Journal of Pediatrics*, July 1953, p. 75.

38. *The Caraka Samhitá*, Vol. 1, *Sarira Sthana*, Chap. 8, verses 52–54 (Jamnagar, India: Shree Gulabkunverba Ayurvedic Society, 1949), p. 434.

39. B. S. Platt and S. Y. Gin, "Chinese Methods of Infant Feeding and Nursing," *Archives of Diseases in Childhood*, Vol. 13 (1938), pp. 343–54.

40. Jelliffe, *Infant Nutrition*, p. 41.

41. Harfouche, "The Importance of Breastfeeding," p. 136.

42. "Milk and Malaria," *British Medical Journal*, Vol. 12 (1952), p. 1405, and Vol. 2 (1953), p. 1210; O. Mellander and B. Vahlquist, "Breast Feeding and Artificial Feeding," *Acta Paediatrica*, Supplement, Vol. 11 (1958), p. 101; "Breast Feeding and Polio Susceptibility," *Nutrition Reviews*, May 1965, pp. 131–33; Leonardo J. Mata and Richard G. Wyatt, "Host Resistance to Infection," *American Journal of Clinical Nutrition*, August 1971, pp. 976–86; and B. S. Platt and A. Moncrieff, in *British Medical Bulletin*, Vol. 5 (1947), p. 117.

43. D. B. Jelliffe, "Breast Feeding in Technically Developing Areas," *Courrier*, April 1966, pp. 191–95.

44. Sylvia Brody, *Patterns of Mothering* (International Universities Press, 1956), p. 65; C. Hoefer and M. C. Hardy, "Later Development of Breast Fed and Artificially Fed Infants," *Journal of the American Medical Association*, Vol. 92 (1929), p. 615; and J. W. B. Douglas, "Breast Feeding in Great Britain in 1946," p. 335.

45. Herman F. Meyer, "Breast Feeding in the United States," *Clinical Pediatrics*, December 1968, pp. 712–13.

46. Helen A. Guthrie and George M. Guthrie, "The Resurgence of Natural Child Feeding," *Clinical Pediatrics*, August 1966, pp. 481–84.

47. Eva J. Salber and Manning Feinlib, "Breast Feeding in Boston," *Pediatrics*, February 1966, pp. 299–303; and Joseph Rivera, "The Frequency of Use of Various Kinds of Milk during Infancy in the Middle and Lower-Income Families," *American Journal of Public Health*, February 1971, pp. 277–80.

48. Meyer, "Breast Feeding in the United States," pp. 713–14.

49. A. I. Ross and G. Herdan, "Breast Feeding in Bristol," *Lancet*, Vol. 1 (1951), p. 630.

50. Interview, Gilbert Martinez, Ross Laboratories, Columbus, Ohio, Jan. 17, 1972.

51. J. Strom, "Falling Rate of Breast Feeding in Sweden," *Acta Paediatrica*, Vol. 45 (1956), p. 453; M. Chajeka and H. Salamon, "Polish Breast Feeding," and M. Chajeka, "Incidence and Duration of Breast Feeding in Polish Infants," *Pediatria*

*Polska,* Vol. 39 (1964), pp. 77 and 85; and D. B. Newton, "Breast Feeding in Victoria," *Medical Journal of Australia,* Vol. 2 (1966).

52. Documented by Jelliffe, *Infant Nutrition;* H. F. Welbourn, in *Journal of Tropical Pediatrics,* Vol. 3 (1958), p. 157; D. S. McLaren, in *Lancet,* Vol. 2 (1966), p. 485; B. E. R. Symonds, in *Journal of Tropical Pediatrics,* Vol. 3 (1958), p. 157; D. B. Jelliffe, B. E. R. Symonds, and E. F. P. Jelliffe, in *Journal of Pediatrics,* Vol. 57 (1966), p. 902; F. DelMondo, *Quarterly Review of Pediatrics,* Vol. 15 (1960), p. 50; and H. A. Guthrie, *Journal of Tropical Pediatrics,* Vol. 10 (1964), p. 65.

53. O. Ballarine, "Effect of Introduction of Infant Foods in Developing Countries" (paper presented at PAHO meeting, Bogotá, November 1970), p. 2.

54. Interview, D. B. Jelliffe, 1968.

55. Burgess and Dean, *Malnutrition and Food Habits,* p. 24. See also F. Viteri, "Weaning Foods for Low-Income Families" (paper presented at PAHO meeting, Bogotá, November 1970), Annex 4, p. 2.

56. Bo Vahlquist, "Occurrence of Nutritional Anemia in Children," in Gunnar Blix (ed.), *Causes and Prevention of Nutritional Anemias,* Symposia of the Swedish Nutrition Foundation, 6 (Stockholm: Almqvist and Wiksell, 1968), pp. 36–46.

57. Gopalan, "Studies on Lactation," p. 97.

58. C. D. Williams, in *Archives of Diseases of Childhood,* Vol. 21 (1946), p. 37.

59. J. D. Call, "Emotional Factors in Breast Feeding," *Journal of Pediatrics,* Vol. 55 (1959), p. 485.

60. Interview, D. B. Jelliffe, 1970; and Boon, Paramathypathy, and Boo, "Breast-feeding in Singapore."

61. Mönckeberg, "Factors Conditioning Malnutrition," p. 29.

62. Interview, D. B. Jelliffe, 1970.

63. C. A. M. Wennen-Van Der May, "The Decline of Breast Feeding in Nigeria," *Tropical and Geographical Medicine,* Vol. 25 (1969), pp. 93–96.

64. Derrick B. Jelliffe and E. F. Patrice Jelliffe, "The Urban Avalanche," *Journal of the American Dietetic Association,* August 1970, p. 116.

65. Mönckeberg, "Factors Conditioning Malnutrition."

66. Davidson, "A Brief History of Infant Feeding," p. 84.

67. Ibid.

68. P. R. Krishnaswami, "Note on Protein" (Bombay, 1968; processed).

69. Alice Gerhard, *Please Breast-Feed Your Baby* (Hawthorn Books, 1970), pp. 109–10.

70. J. P. Sedwick and E. C. Fleischner, "Breast Feeding in the Reduction of Infant Mortality," *American Journal of Public Health,* Vol. 11 (1921).

71. F. H. Richardson, in *Journal of the American Medical Association,* Vol. 85 (1925), p. 668.

72. J. M. Bierman, "Infant Feeding in the USSR," *Quarterly Review of Pediatrics,* August 1957, p. 137.

73. Gerhard, *Please Breast-Feed Your Baby,* p. 110.

74. W. H. Trachsler, "Infant Feeding in Switzerland," *Quarterly Review of Pediatrics,* Vol. 11 (1956), pp. 16 and 202.

75. Federal Office for Social Security, Subdivision for Sickness Insurance, Bern, Switzerland, Nov. 5, 1971.

76. Myron Winick, "Malnutrition and Brain Development," *Journal of Pediatrics,* Vol. 74 (May 1969), pp. 667–79.

77. Derrick B. Jelliffe, Paper Presented at Asian Nutrition Congress, Hyderabad, India, January 1971.

78. Harfouche, "The Importance of Breastfeeding," pp. 157–58.

CHAPTER 8

1. Computer simulation by Indian Institute of Public Opinion; see Alan D. Berg and F. James Levinson, "Combatting Malnutrition: A Working Model," *International Development Review*, June 1968, pp. 16–17.

2. Brock Chisolm, quoted in Anne Burgess and R. F. A. Dean (eds.), *Malnutrition and Food Habits* (London: Tavistock Publications, 1962), pp. 114–15.

3. Burgess and Dean, *Malnutrition and Food Habits*, p. xiii.

4. W. H. Sebrell, "20 Years of Enrichment" (address to the Twentieth Anniversary of Bread Enrichment Meeting, New York City, Feb. 24, 1961; processed).

5. Ibid.

6. Army Medical Nutrition Laboratory, Report No. 71 (1950); and W. B. Bean, R. W. Vilter, and M. A. Blankenhorn, in *Journal of American Medical Association*, Vol. 40 (1949), p. 872.

7. W. R. Aykroyd and others, "Medical Resurvey of Nutrition in Newfoundland," *Canadian Medical Journal*, April 1949, pp. 329–52; G. A. Goldsmith, "Relationship between Nutrition and Pregnancy as Observed in Recent Studies in Newfoundland," *American Journal of Public Health*, August 1950, pp. 953–59.

8. J. Salcedo, Jr., and others, "Artificial Enrichment of White Rice as a Solution to Endemic Beriberi, Report of Field Trials in Bataan, Philippines," *Journal of Nutrition*, Dec. 11, 1950, pp. 501–23.

9. F. A. Arnold, Jr., "The Use of Fluoride Compounds for the Prevention of Dental Caries," *International Dental Journal*, Vol. 7 (1957), p. 56; H. Trendley Dean and others, "Studies on Mass Control of Dental Caries through Fluoridation of the Public Water Supply," *Public Health Report*, Oct. 27, 1950, pp. 1403–8; and Felix Bronner, "Fluoridation or Obsession?" *American Journal of Clinical Nutrition*, October 1969, p. 1346. See also Abraham E. Nizel and Judith S. Shulman, "Interaction of Dietetics and Nutrition with Dentistry," *Journal of the American Dietetic Association*, November 1969, pp. 470–75.

10. S. S. Sooch and V. Ramalingaswami, "Preliminary Report on an Experiment in the Kangra Valley for the Prevention of Himalayan Endemic Goiter with Iodized Salt," *Bulletin of the World Health Organization*, Vol. 32, No. 3, pp. 229–45; and interview, V. Ramalingaswami, 1969.

11. Nevin Scrimshaw and others, "Efecto de la Yodación de la Sal sobre la Prevalencia de Bocio Endemico en Niños Escolanes de Guatemala," *Boletín de la Oficina Sanitaria Panamericana*, March 1966, pp. 222–28.

12. Interview, Sidney Cantor, New Delhi, 1969.

13. F. James Levinson, "Food Fortification in Low-Income Countries: A New Approach to an Old Standby," *American Journal of Public Health*, May 1972, pp. 715–18.

14. For a detailed discussion of salt fortification, see F. James Levinson and Alan Berg, ". . . with a grain of fortified salt," *Food Technology*, September 1969, pp. 70–72.

15. A. L. Dias, Concluding Remarks, *Protein Fortification of Foods* (Proceedings of Seminar at Jadarpur University, Calcutta, Feb. 15–16, 1969), pp. 111–12.

16. P. C. Spensley, D. Halliday, and Elizabeth Orr, "The Prospects for 'Non-Conventional' Protein Resources" (London: Tropical Products Institute, 1970; processed).

17. UN Protein Advisory Group, "Report on the PAG ad hoc Working Group Meeting on Milk Intolerance—Nutritional Implications," Doc. 1.27/g (Nov. 22,

1971); and Michael Latham, "Background Information on Lactose Intolerance" (report to Committee on International Nutrition Programs, Food and Nutrition Board, National Research Council, 1971; processed).

18. UN Protein Advisory Group, "Textured Vegetable Proteins," *PAG Bulletin*, Vol. 2, No. 1 (Winter 1971), pp. 22–26.

19. Uwe Kracht, "Status Reports on Incaparina and Competitors," *Proceedings of Western Hemisphere Nutrition Congress III, Bal Harbour, Fla., September 1971* (Mt. Kisco, N.Y.: Futura Publishing, 1972), pp. 99–102.

20. See Max Milner, "Protein Food Problems in Developing Countries," *Food Technology*, June 1962, p. 51; D. B. Jelliffe, "The Essential Characteristics of Weaning Foods," *Canjanus*, March 1970, pp. 148–57; Albert L. Elder and Samuel M. Weisberg, "High Nutrition–Low Cost Foods: Their Impact in Developing Countries" (paper presented at Third International Congress of Food Science and Technology, Washington, Aug. 9–14, 1970); and Sidney M. Cantor and George E. Shaffer, Jr., "New Protein Foods from Plant Sources: A System for Economic Evaluation" (paper presented at 8th Annual Meeting of Society for Economic Botany, University of Miami, Florida, June 5–8, 1968).

21. Spensley, Halliday, and Orr, "Prospects for 'Non-Conventional' Protein Resources," p. 8.

22. T. A. Mahavan and C. Gopalan, in *Archives of Pathology*, Vol. 80 (1965), p. 123, and Vol. 85 (1968), p. 133; W. H. Butter and J. M. Barnes, in *British Journal of Cancer*, Vol. 17 (1963), p. 699; N. Platonow, *Veterinary Record*, Vol. 76 (1964), p. 589; and W. R. Aykroyd and J. Doughty, *Legumes in Human Nutrition*, Nutrition Studies No. 19 (Rome: FAO, 1964).

23. Jasper Guy Woodroof, *Coconuts: Production, Processing, Products* (Westport, Conn.: Avi Publishing Co., 1970), p. 6.

24. D. R. Strength, "Preparation, Characterization and Evaluation of Coconut Protein," *Proceedings of Third International Congress of Food Science and Technology, Washington, August 1970* (Chicago: Institute of Food Technologists, 1971), pp. 272–79.

25. M. Kantharaj Urs and K. R. Kulsalya, "Studies of Preparation of Edible Grade Meal from Mustard Seeds," Doc. 2.35/5 (UN Protein Advisory Group meeting, Geneva, Oct. 13, 1971); and Rhoda Palter, Jo Kohler, and P. F. Knowles, "Survey for a High-lysine Variety in the World Collection of Safflower," *Journal of Agricultural Food Chemistry*, November–December 1969, pp. 1298–1300.

26. E. J. Bass, "Wheat Protein Concentrates and Related Food Products," in Max Milner (ed.), *Protein-Enriched Cereal Foods for World Needs* (St. Paul: American Association of Cereal Chemists, 1969), pp. 117–28.

27. Statement on single cell protein, *PAG Bulletin* (1968), p. 15. Also see Steven R. Tannenbaum, "Single-Cell Protein, Food of the Future," *Food Technology*, Vol. 25, No. 9, pp. 98–103; and R. I. Mateless and S. R. Tannenbaum, *Single-Cell Protein* (MIT Press, 1968).

28. Arthur E. Humphrey, "Single-Cell Protein (SCP)" (report prepared for U.S. Agency for International Development, New Delhi, Jan. 14, 1969).

29. M. S. Iyengar, "Protein from Petroleum as a Potential Source for Fortification of Food," in *Protein Fortification of Foods*, pp. 31–40.

30. A. E. Humphrey, "Starvation: Chemical Engineering Can Help Fight It," *Chemical Engineering*, 1966, p. 149.

31. William J. Oswald and Clarence G. Golveke, "Large Scale Production of Algae," in Mateless and Tannenbaum, *Single-Cell Protein*.

32. Bernal Diaz del Castillo, *The Discovery and Conquest of Mexico*, ed. Genaro Garcia; trans. A. P. Maudslay (Grove Press, 1956).

33. D. M. Hegsted, "Nutritional Value of Cereal Proteins in Relation to Human Needs," in Milner, *Protein-Enriched Cereal Foods*, p. 42.

34. "The Potential of Fish Protein Concentrate for Developing Countries," agenda item 1/G (FPC Working Group, UN Protein Advisory Group, London, November 1970).

35. R. Devadas, *Problems and Prospects in Alleviating Protein Malnutrition in India* (paper presented at 8th Pugwash Symposium, Frankfurt, Germany, May 12–23, 1970).

36. Letter to PAG Secretariat from F. J. Moss, April 13, 1970.

37. "PAG Statement on Leaf Protein Concentrate," Doc. 3.14/8, Appendix F (UN Protein Advisory Group meeting, New York, May 1970), p. 35.

38. Hoffman LaRoche data, 1971; and Daniel Rosenfield, "Breeding and Fortification Workshop: Wheat Fortification" (paper presented at Amino Acids Workshop, Annapolis, Md., Dec. 8, 1970).

39. Hegsted, "Nutritional Value of Cereal Proteins," pp. 38–48.

40. Nevin S. Scrimshaw and Aaron M. Altschul, *Amino Acid Fortification of Protein Foods* (MIT Press, 1971); and Sheila M. Pereira and others, "Lysine Supplemented Wheat and Growth of Preschool Children," *American Journal of Clinical Nutrition*, Vol. 22 (May 1969), pp. 606–11.

41. Uwe Kracht, "Economic Aspects of the Supplementation of Cereals with Lysine" (report presented to Ad Hoc Group on Amino Acid Fortification, FAO/WHO/UNICEF/PAG, Rome, May 7–8, 1969), p. 31.

CHAPTER 9

1. Alan Berg, "Industry's Struggle with World Malnutrition," *Harvard Business Review*, January–February 1972, pp. 130–41.

2. Lester R. Brown, *Seeds of Change* (Praeger, 1970), pp. 149–53.

3. Letter to Agency for International Development from H. M. Connelly, Kraft Foods, July 8, 1969.

4. "Fortified Foods: The Next Revolution," *Chemical and Engineering News*, Aug. 10, 1970, pp. 138–41.

5. D. Zenoff, "The Latest Weapon in the Fight Against Malnutrition," *Columbia Journal of World Business*, November–December 1968, pp. 67–71.

6. Uwe Kracht, "Status Reports on Incaparina and Competitors," *Proceedings of Western Hemisphere Nutrition Congress III, Bal Harbour, Fla., September 1971* (Mt. Kisco, N.Y.: Futura Publishing, 1972), pp. 99–102.

7. Bo Wickstrom, "Marketing of Protein-Rich Foods to Vulnerable Groups: From Pre-Appraisal to Post-Evaluation" (paper presented at Dag Hammarskjöld Seminar on Nutrition as a Priority in African Development, Uppsala, Sweden, July 1971).

8. J. K. Roy, "A Social Custom Associated with the Feeding Practice Profoundly Affecting the Protein Intake . . . ," *Proceedings of the Nutrition Society of India*, No. 6 (1968).

9. Interview with Derrick B. Jelliffe; see also Derrick B. Jelliffe, "Commerciogenic Malnutrition?" *Food Technology*, February 1971, pp. 55–56.

10. Letter to the author from C. W. Cook, 1971.

11. Letter to the author from K. J. George, Joint-Secretary of Industrial Development, April 14, 1969.

12. John C. Abbott, "Marketings of New Protein Foods" (paper prepared for Food and Agriculture Organization [FAO], n.d., processed).

CHAPTER 10

1. Alan Berg, "Supplemental Feeding Programs" (paper presented at meeting of UN Protein Advisory Group, Paris, June 1972; processed).

2. *Administrative Policies for International Food and Nutrition Programs* (National Academy of Sciences, April 1964).

3. Cicely D. Williams, "Self-Help and Nutrition: Real Needs of Underdeveloped Countries," *Lancet*, Feb. 13, 1954, pp. 323–25; and Fernando Mönckeberg, "Factors Conditioning Malnutrition in Latin America with Special Reference to Chile: Advices for a Volunteers Action," in Paul György and O. L. Kline (eds.), *Malnutrition Is a Problem of Ecology* (S. Karger, 1970), pp. 29–30.

4. This section benefits from a history by Majorie L. Scott, *School Feeding, Its Contribution to Child Nutrition*, FAO Nutrition Studies No. 10 (Rome: FAO, 1953); see also Rajammal P. Devadas and A. Rodharukamani, *The School Lunch Programme, Organization and Outcomes*, Publication 753 (Faridabad: Government of India, Ministry of Education, 1969); and Toshio Oiso, "Problems in Organization and Implementation of School Meal Programs" (paper presented at First Asian Congress of Nutrition, Hyderabad, India, Jan. 28, 1971; processed).

5. F. James Levinson, "Our Child Feeding Overseas," *Journal of the American Dietetic Association*, December 1970, p. 503.

6. Data from CARE, 1971.

7. Charles L. Schultze, *The Distribution of Farm Subsidies* (Brookings Institution, 1971), p. 1.

8. Frank Ellis and Alan Berg, "Meeting Nutrition Needs" (report of Sub-Group on Nutrition, Interagency Task Force on Food and Agricultural Assistance to Less-Developed Countries, March 3, 1965; processed).

9. *Ambassador's Journal* (Houghton Mifflin, 1969), p. 399.

10. P. R. Crowley, "Bal Ahar Case Study," in *Development and Introduction of New Donated Foods* (AID, forthcoming).

11. David Coursin, "Report on Nutrition, Brain Development and Behavior" (paper presented to Committee on International Nutrition, Food and Nutrition Board, National Academy of Sciences, 1972; processed).

12. Leon G. Mears, "Changing Food Preferences in Japan Spur Imports of U.S. Farm Items," *Foreign Agriculture*, Jan. 11, 1971, p. 4.

13. Devadas and Rodharukamani, *The School Lunch Programme*, pp. 108–9.

14. Scott, *School Feeding*, pp. 63–64.

15. Ibid., p. 63.

16. Internal report prepared by Office of International Research, Nutrition Section, National Institutes of Health, for Agency for International Development, 1969, pp. 7–8; and Nevin Scrimshaw and Miguel A. Guzmán, "The Effect of Dietary Supplementation and the Administration of Vitamin $B_{12}$ and Aureomycin on the Growth of School Children," *Current Research on Vitamins in Trophology*, Nutrition Symposium Series No. 7 (National Vitamin Foundation, 1953), pp. 101–17.

17. David Mathiasen, "Measuring Children as a Means of Evaluating Public Nutrition Programs: A Study of the Indian School Feeding Program in the State of

Orissa," and Paul Jonas, "Demographic Effects of Development Programs: A Statistical Model of the Orissa School Feeding Project" (papers presented at annual meeting of American Statistical Association, Detroit, Dec. 28–30, 1970; processed); and Prodipto Roy and Radha Nath Rath (eds.), *The School Lunch Program in Orissa* (New Delhi: Council for Social Development, 1971).

18. Prodipto Roy, "School Lunch Evaluation" (paper presented at International Symposium on Social Welfare Research, Brookings Institution, May 23, 1971; processed).

19. See Vitoria García de Yazigi, quoted in Anne Burgess and R. F. A. Dean (eds.), *Malnutrition and Food Habits* (London: Tavistock Publications, 1962), p. 141; R. P. Devadas, "Better Food Utilization and Changing the Food Habits," *Indian Journal of Home Science*, January 1968, p. 4; Derrick B. Jelliffe, *Infant Nutrition in the Subtropics and Tropics*, Monograph Series No. 29 (2nd ed., Geneva: WHO, 1968), p. 77; and Mönckeberg, "Factors Conditioning Malnutrition," pp. 28–33.

20. Paul Johnson, "Keeping Pests out of Food for Peace," *War on Hunger*, November/December 1969, pp. 9–11; and Paul E. Johnson, William H. Schoenherr, and John H. Dively, *Evaluation of Dry Cereal Shipments to India and the Philippines* (U.S. AID, Office of Food for Peace, Feb. 25, 1970), p. 21.

21. Levinson, "Our Child Feeding Overseas," p. 504.

22. Report on Operation of Child Feeding Program, Kirloskar Consultants Ltd., Poona, India, for U.S. AID, India, 1969.

23. Scott, *School Feeding*, pp. 57, 122; and *Food and Nutrition Education in the Primary School*, FAO Nutritional Studies No. 25 (Rome: FAO, 1971).

24. Irwin H. Rosenberg, "Draft Position on Antibiotic Field Trials" (report presented to Committee on International Nutrition Programs, Food and Nutrition Board, National Academy of Sciences, Nov. 11, 1971; processed); Norbert Hirschhorn, "Can small daily doses of antibiotics prevent the cycle of diarrhea, malabsorption and malnutrition in children?" *American Journal of Clinical Nutrition*, July 1971, pp. 872–75; "Control of Ascariasis," WHO Technical Report Series No. 379, RNTP/RFNS/19 English (Geneva: WHO, 1967), p. 5; Herbert Pollack, "Disease as a Factor in World Food Problem," *American Journal of Clinical Nutrition*, August 1968, pp. 868–74.

25. M. A. Church, "Educational Methods, Cultural Characteristics and Nutrition Rehabilitation: Experience in Kampala Unit, Environmental Child Health," *Journal of Tropical Pediatrics*, March 1971.

26. Parvaghi K. Rao, "Socio-Cultural Factors and Malnutrition in Telengana Region of Andhra Pradesh," *Proceedings of the Nutrition Society of India*, No. 6 (1968), p. 38.

27. Department of Food and Nutrition, "Report of the School Lunch Programme and Associated Activities in Raipura" (Baroda, India: Department of Food and Nutrition, n.d.; processed), App. 1.

28. Hermann M. Southworth and Bruce Johnston (eds.), *Agricultural Development and Economic Growth* (Cornell University Press, 1967), p. 353.

29. Bunker Roy, *Times of India*, Oct. 31, 1971.

30. Fred Sai, in discussion at Dag Hammarskjöld Seminar on Nutrition as a Priority in African Development, Uppsala, Sweden, July 1971.

31. Philip Harvey, "Famine in India" (report prepared for CARE, 1969; processed).

32. Annex O, Annual Program Memorandum, U.S. Agency for International Development, New Delhi, July 1968.

CHAPTER 11

1. C. Gopalan, in discussion at Technical Session 3, International Symposium on Protein Foods and Concentrates, Central Food Technological Research Institute, Mysore, India, June 1967.

2. C. Subramaniam, speech, reported on U.S. Information Service Wireless File, MEF X-1, March 20, 1968.

3. W. Ladejinsky, "The Green Revolution in Punjab," *Economic and Political Weekly* (India), June 28, 1969, pp. A73–A82.

4. See Marketing Research Corporation of India, "Survey Report on the Bakery Industry in India" (Marketing Research, 1969); Operations Research Group, *Food Habits Survey* (Bombay: Protein Foods Association of India, 1969); Hindustan Thompson, Ltd., *Food Habits Survey* (Calcutta: Hindustan Thompson, 1971); and "Growing Bakery Production Boosts Flour Consumption in India," *Foreign Agriculture*, June 28, 1971, p. 10.

5. Concluding Remarks, at Seminar on Protein Fortification of Foods, Calcutta, Feb. 16, 1969 (processed), p. 3.

6. P. K. Kymal, "Fortification of Atta," and S. K. Gupta, "Protein Enrichment of Bread," in *Protein Fortification of Foods* (Proceedings of Seminar at Jadavpur University, Calcutta, Feb. 15–16, 1969), pp. 84–89.

7. F. James Levinson and Alan D. Berg, ". . . with a grain of fortified salt," *Food Technology*, September 1969, pp. 70–72.

8. Operations Research Group, *Food Habits Survey*; and Hindustan Thompson, Ltd., *Calcutta Food Habits Survey* (Hindustan Thompson, 1972).

9. Research and Marketing Services, "A Study of Tea as a Fortification Carrier" (report prepared for U.S. Agency for International Development [USAID], Bombay, May 14, 1970; processed), Vol. 1, p. 11.

10. Mansinghal Associates, "Report on Identifying Regions of India Suitable for Introduction of Fortified Rice" (report prepared for USAID, New Delhi, March 1969; processed), Vol. 3; and Clinton L. Brooke, "Rice Fortification," in *Protein Fortification of Foods*, pp. 70–71.

11. S. B. Deb, "Fortifying Tea with Lysine Hydrochloride," and R. Choudhury, "Tea as a Vehicle for Lysine Fortification," in *Protein Fortification of Foods*, pp. 74–79.

12. Clinton L. Brooke and W. M. Cort, "Vitamin A Fortification of Tea," *Food Technology*, Vol. 26 (June 1972), p. 50.

13. F. James Levinson, "Food Fortification in Low Income Countries: A New Approach to an Old Standby," *American Journal of Public Health*, May 1972, pp. 715–18.

14. *The Protein Emergency* (Ahmedabad: Indian Institute of Management, 1967); and *New Foods for National Development* (Ahmedabad: Indian Institute of Management, 1967). Also see *The Protein Crisis* (Bombay: Protein Foods Association of India, n.d.).

15. Research and Marketing Services, "A Project Outline for the Effectiveness of the 'Protein' Pilot Communication Programme in Maharastra" (Bombay: Lintas Ltd. for Protein Foods Association of India, May 11, 1970; processed); Protein Foods Association of India, "A Mass Media Nutrition Education Programme, Results of a Pilot Operation and Proposal for Extension" (Protein Foods Association, n.d.; processed), and "Highlights of Communication Research" (Protein Foods Association, n.d.; processed). Also, letter to the author from Gerson da Cunha, Nov. 13, 1971. For additional detail, see *A Movement Gains Momentum: New Hope for Nutrition*

(Bombay: Protein Foods Association of India, 1970); and reports of general meetings of the Protein Foods Association of India, Bombay, March 3, 1969; March 30, 1970; and March 26, 1971.

16. R. Balasubramaniam, *Report of the Committee on Rational Development of Food Industries* (Government of India, Directorate General of Technical Development, 1971; processed).

17. Prodipto Roy and Radha Nath Rath (eds.), *The School Lunch Program in Orissa* (New Delhi: Council for Social Development, 1971).

18. Operations Research Group, *Food Habits Survey.*

19. "Comprehensive Nutrition Plan" (Government of India, Ministry of Health, Office of Nutrition Adviser, 1968; processed); and Alan D. Berg and F. James Levinson, "Combatting Malnutrition: A Working Model," *International Development Review*, June 1968, pp. 15–17.

20. *Fourth Five Year Plan, 1969–1974* (New Delhi: Government of India Planning Commission, 1970).

21. Economic and Social Policy Resolution, 73rd session of Indian National Congress party.

22. "National Cess Proposed for Child Welfare," *Hindustan Times*, Dec. 21, 1969.

23. "Congress N Manifesto," *Hindustan Times*, Jan. 25, 1971.

24. "Golden Jubilee Celebrations of the Nutrition Research Laboratories," New Delhi.

25. Quoted in *Nutrition* (Hyderabad, India), January 1967, inside cover.

26. Quoted in *Yojana* (New Delhi), Jan. 26, 1969, contents page.

CHAPTER 12

1. Martin J. Forman, "Supplemental Feeding for Preschool Children," in *Proceedings of the Third Far East Symposium on Nutrition, Manila, Philippines, Feb. 14–21, 1967* (GPO, 1967), pp. 119–25.

2. UN Economic and Social Council, *Increase in the Production and Use of Edible Protein: The Protein Problem*, Doc. E/4829, June 8, 1970.

3. List from Sol Chafkin, James Pines, Alan Berg, and Richard Longhurst, *A Review of Possible World Bank Actions on Malnutrition Problems* (American Technical Assistance Corp., 1972).

4. F. James Levinson, "Investment in Nutrition: Objectives Redefined" (January 1972; processed).

5. Sidney Cantor Associates, Inc., "Commercial Feasibility of Fish Protein Concentrate in a Developing Country" (prepared for U.S. Agency for International Development, October 1969; processed), Vol. 1.

6. Demissie Habte, in discussion at Eastern African Conference on Nutrition and Child Feeding, Nairobi, Kenya, May 19–23, 1969.

7. A. P. Vamoer, "Nutrition, Planning and Coordination," *Proceedings of the Eastern African Conference on Nutrition and Child Feeding* (GPO, 1969), pp. 274–82.

8. Letter to the author from B. Venkatappiah, July 2, 1970.

9. Morton H. Halperin, "Why Bureaucrats Play Games," *Foreign Policy*, Spring 1971, pp. 70–90 (Brookings Reprint 199).

10. Ibid.

11. Vamoer, "Nutrition, Planning and Coordination."

12. See "Documentation and Information in the Edible Protein Field," FAO/WHO/UNICEF/PAG, Doc. 1.4.4/3 (Dec. 28, 1970); "Information Services in the Field of Edible Protein," Doc. 3.14/14, Appendix J (UN Protein Advisory Group meeting report), pp. 84–88; and H. W. Kay and J. Krautwurst, "Electronic Retrieval System for a Dairy Research Center," and E. J. Mann, "The International Food Information Service" (papers presented at Third International Congress of Food Science and Technology, Washington, Aug. 9–14, 1970; processed).

13. Alan D. Berg and F. James Levinson, "A New Need: The Nutrition Programmer," *American Journal of Clinical Nutrition*, July 1967, pp. 893–95.

14. J. B. Cordaro and F. James Levinson, "A Curriculum for the Nutrition Programmer," *American Journal of Clinical Nutrition*, November 1971, pp. 1352–53.

15. Interview, B. L. Taneja, 1968.

16. Conclusion of Nutrition Policy Roundtable, Brookings Institution, Washington, Sept. 10, 1970.

## APPENDIX A

1. Report on the Bihar Famine, Indian Ministry of Food and Agriculture, 1966 (processed), p. 6.

2. Headlines from *Economist*, April 13, 1968, p. 34, and *Reader's Digest*, August 1968, p. 137.

3. Bernard D. Nossiter, "Bihar's Famine Relief Viewed as Model," *Washington Post*, Nov. 6, 1967.

4. For a manual on the conduct of famine relief programs, see G. B. Masefield, "Food and Nutrition Procedures in Times of Disaster," Nutrition Studies 21 (Rome: Food and Agriculture Organization, 1967).

5. William W. Hunter, *Annals of Rural Bengal* (London: Smith, Elder, 1868); and B. M. Bhatia, *Famines in India* (London: Asia Publishing House, 1967).

6. "India Starves," *Newsweek*, Oct. 4, 1943, pp. 38–39.

7. All India Radio, Nov. 18, 1966.

8. B. G. Verghese, *Beyond the Famine* (New Delhi: Bihar Relief Committee, 1967), p. 4.

9. Letter to the author from F. C. Gera, Nov. 24, 1966.

10. Paul Crowley, Acceptability Studies on Bal Ahar (reports prepared for U.S. Agency for International Development, New Delhi, 1970).

11. Lester Brown, *Seeds of Change* (Praeger, 1970), p. 7.

12. For added detail on this and other political aspects of the famine, see Alan Berg, "Famine Contained: Notes and Lessons from the Bihar Experience," in Gunnar Blix, Yngve Hofvander, and Bo Vahlquist (eds.), *Famine: Nutrition and Relief Operations* (Uppsala, Sweden: Swedish Nutrition Foundation, 1971).

13. C. Subramaniam, Indian Minister of Food and Agriculture, in discussion at Nutrition Policy Roundtable, Brookings Institution, February 1971.

14. Verghese, *Beyond the Famine*, p. 2.

15. Philip Harvey, "Development Potential in Famine Relief: The Bihar Model," *International Development Review*, December 1969, pp. 7–9.

16. All India Radio, March 1967.

17. See M. C. Swaminathan, K. V. Rao, and D. H. Rao, "Food Situation in the Drought Affected Areas of Bihar," *Journal of Nutrition and Dietetics* (In-

dia), No. 6 (1969), pp. 209–17; V. Ramalingaswami and others, "Studies of the Bihar Famine 1966–67" (All India Institute of Medical Sciences, 1970; processed).

18. V. Ramalingaswami, in discussion at Famine Symposium, Uppsala, Sweden, February 1967. For information on the nutritional effects of starvation, see Blix, Hofvander, and Vahlquist, *Famine*; Vernon R. Young and Nevin S. Scrimshaw, "The Physiology of Starvation," *Scientific American*, October 1971, pp. 14–20; and Ancel Benjamin Keys and others, *The Biology of Human Starvation* (University of Minnesota Press, 1950).

19. Verghese, *Beyond the Famine*, p. 42.


## APPENDIX C

1. C. Gopalan, "Studies on Lactation in Poor Indian Communities," *Journal of Tropical Pediatrics*, December 1968, p. 92.

2. John McKigney, "Economic Aspects," *American Journal of Clinical Nutrition*, August 1971, pp. 1005–12.


## APPENDIX D

1. "Seasonal Hunger in Underdeveloped Countries," *Nutrition Reviews*, May 1968, pp. 142–45. See also Sue Schofield, "The Nutrition Status of Children, Evidence from Village Studies" (Sussex, England: Institute of Development Studies, May 7, 1972; processed).

2. For an example of the interview-cum-survey technique, see *Nutrition Research Profile* (U.S. Agency for International Development [USAID], New Delhi, 1967).

3. For material related to nutrition objectives, see J. Hrubý and O. Šmrha, "Food Policy in Czechoslovakia" (Prague: Institute of Human Nutrition, 1969; processed); F. James Levinson, "Nutrition Intervention in Low Income Countries: Its Economic Role and Alternative Strategies" (master's thesis, Cornell University, 1971); Patrick J. François, "Nutrition—a New Operational Technique in National Planning," *Food and Nutrition in Africa*, July 1969, pp. 65–72; and Dana G. Dalrymple, *Economic Aspects of Nutrition Improvement in Tunisia* (U.S. Department of Agriculture, Foreign Economic Development Service, July 1970).

4. J. M. Bengoa, "Significance of Malnutrition and Priorities for Its Prevention," and Douglas Wilson, "The Economic Analysis of Malnutrition," in Alan Berg, Nevin Scrimshaw, and David Call (eds.), *Nutrition, National Development and Planning* (MIT Press, forthcoming).

5. Sol Chafkin, "An Operations Oriented Study of Nutrition as an Integrated System of Tamil Nadu" (report prepared for Food and Nutrition Division, U.S. Agency for International Development/New Delhi, Feb. 11, 1970); C. Subramaniam, report presented to the United Nations Secretary-General's Panel to Formulate a United Nations Strategy on the Protein Problem Confronting the Developing Countries, 1971; Asok Mitra, "The Nutrition Movement in India," in Berg, Scrimshaw, and Call, *Nutrition, National Development and Planning*; and interviews, Sidney M. Cantor, 1969–71.

6. Charles J. Hitch, *Decision-Making for Defense* (University of California Press, 1965), p. 54. Also see Allen Schick and others, "Planning-Programming-Budgeting System: A Symposium," *Public Administration Review*, December 1966, pp. 243–310; Charles L. Schultze, *The Politics and Economics of Public Spending*

(Brookings Institution, 1968); Robert H. Haveman and Julius Margolis, *Public Expenditures and Policy Analysis* (Markham, 1971).

7. For a different categorization of profiles, see Karl Eric Knutsson, "Malnutrition and the Community" (paper presented at 1971 Dag Hammarskjöld Seminar on Nutrition as a Priority in African Development, Uppsala, Sweden, July 1971).

8. David Mathiasen, "Some Comments on Nutrition" (memorandum, USAID, New Delhi, Feb. 18, 1969; processed). Also see Hans Heinrich Thias and Martin Carnoy, *Cost-Benefit Analysis in Education: A Case Study of Kenya* (International Bank for Reconstruction and Development, 1972); and Arnold C. Harberger and others, *Benefit Cost Analysis, 1971* (Aldine, 1972).

9. Alice M. Rivlin, *Systematic Thinking for Social Action* (Brookings Institution, 1971), p. 2.

10. J. D. Wray, "Evaluation: Everybody Talks About It . . . ," in Paul György and O. L. Kline (eds.), *Malnutrition Is a Problem of Ecology* (S. Karger, 1970), pp. 144–52.

11. Rivlin, *Systematic Thinking for Social Action*, p. 85.

12. Letter to the author from Asok Mitra, Nov. 3, 1970.

13. Aaron Wildavsky, "Does Planning Work?" *Public Interest*, Summer 1971, pp. 95–104.

14. Hitch, *Decision-Making for Defense*, p. 76.

# Index of Names

277

# General Index

Aflatoxin, 127–28
Africa, 46–47, 74, 80, 81, 128, 134
Agency for International Development (AID), 23, 37, 164, 178
Agriculture: back yard programs, 57, 67–68; credit need, 22, 57–58; export demands, 72; extension services, 57; fertilizer, 53; food waste, 70–71; green revolution, 53–63; high-yield seeds, 53–61; import tariff effect, 58; irrigation effect, 53, 57; laborers, 57–58; multiple cropping, 57; and nutrition, 6, 43–45, 71–73, 196; price supports, 57; pulse production, 58–59, 61; seasonal unemployment, 20; small farmer, 55, 57; subsistence vs. cash, 43–45; tenant farmer, 57. *See also* Livestock production; Rural areas
AID. *See* Agency for International Development
Alfalfa, 138–39
Algae, 134
Algeria, 119
Amino acids, 124, 129; lysine, 52, 131, 139–40, 157, 182, 186; synthetic, 139–41; threonine, 52, 140; tryptophan, 52, 140
Andhra Pradesh, India, 174
Anemia. *See* Iron deficiency anemia
Animal feed: fish meal, 135; food industry, 145; LPC, 139; mill feed, 131–32; oilseeds, 124–25, 127, 129, 145, 188; SCP, 133–35; synthetic nutrients, 139–40
Applied nutrition programs, 76–77. *See also* Education in nutrition
Argentina, 130
Ascorbic acid, 115
Atta, 116–17, 157, 183
Australia, 98, 182

Bal Ahar, 84, 119, 125, 155, 165, 167–68, 186–87. *See also* Food, formulated

Balwadi, 79–80
Bangladesh, 74, 111
Bataan, Philippines, 110
Beans, 46. *See also* Pulses
Beriberi, 15, 45, 109–10
Bihar, India: family size, 33; famine, *1966*, 37, 170, 180–81, 185–86, 189
Birthrate, 32–34, 39
Birth weight, 9
Black market, 161, 164–65
Blindness, 2, 16, 26, 197. *See also* Vitamin A
Bolivia, 26, 44, 46, 144
Bombay, India, 182–83
Brain size, 9, 24. *See also* Mental development
Brazil, 152; breast feeding, 98; child feeding programs, 94–95, 163–64; child mortality, 4; food fortification, 117, 136; food habits, 74; formulated food, 119, 121, 133, 149; malnutrition effect, 11; meat production, 66; oilseed production, 127; productivity study, 13–14
Bread, 44; fortification, 109, 117; Modern Bread, 140, 182–83, 186–87, 191. *See also* Wheat
Breast feeding, 7, 24; advertising techniques, 103–04; vs. bottle feeding, 94–95; and child mortality, 104–06; and communications media, 102; and contraceptive use, 38–39; cultural inhibitions, 102–03; decline in, 90–93, 97–98; and disease, 97; economics of, 89–97; and family planning, 93; and fecundity, 39; and food supplements, 89; government campaigns, 100–05; health workers, 105; history of, 95–96; and income level, 45, 97–100; iron effect, 97; lactation failure, 105–06; and malnutrition, 95; maternal diet, 91–92; maternity leave, 104; and milk distribution programs, 105; milk quality, 89, 96–97; nutrition educa-

283